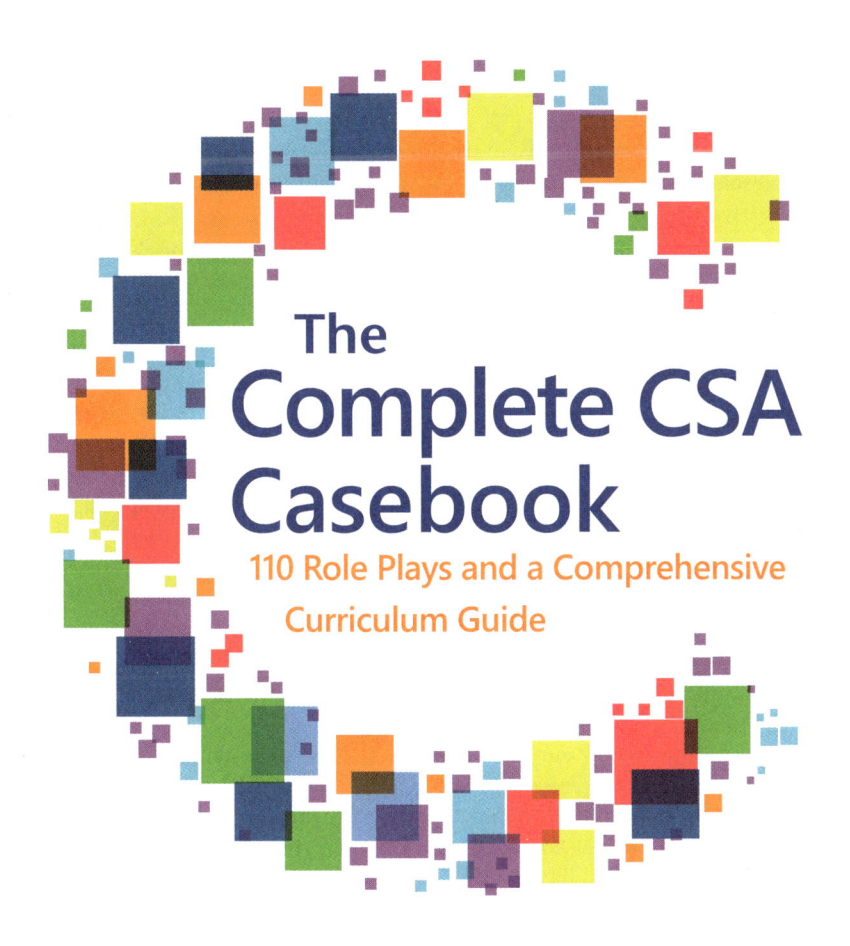

The Complete CSA Casebook

110 Role Plays and a Comprehensive Curriculum Guide

It's a truism that the best way to prepare for the CSA exam is to consult with patients. But for 'spare time' preparation, when there are no patients handy, role play with realistic cases and informed, constructive feedback is the next best thing. And *The Complete CSA Casebook* will provide CSA aspirants and their educators with all the material they need. This excellent and comprehensive resource ticks all the required boxes but goes over and above by providing detailed 'ideal' consultation answers plus a ring-binder format enhancing sharing and interaction. Every trainer should have one.

—**Dr Keith Hopcroft, associate GP trainer and clinical advisor,** Pulse

How easy would it be if all the materials you needed for the CSA were in one book, and the curriculum was distilled into a usable guide for you? Here it is. *The Complete CSA Casebook* is a one stop shop of excellence, combining cases with exemplary consultations and background knowledge for those tricky scenarios. The absolute mastery of *Complete CSA* is the way it is so comprehensive without overwhelming. A must-have revision aid.

—**Dr Laura Armitage, GP and Past AiT Committee Chair,** RCGP

A treasure trove of CSA cases. Well laid out in line with the RCGP Curriculum with well referenced learning points and plenty of practical advice.

—**Dr Simon Huins,** FRCGP, **CSA Examiner and Somerset Training Programme Director**

I have been a CSA examiner since its inception and have worked on the Bristol CSA Study Course since it came into being. The *Complete CSA Casebook* uses Liz Moulton's approach to the consultation to best effect. The section on assisting the approach to passing the cases is well worked up and the tips and referencing are up to date with the latest references and thinking. The cases are usefully grouped in curriculum sections. My assessment of the cases having worked through them with my GPRs (all of whom are planning to take the CSA in the next three months) is that they represent a level of complexity and difficulty slightly above the CSA cases themselves which some consider an advantage. Overall we feel this book will prove to be a very valuable resource for groups working for the CSA.

—**Tony Wright,** FRCP FRCGP Cert Med Ed

This book covers all aspects of the RCGP curriculum to an extremely high standard with the latest guidelines summarised in a superbly convenient, easy access way. During revision you end up with so many resources for the different aspects of curriculum that to have them all to hand while role playing is priceless. The layout is enjoyably logical, coordinated and allows a consistent safe approach to the exam, as well as for GP training and real life consultations. The colour coordination is a particular highlight, and the patient / doctor cards allow effortless CSA exam style case practice. The book would also remain extremely useful once qualified for refreshing memory of guidelines and brushing up on essential GP skills and knowledge.

—**Dr Rachel Ruddock,** MRCGP DRCOG MBChB,
GP at Vere Foster Medical Group, Belfast, Northern Ireland

This book is an excellent resource for any GP trainee preparing for the CSA. The authors provide useful hints and tips on a large number of important areas as well as over 100 cases covering all aspects of the RCGP Curriculum. The cases are a good representation of what you will encounter on the day and the ring binder format will make for easy role play when revising. A great book for GP trainees and trainers alike.

—**Dr Lara Khoury,** MRCGP, MBBS, BSc Hons,
GP at Ellison View Surgery, South Tyneside

Complete CSA Casebook
110 Cases and a Complete Curriculum Guide

110 cases
- 110 paired role play cards so no need to pass around a book!
- Seamlessly aligned with the RCGP curriculum.
- Five cases for each module of the curriculum.
- Includes even the 'difficult' modules: intellectual disability and genetics cases.
- Helps build confidence that you are on the right track.
- Women's Health has 10 cases, to cover maternal health and gynaecology.

Example answers
- For every case.
- Example consultations written in prose, word for word – how we would do it.
- See how it can be done … in 10 minutes!
- How to give quick and jargon-free explanations.

Easy to use generic feedback cards
- Marking schemes can be hard to follow if you are not a trained examiner. We have a single easy-to-use marking scheme and tick lists for each consultation example.

Guideline summaries
- For every case.
- Revision cards and up-to-date guidelines.
- Including useful information and web links we have collected.

> The web links will be stored and updated at the **Link Hub on CompleteCSA.co.uk**
> The treasure chest symbol means there is relevant information on the Link Hub.

The ring binder
- Colour-coded RCGP Curriculum Modules.
- Easy-to-use ring binder.
- Helps you remain organised and keep the cases in order.

Helpful advice
- Tips based on our experience of the CSA exam.
- A summary of consultation models.
- Useful phrases and jargon switch.

Physical Examination Cards
- Stepwise guides to slick and thorough examinations.

Complete CSA's FOCUS Consultation Model
- A consultation model created specifically for the CSA – practical, straightforward and easy to remember under stress.

Written by two newly qualified GPs who have done the CSA and an experienced GP educator.

Introduction from the **Complete CSA** Team

The challenge of the CSA exam is being able to synthesise 10 years of medical education competently, sensitively, quickly and safely, to manage any medical problem presented by any patient who walks through the door. This is also the challenge faced every day by busy GPs in clinical practice.

Whilst revising for the CSA, it became apparent to us that there was no single resource that provided loose-leaf role play cards, together with realistic examples of how cases can actually be completed competently in 10 minutes and a summary of relevant guidelines. The *Complete CSA* aims to create this practical and organised approach, seamlessly linked to the RCGP curriculum.

To help show you what can be achieved, the *Complete CSA* breaks down the consultation into elements. We have also grouped these into our FOCUS Consultation Model, which may help you revise whilst developing your own unique consulting style.

Whatever consultation model(s) you use, we strongly advise that you have a fluid approach, adapting to meet the needs of each individual consultation. When you meet a new acquaintance in any setting or an old friend, demonstrating courtesy and respect for the person in front of you and showing a genuine curiosity and interest in their life will enable rapport and storytelling to come naturally – there is no need to follow a rigid formula.

We appreciate that some readers may have specialist knowledge in particular areas and may well approach some problems differently. The authors are conscientious generalists and this is reflected in our approach to the cases. We hope you find our example consultations helpful – but would remind you that there are many ways to deliver a good consultation, and to pass the CSA!

The Learning Points for each case also extract pieces of information from the relevant resources or guidance, and we strongly advise referring to the full text.

See our website **www.completecsa.co.uk** for the Link Hub and further resources. Look out for dates for **Complete CSA Courses** created by the authors. You may also wish to look at 'The Naked Consultation – a practical guide to primary care consultations' which will help you develop and hone your consultation skills further.

Whilst role playing cases we encourage the doctor to remember Complete CSA's motto:

'Common things are common! … But what mustn't I miss?'

Finally, the responsibility of making frequent and fast decisions whilst holding risk, the urge to always get it right (with the fear of getting it wrong), the pressure to not waste NHS resources, whilst managing complexity, with a high patient load and the medico-legal need to document it all within too little time can feel overwhelming. However, take every opportunity to remember your own loved ones and just do your best for the person looking to you for help. Keep faith in General Practice and remember the unique, professional and supportive work ethos we share.

We wish you all the best.

Emily, Helen and Liz

The Authors

The authors

Dr Emily Blount

MBBS (merit) DRCOG DFSRH MRCGP

A GP since August 2014 after completing the CSA exam in 2014, scoring in the top 3% of candidates. Emily is now a GP and a GP Training Programme Director in Oxford.

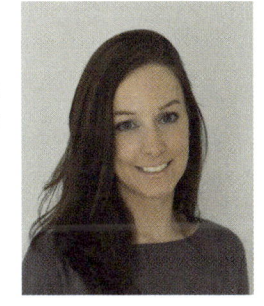

Dr Helen Kirby-Blount

MB ChB (hons) DRCOG MRCGP

Helen sat the CSA exam in 2013 and is now a mother and salaried GP in Nottinghamshire. Helen is the clinical lead for patients with Intellectual Disability within her practice. Helen created the FOCUS Consultation Model.

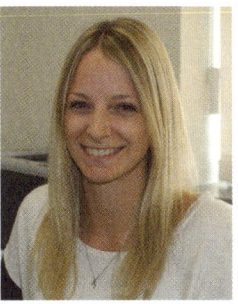

Dr Liz Moulton MBE

MB ChB DRCOG FRCGP MMEd (distinction)

A GP trainer for 25 years, with a wealth of experience of preparing candidates for the MRCGP, Liz has also undertaken most roles within HEE Yorkshire and the Humber and was Deputy Director of Postgraduate GP Education. Liz was a GP advisor to Leeds Health Authority and to the Department of Health. She currently works as a freelance GP and appraiser as well as working for the RCGP practice support unit and as an Honorary Lecturer at the University of Leeds where she teaches on the Masters' programme for medical education. Liz is the author of *The Naked Consultation*.

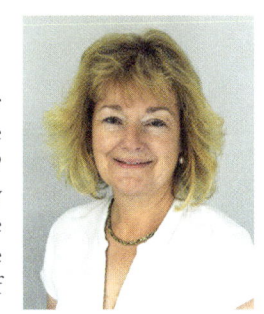

With thanks to contributors

Dr Rachel Ruddock, Dr Richard Wood, Dr Ros Lloyd-Rout and Dr Lynnette Peterson who helped to brainstorm this book and whose voices and wise words are hidden within.

Mr William Britnell for your expertise in urology.

Dr John J. Featherstone and Dr Justin Amery for your time, enthusiasm and helpful advice.

Alice Oven for your guidance and encouragement throughout the process.

Dedications

This book is dedicated to our wonderful family.

Your health and happiness are all that matters. We thank you for all your love and devoted support.

Contents

Complete CSA Casebook v
Introduction from the Complete CSA Team vi
The Authors vii

Introduction (Chapter 1)

How to Use the Book 1
Symbols in the Book 2
RCGP Curriculum 3
Consultation Models 6
Complete CSA's FOCUS Consultation Model 11
Easy to Use Generic Feedback Card 14
Practising the Skills within FOCUS 16
Top Tips 17
Useful Phrases 22
Jargon Switch 26
Resitting the Exam 27
Abbreviations 28
Disclaimer 32

Cases within the RCGP Curriculum (Chapters 2–23)

2	Healthy People	33
3	Genetics in Primary Care	61
4	Acutely Ill People	83
5	Children and Young People	105
6	Older Adults	127
7	Maternal Health	149
8	Gynaecology	173
9	Men's Health	199
10	Sexual Health	223
11	End-of-Life Care	247
12	Mental Health	269
13	Intellectual Disability (ID)	291
14	Cardiovascular Health	313
15	Digestive Health	337
16	Drug and Alcohol Abuse	359
17	ENT, Oral and Facial	381
18	Eye Problems	405
19	Metabolic Problems	429
20	Neurological Problems	453

21	Respiratory Health	475
22	Musculoskeletal Problems	499
23	Skin Problems	521

Examination Checklists (Chapter 24)

Informed Consent	543
Cardiovascular	544
Respiratory	545
Abdominal	546
Cranial Nerves	547
Neurological	548
Thyroid/Neck	549
Shoulder/Cervical Spine	550
Elbow	551
Hands/Wrists	552
Hips/Lumbar Spine	553
Knee	554
Foot/Ankle	555
ENT	556
Peripheral Vascular	557

Appendix

Useful Resources	559
Index	561

CHAPTER 1 INTRODUCTION

How to Use the Book

We have organised a selection of core cases into modules, aligned to the RCGP curriculum.

The book is designed for groups of two or three: a doctor, a patient and, if available, an examiner.

Each core case has one card for the Doctor (Doctor's Notes) and another card for the Patient (Patient's Story).

Once you've completed your 10-minute consultation, turn your cards over to find our suggested Example Consultation and Learning Points, which cover the important facts or guidelines relevant to the case.

Where we have extracted learning points, always refer to full guidance.

Where a medication is mentioned, always refer to the BNF.

Instructions for the patient	The Presenting Complaint (PC) is the *'opening gambit'*. You should freely give the doctor anything in quotation marks. Further information should be given only if the doctor asks relevant questions.
Instructions for the doctor	We suggest using our **FOCUS Model**, which has been broken down into elements on each Example Consultation, as a guide. Include all these elements and you have an excellent consultation; however, flexibility is often needed.
Instructions for the examiner	Mark the Giving Feedback Card. We have also provided tick boxes on each Example Consultation page.

Clinical Examinations: There are three options:
1. Allow the doctor to examine and then state the examination findings.
2. Write the examination findings on a separate sheet to be given to the doctor.
3. Verbally tell the doctor the findings once they have moved to examine.

Only give what has been requested and practise all three of these scenarios.

Constructive criticism is essential. Be honest and agree to the rules before you start!

Symbols in the Book

Face to Face

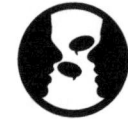

Home Visit

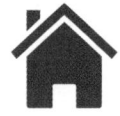

Telephone Call

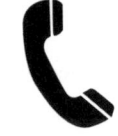

Child Consultation

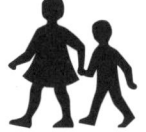

Examination Card

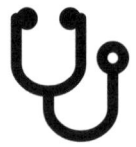

See the Link Hub

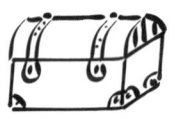

RCGP Curriculum

The RCGP defines and describes the GP curriculum – the competencies and capabilities that you need to develop (and evidence!) to become an effective and safe GP. The curriculum can be found on the RCGP website, but we describe it here for convenience and to explain which areas are tested by the CSA and are therefore particularly relevant to this book.

The RCGP **core statement** 'Being a general practitioner' is divided into five areas of capability and each of these is subdivided:

1. Knowing yourself and relating to others
   a. Fitness to practise
   b. Maintaining an ethical approach
   c. Communication and consultation
2. Applying clinical knowledge and skill
   a. Data gathering and interpretation
   b. Making decisions
   c. Clinical management
3. Managing complex and long-term care
   a. Managing medical complexity
   b. Working with colleagues and in teams
4. Working well in organisations and systems of care
   a. Maintaining performance, learning and teaching
   b. Organisation, management and leadership
5. Caring for the whole person and wider community
   a. Practising holistically and promoting health
   b. Community orientation

The RCGP website gives detailed descriptions and explanations of each of these areas and can be accessed at: http://www.rcgp.org.uk/training-exams/gp-curriculum-overview/~/media/Files/GP-training-and-exams/Curriculum-2012/RCGP-Curriculum-1-Being-a-GP.ashx

As well as capabilities, four **professional modules** are listed:

A. The GP consultation in practice
B. Patient safety and quality of care
C. The GP in the wider professional environment
D. Enhancing professional knowledge

Then there are 21 **clinical modules**, and these form the main content of this book, with five cases illustrating each one (10 for women's health). However, as well as assessing your clinical knowledge in these areas, the CSA exam tests your ability to apply many, though not quite all, of the above capabilities.

The remaining areas are tested through the AKT and the various tools of workplace-based assessment.

RCGP Curriculum

Specifically, the RCGP maps the following aspects of the capabilities to the CSA:

1a – Fitness to practise
Develop the attitudes and behaviours expected of a good doctor

1b – Maintaining an ethical approach
Treat others fairly and with respect, acting without discrimination
Provide care with compassion and kindness

1c – Communication and consultation
Establish an effective partnership with patients
Maintain a continuing relationship with patients, carers and families

2a – Data gathering and interpretation
Apply a structured approach to data gathering and investigation
Interpret findings accurately to make a diagnosis
Demonstrate a proficient approach to clinical examination
Demonstrate a proficient approach to the performance of procedures

2b – Making decisions
Adopt appropriate decision-making principles
Apply a scientific and evidence-based approach

2c – Clinical management
Provide general clinical care to patients of all ages and backgrounds
Adopt a structured approach to clinical management
Make appropriate use of other professionals and services
Provide urgent care when needed

3a – Managing medical complexity
Enable people with long-term conditions to improve their health
Manage concurrent health problems in an individual patient
Adopt safe and effective approaches for patients with complex health needs

3b – Working with colleagues and in teams
Work as an effective team member
Coordinate a team-based approach to the care of patients

4b – Organisation, management and leadership
Make effective use of information management and communication systems

5a – Practising holistically and promoting health
Demonstrate the holistic mindset of a generalist medical practitioner
Support people through individual experiences of health, illness and recovery

5b – Community orientation
Understand the health service and your role within it

RCGP Curriculum

When practising for the CSA and using our example consultations, remind yourself about the above capabilities and remember to demonstrate them appropriately. You may also find it helpful to refer to this list and use it to analyse some of your everyday consultations, thinking about which capabilities you applied effectively and which ones need further development. You could make use of this list when watching your own videoed consultations with or without your trainer.

Ask yourself the following questions, which are directly derived from the above list and are grouped together within the three CSA assessment domains:

Data gathering
- Did I correctly interpret the clinical findings and use these to inform the diagnosis?
- Was my clinical examination / any procedure proficient?
- How did I make my decision? Did I apply decision-making principles?

Clinical management
- Was my management evidence based and scientific?
- Did I think of others in the team and use their skills appropriately?
- Did I work effectively as a team member and coordinate the roles of others in the team?
- If the patient had a long-term condition, did I use the consultation to help him improve his health?
- Did I manage the patient's concurrent health problems as well as her presenting complaint?
- For patients with complex needs, was my approach safe and effective?
- Did I use information management (IM) resources effectively (sharing results with the patient, accessing web material together, finding and printing a patient information leaflet)?
- Did I support this patient, as an individual, through his experience of health, illness or recovery?
- Did I demonstrate that I understand how the health service works (e.g. local community services, referral pathways, secondary care resources etc.).

Interpersonal skills
- Did I treat this patient fairly, with respect and without discrimination?
- Was I compassionate and kind?
- Did I work in partnership with this patient?
- Did I work towards building a continuing relationship with this patient, their family or carer?
- Did I demonstrate that I have a holistic approach – thinking about more than the patient's symptoms and illness, i.e. the context of his or her life, relationships, work, home, psychosocial aspects etc.

Other
- Did I display the behaviours and attitudes expected of a good doctor?
- Was my consultation well structured?

Consultation Models

You may well have been taught a framework or model for your consultations. Using a tried and tested structure can help to ensure that you remember all the key phases and don't leave anything out. The CSA is marked in three different domains, and we will explore how some of the common models fit with this and which skills contribute to each domain. Although the individual models differ in their detail, most conform broadly to the following five-stage structure:

- Find out why the patient has come
- Work out what's wrong
- Explain the problem(s) to the patient
- Develop a management plan and share this with the patient
- Use time well and efficiently

Some also have a sixth stage – take care of yourself. Very important both in the CSA and in your consulting room.

The CSA marking domains are:

Data gathering (find out why the patient has come and work out what's wrong)
Clinical management (explain the problem to the patient, develop a management plan and share it with the patient)
Interpersonal skills (evidenced throughout the consultation from the moment the patient walks in until the door closes).

Using time well and efficiently is essential because, if you run out of time before you get to the management plan, you will score no marks in that area – a recipe for failure.

Looking after yourself in the 2 minutes between each consultation is vital – otherwise one 'bad' consultation will lead to another. Videotapes of the CSA reveal that, after a difficult or dysfunctional consultation, some candidates use their 2 minutes between patients to pore over the previous notes. They try to work out what went wrong rather than putting it out of their mind and spending those precious moments reading and thinking about the next patient. Don't let this happen to you!

Let's look at some common models and see where the different stages fit within the CSA marking structure.

Consultation Models

Pendleton (1984). One of the first patient-centred models.

Seven tasks:

A. Data gathering
1. Find out why the patient has come, including the problem (cause, effects, history) and the patient's ideas, concerns and expectations.
2. Consider other problems.

B. Clinical management
3. Choose (with the patient) an appropriate action for each problem.
4. Achieve a shared understanding of the problems.
5. Involve the patient in the management and encourage them to accept appropriate responsibility.
6. Use time and resources appropriately.

C. Interpersonal skills
7. Establish or maintain a relationship with the patient which helps to achieve the other tasks.

Helman (1981)
Although this isn't a model of the consultation, Cecil Helman, a medical anthropologist, described six questions that any patient might have in his head when coming to see the doctor. It is well worth bearing these in mind when data gathering, particularly around ICE (ideas, concerns and expectations) and in clinical management, when you are explaining to the patient. Armed with the patient's own thoughts, fears and hopes, the answers to these questions could provide a useful framework for your explanation.

1. What has happened?
2. Why has it happened?
3. Why to me?
4. Why now?
5. What would happen if nothing was done about it?
6. What should I do about it or whom should I consult for further help?

Consultation Models

Neighbour (1987)

A five-part model 'anchored' to the fingers of the left hand, so relatively easy to remember even when you are stressed in the exam.

A. Data gathering

1. **Connecting**   This stage is about rapport building (interpersonal skills) as well as gathering data. 'Connection' starts the moment the patient walks through the door. Look at the patient, what do you notice? How do they seem? What is this telling you? Tune in to the patient to get on their wavelength. Explore their story until you have enough information to summarise.

2. **Summarising**   Some candidates think that summarising wastes precious moments in the time-limited CSA but we disagree! Summarising the patient's story back to them 'So, what I've heard you say is ….,<the problem>….<how it started>…. <how it's affecting you at home/work> ….<what you're worried about>' will ensure that you know you are on the right track. If you take 30 seconds to summarise, it will be clear from the patient's verbal or non-verbal communication whether or not you have got it right. If you've missed something important, much better to find it out now, midway through the consultation, rather than right at the end or even not until you read your disappointing CSA results. If you are unsure, or even in a consultation 'hole' where you are struggling, summarising is the best tool to get you back on track again.

B. Clinical management

3. **Handing over**   This is where doctor and patient negotiate and agree upon a management plan and empower the patient by 'hand over' of control.

4. **Safety netting**   Safety netting ensures there are safe contingency plans. Neighbour describes a really robust structure for a three-point safety net. A vague 'come back if you're no better' is unlikely to score you any marks in the CSA, so learn and use this structure:

    i. This is what I expect to happen.

    ii. This is how you [the patient] will know if I'm wrong.

    iii. If that happens, this is what you should do.

    Easy and safe!

C. Interpersonal skills

As with other models, these run as a thread from beginning to end of the consultation.

Neighbour's fifth stage is 'Housekeeping'. In his book, he describes a number of quick and easy ways to deal with stress and negative feelings that have arisen during the consultation so that you can ensure you are in the best shape ready for the next patient. Well worth a read. These techniques are easy to learn and applicable to all your future consultations.

Consultation Models

Calgary Cambridge

This is a very comprehensive and evidence-based approach to the consultation – another five-stage model which includes specific detail of tools and techniques.

A. Data gathering

1. Initiating the session

    Introductions

    Establishing rapport

    Finding out the reason for the consultation

2. Gathering information

    Exploring the patient's perspective using a range of verbal and non-verbal communication skills including open and closed questions, ICE, clarification, summarising etc. Finding out 'Why now?' – the universal question of the consultation is 'Why has this patient come today with this problem?' If you can't answer this by the end of the consultation, you have missed something important!

B. Clinical management

3. Explanation and planning

    Finding out what the patient knows

    Asking what the patient wants to know

    'Chunks and checks' – information in digestible chunks

    Careful timing of explanations – not too soon

4. Closing the session

    Safety nets and follow-up

C. Interpersonal skills

5. Building the relationship

    Developing rapport

    Accepting the patient's views as legitimate

    Using non-verbal behaviour

    Involving the patient (e.g. thinking aloud, explicitly describing examination process and findings)

Calgary Cambridge also explores the very important feature of providing structure to the consultation by approaching it logically, using mini-summaries and keeping to time. All very important – a messy disordered consultation is inefficient.

Consultation Models

6 S for success

A relatively new model developed in 2013 by Alex Watson with an easy to remember alliterative '6 S' model.

Story, Summarising, Sharing, Securing, Status, Sanity

A. Data gathering

1. **Story** – connecting with the patient, being attentive, letting him tell his story, demonstrating verbally and non-verbally that you are listening to what he is saying. Find out thoughts, hopes and fears. Find the subplot if there is one.
2. **Summarising** – an opportunity to review what has been said so far, non-judgementally. The patient feels listened to and there is opportunity to clarify, add additional information and correct any misunderstandings before moving on.

B. Clinical management

3. **Sharing** – moving from listening to discussion about management, including the patient's thoughts, fears and hopes and incorporating the doctor's view. Any risks can also be discussed and shared between doctor and patient.
4. **Securing** – Safety netting the consultation, securing the evidence by making notes. (Written notes are not needed in the CSA!)

C. Interpersonal skills

5. **Status** – again, something that overarches and underpins the consultation: how we behave with others, how they perceive us and we perceive them and how this affects the consultation for good or bad.

    A mid-level point is the most helpful so that the clinician takes care to be warm, interested and on a level with the patient, avoiding the unhelpful extremes of arrogance/aloofness and timidity/being apologetic.

Watson's sixth stage is 'sanity' – similar to housekeeping described by Neighbour. Making sure that you are in good shape for the next patient and for your future in general practice.

Complete CSA's FOCUS Consultation Model

The **FOCUS Consultation Model** groups the key elements of the consultation.

FILTER
Open	Ask as many open questions as possible to collect the story.
Flags	Use focused questions. Check for red flags and whittle down differentials.
Risk	Ask about risk factors for your suspected diagnosis.
History	Take the history: past, systemic, family, medicines and social.
O/E	Explain exactly what you would like to examine and gain informed consent.

OPPORTUNITY
Sense — Reflect what you sense from non-verbal cues.
E.g. *'I feel/can see that (fidgeting/breathless/distracted/in a rush) …'*

ICE — Explore ideas, concerns and expectations.

Impact — Find out how the problem has affected the patient.

Curious — Respond to verbal cues.
E.g. *'You mentioned your friend. What is their experience of …?'*

CONTEXT
Summary — Demonstrate you have listened by summarising the ICE.

Empathy — Show you have put the problem into the context of their life.
E.g. *'I can see your past experience of … can lead you to consider …'*

Impression — State your impression!

Experience — Check their understanding or experience of what you have diagnosed.

Explanation — Provide a concise and jargon-free explanation.

UNITE
Options — Provide an organised list of options. Confirm their understanding and interest.
E.g. *'Things that you can do …, I can do …, others can help with …'*

Empower — Suggest what the patient can do themselves to help the problem.

Future — Explain what you believe should or is likely to happen at the next steps.
E.g. *'Thinking ahead … Return to the GP in …'*
E.g. *'At the hospital you can expect to …'*

SAFETY
Safety net — Give clear instructions about when to re-present to a doctor.

Remember to ask:

Paediatrics:	Gestation, delivery, postnatal, immunisations and development.
Women's:	Last menstrual period, cycle, post-coital bleeding, intermenstrual bleeding, discharge, smears, parity and operations.

Complete CSA's FOCUS Consultation Model

FOCUS Consultation Model explained

We don't expect you to learn and remember all the elements, and a formulated approach is not natural. However, this can be a useful list to see what can be achieved in a consultation. If you need help under exam conditions, the **FOCUS model** may help you, but find your own style.

The more you practise, the more likely you are to have good consultations with greater depth.

Not every consultation will need every element and the order will change. Be flexible.

Consider how many seconds you will allow yourself for each element. If an element requires longer, keep bringing the patient back into the discussion, e.g. checking their understanding or reaction.

FILTER

Here you should gather information from the patient and gradually filter the data to help you move towards a diagnosis. Identify risk factors and red flags to formulate your differential diagnosis. Check history: past medical history (PMH), drug history (DH), family history (FH) and social history (SH) to look for relevant information which will ultimately affect diagnosis and management.

OPPORTUNITY

Use identified cues to give the patient the opportunity to discuss their ICE (ideas, concerns and expectations). Be curious, sense how they are feeling and assess the impact of their symptoms on their life.

CONTEXT

Combine the information gathered to put the presenting problems into their psychosocial context. Illustrate this to the patient and examiner by forming a concise summary. Share your impression which is always followed by checking the patient's experience and understanding of the diagnosis you have stated.

UNITE

Share the management plan to unite doctor and patient. Discuss options; what can the patient do (empower) ... what can I do ... what can others (specialists/family) do and finally what resources (websites, support groups, patient information leaflets) are available?

SAFETY

Always offer a safety net. Be specific – what do they need to look out for? How long should they wait before returning? What should they do if they feel they are getting worse?

The diagrammatic model opposite illustrates how the model links to the CSA mark scheme.

Complete CSA's FOCUS Consultation Model

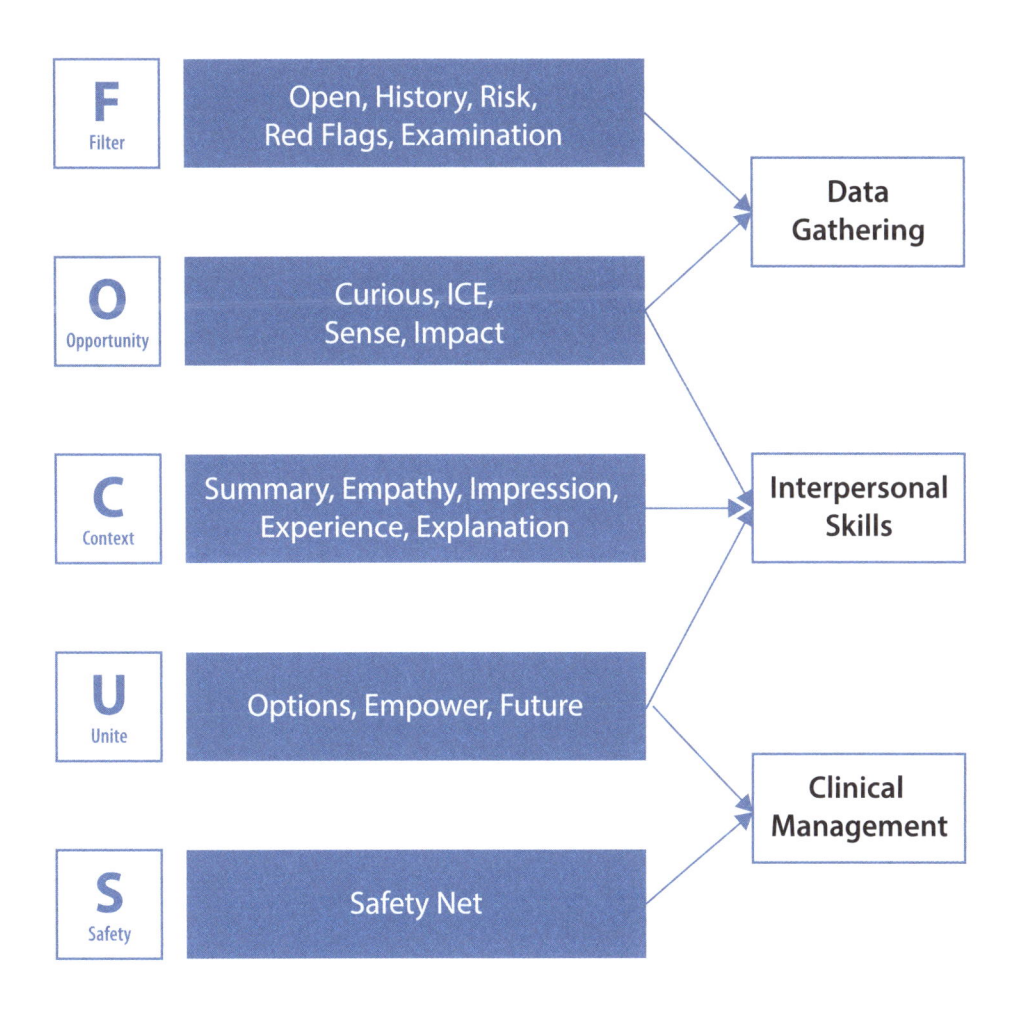

F — Filter: Open, History, Risk, Red Flags, Examination → Data Gathering

O — Opportunity: Curious, ICE, Sense, Impact → Data Gathering

C — Context: Summary, Empathy, Impression, Experience, Explanation → Interpersonal Skills

U — Unite: Options, Empower, Future → Interpersonal Skills / Clinical Management

S — Safety: Safety Net → Clinical Management

Easy to Use Generic Feedback Card

Below are some pointers which you can look out for when marking each other's cases. On the next page there is a blank grid which you could photocopy to make marking easier. Look for what the doctor has done well and what could be improved in each domain.

Data gathering:
- Was the main reason for attendance established? Were relevant red flags checked?
- Was an organised system used for gathering background information: PMH, DH, FH, SH?
- Were cues in the history detected? Were ideas, concerns and expectations elicited?
- Was there an appropriate and slick examination where necessary?
- Were any instruments required during the examination used proficiently?

Clinical management:
- Was an appropriate working diagnosis made?
- Was an appropriate management plan discussed with the patient including appropriate tests, medication, referrals, follow-up etc?
- Were opportunities to tackle health promotion found?
- Did the doctor appropriately safety net?

Interpersonal skills:
- Did the doctor adopt a sensitive approach?
- Did the doctor use appropriate language and avoid jargon?
- Did the doctor share the management plan?
- Did the doctor demonstrate active listening skills?
- Did the doctor put the problem in the psychosocial context relevant to the patient?
- Did the doctor appear genuinely interested in the patient?

Possible negative descriptors for feedback and to discuss:
- The consultation appeared disorganised.
- A significant agenda, abnormal result or red flag was missed.
- Failure to examine (if appropriate).
- Poor time management.
- The focus of the consultation was on the wrong agenda/complaint.

Easy to Use Generic Feedback Card

Case

Data Gathering	
POSITIVE	NEGATIVE

Clinical Management	
POSITIVE	NEGATIVE

Interpersonal Skills	
POSITIVE	NEGATIVE

Overall Impression

Practising the Skills within FOCUS

Recognise your strengths! Then consider which elements you find the most challenging.
Target your revision. Analyse and fine tune each micro skill a day at a time …

FILTER   Be assertive and sharpen your history.

Non-verbal   Use videos to analyse non-verbal communication.

Open   If you often dive in too soon, concentrate on routinely asking a series of encouraging/open questions – at least three before you move to semi-closed or closed questions.

History   Think about your management whilst taking the history. Practise actively, not subconsciously, taking a history to: filter, hypothesise, confirm hypothesis (by ruling out other differentials) then **asking the questions which actually change your management**!

Do not ask irrelevant questions (e.g. allergies may not be necessary).

Examination   Have study sessions practising only your examinations so they are slick.

OPPORTUNITY

Curious   Work on those cues, e.g. repeating phrases back to patients.

Impact/Sense   Put a Post-it note on your desk to remind you in your surgery.

CONTEXT

Empathy   With every patient you see, practise summarising their ICE followed by a statement which links the ICE to their background, experience or situation.

Impression   The words (or equivalent) 'I believe the diagnosis is … What do you know about …? Let me explain …' should be rolling off the tongue at 6 minutes.

Explanation   For each diagnosis practise a sentence. Without jargon!

UNITE

Options   To remind yourself, try using 'Let's decide on some options together.'

SAFETY

Safety net   Practise excellent documentation to reinforce this. Remember, be specific. Watching back video consultations can help you check how clear your safety netting is.

Top Tips – on the day

The day will feel like a typical surgery

It is a fair and realistic exam and you should do what you normally do. You are a locum GP, so you are not expected to have seen the patient before and, similarly, when safety netting remember that you will not see them again. Any emotions displayed by the patient, e.g. anger, will not be targeted at you (because you have never seen the patient before). Remember not to criticise real or imaginary colleagues, e.g. the last doctor who treated the patient.

Why this day is easier than the rest …

The patient will have only one problem (unless the case is about managing multiple agendas).

The actor will give you the answers quickly if you ask the right questions!

There is no need to document so you have the full 10 minutes for the consultation … Bliss!

Why the day is harder than the rest …

As a trainee, you know this is the day you have been working towards for 3+ years.

You have spent £1500 on this day. Along with the rest! It is the final hurdle of training.

What you need to say to yourself on the morning …

You have been listening to patients and managing problems for at least 5 years.

Ask the right questions and you will not go down the wrong track because you will be guided by their answers.

You will be nice, you will be curious and you will be interested.

You can make a few suggestions (even if you miss out a few things).

So the hardest parts of this exam are …

Overcoming nerves. Housekeeping (forgetting the last one if it went terribly!).

Remembering all the elements. So use the **FOCUS Model**! You could write this down as a prompt on your whiteboard (the examiner doesn't look at this).

Suggested time management:

History and Examination within the first 6 minutes.

By 6 minutes you should be stating your Impression.

Future (follow-up) and Safety Net at 9 minutes.

If the buzzer is about to go … squeeze in that safety net!

Top Tips – consultation scenarios

Child consultation
The RCGP have now introduced child actors. Remember to acknowledge him/her and aim to get as much history as you can from the child. The parent may wish to lead, but keep asking and including the child using language appropriate to their stage of development.

Telephone consultations
Telephone calls can be challenging. Non-verbal clues are gone, although you can often get a feel by listening to how they speak or sound. Are they breathless? Do they sound distressed? You will still be able to sense, e.g. from the patient's tone of voice, how concerned they are and consider reflecting this to the patient or commenting on non-speech sounds. If speaking to a friend or relative, ask them to describe what they see. How worried is the carer? If they are concerned, you should be too.

To help decide how urgently to see a child, ask Mum what they are doing at that particular moment. A child lying in Mum's arms is likely to need more urgent attention than one who is happily playing. Most parents know intuitively what is usual for their child and what is not.

If an examination is required, bring them in! Can you use the skill set in the team, e.g. the asthma nurse or the nurse practitioner, instead of, or before, seeing them yourself?

If the patient has difficulty with the language or is vulnerable (adult or child), have a lower threshold for seeing them face to face.

If a relative asks to collect something for a patient (e.g. her daughter's pill), remember you **do not have the patient's consent to disclose any information** (e.g. to confirm a medication). Ask the relative to tell the patient they need to speak to you, then call the patient yourself. Never confirm or imply that the patient is registered at the practice unless you are certain that it would not put the patient at risk.

Within your practice, make sure you have safe systems you can trust and that all the staff comply. E.g. the front desk confirms the telephone number, all patient contact is documented in the notes or on the appointment system and that the triage system is safe.

Some practical tips:
- Always check the identity of the person to whom you are speaking on the phone.
- If the patient called you, ask for and note down their contact number in case you get cut off.
- If you are phoning a patient and there is no answer, remember there may be a good reason for this. Consider how many times you will call again and the interval between calls.
- If there is no response to a reasonable number of calls (e.g. three), leave a clear and detailed voice message, e.g. *'It is Doctor Blount calling from the surgery. The time is 3.23 pm. Please call the surgery as soon as you receive this message and the receptionist will inform me that you are available. If the surgery has closed and you still need to speak to a doctor, please call 111.'*
- Remember to note each attempt in the medical record, e.g. 'Failed telephone encounter'.
- If you are worried (e.g. elderly patient), think about asking the police to do a welfare check.
- Think about which diagnoses you are willing to manage over the phone: never take short cuts.
- If you are managing the problem over the phone, detailed safety netting and ensuring the patient understands contingency plans are essential.
- Always ensure you can justify your actions.
- Always let the patient put the phone down first.

Home visits
You may be led to another room to simulate a home visit.

Top Tips – in the consultation

Investigations
Consider resources and avoid over-investigating. It is good practice to explain which tests you believe are necessary and this also tells the examiner.

Prescribing in the exam
It is likely that you will be asked to write a prescription. The examiners do not want you to suggest the patient collects the prescription later. The medication is usually something simple but, unless you are 110% sure, check the drug and the dose in the BNF. However, use your time wisely. You may prefer to wait until you have finished the consultation rather than spend time writing a prescription in the middle of the consultation when you could be gaining many marks for the other elements.

When you mention a medicine you should provide the following:
The name of the medicine and how to take it.
Why it is indicated and a simple statement about how it works.
What the risks and potential side effects are.
Check whether the patient is happy to proceed or offer an alternative.

Providing answers to test results
First, establish what the patient understands about why a test was requested. This may help you break bad news sensitively and prevent you putting your foot in it! E.g. a patient expects a CXR to show pneumonia but you suspect cancer.

If the patient tries to move the consultation ahead before you are ready, acknowledge their anxiety or question (e.g. blood test or diagnosis of CKD3) straight away and give them the answer. However, do not be thrown by a patient asking for their management options and go back to the beginning. It is difficult to score marks for Data Gathering if you gather no data!

E.g. *'I can see you are keen for your results. The blood tests show your blood sugar is raised. I'm sure you are keen to know what that means and where we go from here but, to put this result into the context of you, I need to go through your medical history in detail.'*

Parking information
If the patient mentions a new problem, instead of *'We'll come back to that'* … *'Okay so … is important to you, but do you mind if I come back to that?'* So park it but remember to return! This can be used when the two problems aren't connected. Use your whiteboard to make a note of this if you are worried you will forget.

Do remember that if the patient has given you information, there may be more important clues to find. So be curious. E.g. a patient presents with breathing problems but leads you onto his depression. This is hugely important, whether or not it turns into a depression consultation.

Establish the main reason for the consultation, e.g. medical risk or psychosocial. Remain organised and risk assess for each problem, agree where to focus your remaining time then signpost what you could discuss in future.

Top Tips – when a case feels like it's going wrong

If you worry that you might lose your way, remember that you are given a whiteboard where you can write your consultation structure. It can give you added confidence knowing that you may refer to it if necessary.

If you do lose your way in a consultation, try summarising. This should help collate the information you have and help identify areas you have yet to cover.

Remember your structure and the **FOCUS model**.

Check ICE again.

Have you missed a cue? E.g. have they mentioned a friend/relative? In an exam this will be for a reason. Explore this – what do they think? Or has this person had a similar experience? – So be curious!

Has the patient said he/she has been feeling worried?

Try not to guess what the examiner wants you do to. Just do what you would do in a normal surgery. If the patient's demands are unreasonable, negotiate rather than saying no.

Remember you don't have to pass every case.

If you feel that things are going wrong, take a deep breath and try to put it behind you.

The next examiner will have no idea how the last case went and so will not be influenced by it.

If it feels as if a consultation is not going smoothly, don't be afraid to share your feelings with the patient. *'I feel I am not being as helpful as I could be. I'm sorry. Can we take a step back to … and go from there so I can do a better job?'*

Top Tips

Medical complexity

It is unlikely that you will have to approach more than one problem within each CSA case although, as this is the everyday (nearly every patient) reality, it would be fair to be given such a case. Therefore, consider how you will approach it. First, consider how you come across to the patient (and in this case the examiner) when the patient mentions a symptom that you know requires time to safely explore. You appreciate it is likely to require another consultation and therefore their comment instantly increases the demands of the 10-minute consultation. You may feel frustrated and under pressure, but you need to appear calm. E.g. the patient mentions another unrelated symptom (e.g. headaches) when you have only just started discussing their breathlessness …

Phrases which may help: *'Tell me more about that.'* This gives you time to consider if they could be related. (Potentially a rare condition.) Or *'We need to give each problem, the breathlessness and the headache, the time it deserves. Which do you feel we need to concentrate on today?'*

Risk assess! Ask them the **red flags** for both problems. You can then reassure the patient and yourself why you have not explored it further today. If the patient is being vague, you may need to say, *'I need to ask you some specific questions* (red flags) *that will help me to rule out* (e.g.) *a blood clot on the lung.'* Then thank and reassure. If the patient selects the symptom which you feel is less important, e.g. tension type headache over breast lump or haematemesis, explain your concern to the patient and ask their permission to redirect the consultation. *'Would you mind if we discuss … first as I am concerned about …?'*

Grey areas

There are many grey areas in General Practice! Holding the responsibility of potential risk is the greatest challenge. Diagnosis and management plans don't always fit into boxes or guidelines. You are likely to be given a case to see how you approach this. Use present AND ABSENT red flags to help direct your management or possible referral. Provide a pragmatic and safe suggestion and then reach an agreement. Consider if you can tailor the management plan specifically to their history, wishes or needs.

It is okay to share uncertainty, share guidelines, offer choices and provide the patient with the opportunity to make an informed decision. This shares the responsibility; however, be aware some patients do not want the emotional burden of making a decision and turn to the doctor for full direction. A doctor should never share responsibility to make themselves feel better or lighten the weight of responsibility.

Remember, when explaining the options to patients, do not confuse them. Be organised with how you present the dilemma.

Useful Phrases

Useful Phrases: FILTER

Clarify understanding ... *'Can you describe what you mean by wheeze/palpitations?'*

Instead of the vague *'Tell me more'* which will waste time because the patient will ask you what you want to know, try ... *'Tell me the story of (your headaches) from the beginning.'*

If they've had the symptom for months ... *'What prompted you to come now?'*

Checking past history and investigations etc. ... *'As we haven't met before, would you mind telling me ...'*

Useful Phrases: OPPORTUNITY

ICE, ICE, ICE. It is vital that these questions come across naturally and do not sound robotic, so consider what information you need. To understand a patient and, more importantly, for the patient to feel understood, the GP needs to explore their **health belief**; this means their thought process, what is on their mind, their fear, where this has come from, their **experience** of a 'similar' problem or what they have read, who they have spoken to and why they have presented now. Be **curious**! Being aware of what is going through the patient's mind will lead you towards what they may be assuming you will do.

If you miss any (or all!) of this, the patient may feel you have missed something crucial and they may be right.

Try variations on the following:

'Is there anything else that you have been wondering?'

'Have you had any thoughts about what might be causing your symptoms?'

'Is there anything else that has been on your mind?'

'Do you have any thoughts about what you would like us to do?'

'What is important to you when considering what needs to be done today?'

Useful Phrases

Useful Phrases: CONTEXT

Now summarise ICE ... this is a powerful way to show you understand the patient.

'Am I on the right track?' or *'Have I understood you correctly so far?'*

ICE and empathy help address health beliefs in the context of the individual.

Incorporate their thoughts and experience together with their background (social history) to help you empathise.

'I can see that because your father had ... you are worried this could be ... and because you are under a lot of pressure at the moment with ... I can see you have been frightened for what this could mean and had fears of ... but I think what is going on here is ....'

The Result   The patient feels listened to and understood.
                 The doctor understands the patient's health beliefs and can educate.

You can only genuinely empathise when you have understood the person's experience.

Another example ...

'You wonder if it could be ... I see why you would think that, especially when you have experience of/have gone through/your mother has gone through ... However, my impression is ... which may have been caused by ...'

You could use the positive and negative red flags to help you here, explaining why you have reached that conclusion,

Check experience (understanding). *'What do you know about ...?'*

Then educate. *'... is ... and the course of the problem is often ...'*

Useful Phrases

Useful Phrases: UNITE

An inappropriate request … *'Have you thoughts about any problems with that?'*

'Let's think through this together.'

Acknowledge their expectation before giving options. *'I understand you were hoping for … My suggestion of options for where we go from here includes …'*

Remember **you are the doctor** … *'My recommendation would be …'*

But include the patient in the management plan, especially if there are a couple of appropriate options … *'What do you believe is best for you?'* Or *'What is your preference?'*

Structure your management plan:

'What you can do … We can do … What other people can do ….'

If you give a patient an information leaflet, you must explain its contents.

Useful Phrases: SAFETY

'If you find your child is not able to keep down fluids, they are at risk of becoming dehydrated, so please contact us at the surgery. If the surgery is closed, dial 111 to speak to an on-call GP.'

'If you find you require more than 10 puffs of your inhaler over four hours, please call the surgery. However, if you require 10 puffs at the same time, please call 999.'

Useful Phrases

The motivational interview

Fantastic for health promotion cases ...

'How do you think your general health is?'

'What could be improved?'

'Do you want ... to change?'

'Do you feel confident you can change ...?'

'How could you improve ...?'

'What challenges might you encounter with this?'

'How could you overcome these obstacles?'

'What steps do you think you may take?'

'In what time frame should this change happen?'

'When do you want to meet again to discuss this?'

Jargon Switch

Consider the patient in front of you. You may need to change your language.
You may decide to tell your revision partner to tap their pen on the table whenever you use jargon.
For example …

'2 week wait'	Urgent suspected cancer referral
'Abdomen'	Tummy
'Acute'	New symptom
'Benign'	Harmless
'Cervix'	The neck of the womb
'Chronic'	Symptoms you have had a long time
'Cyst'	Fluid-filled lump that is usually harmless
'DNA'	The genetic information passed down from our parents
'ECG'	Test where we put stickers on the chest to see a tracing of the heart, which we call an ECG
'Fracture'	Broken bone
'Inflammation'	Swelling/redness
'Observations'	Heart rate and blood pressure
'Over the counter'	From the pharmacy
'Positive/negative'	Test result. Avoid using this term and explain exactly what the test shows. Patients may believe positive means good, negative means bad which may not actually be the case!
'Ultrasound'	Jelly scan called an ultrasound
'Vital signs'	Heart rate and blood pressure

Resitting the Exam

What may have gone wrong ...

Too slow – you do not reach the management plan. Practise your time management. You may be spending too much time on data gathering (for fear of missing something) to the detriment of the rest of your case.

The doctor talks more than the patient. Consider the many opportunities within the FOCUS model to **engage** and involve your patient before giving information.

Missing the subtleties of the consultation and hence the reason for the patient's attendance. Focus your cases on Opportunity within the **FOCUS Model**.

The patient leaves not knowing the diagnosis. Even if you are unsure, you should reassure yourself and the patient with the important negatives, e.g. why it is not a sinister/serious diagnosis. Or share what you need to do to rule out a sinister/serious diagnosis and how you will get more information (tests, referral, and colleague advice) to make the diagnosis.

You do not produce a safe management plan. Consider whether this is because you have not considered the sinister/serious causes of their symptoms.

Poor organisation. Disorganised consultations don't give a good impression to the examiner or patient. Try to stick to your consultation model and don't jump between history/examination/information giving.

Still not sure? Think about the basics – whose needs aren't being met?

PATIENT NEEDS
- Wants to feel understood.
- Wants to share everything they have noticed:
  - To offload anxiety and hand over responsibility.
  - Just in case it may be relevant.
- Wants to know what is wrong.
- Wants reassurance.
- Wants to get better.

DOCTOR AGENDA
- To know the facts that will change the management.
- Wants clear information so they can make the diagnosis and plan ... within 10 minutes.
- Wants to fix the problem.
- Wants the patient to be satisfied with the plan.

Abbreviations

\# = fracture
°C = degrees centigrade
♀ = female
♂ = male
1/12 = 1 month
20/40 = 20 weeks' gestation
2WW = 2 week wait
3/7 = 3 days
αFP = α fetoprotein
A&E = accident and emergency department
AA = Alcoholics Anonymous
AAA = abdominal aortic aneurysm
ABCD2 score = age, BP, clinical features, duration of symptoms and diabetes
ABPI = arterial brachial pressure index
ACEI = ACE inhibitors
ACL = anterior cruciate ligament
ACR = albumin creatinine ratio
ACS = acute coronary syndrome
ACTH = adrenocorticotropic hormone
ADHD = attention deficit hyperactivity disorder
ADL = activities of daily living
AF = atrial fibrillation
AKA = also known as
AKI = acute kidney injury (acute renal failure)
ALP = alkaline phosphatase
ALT = alanine aminotransferase
AMTS = abbreviated mental test score
Anti-D = anti-D (Rho) Immunoglobulin
APQ = alcohol problems questionnaire
APTT = activated partial thromboplastin time
ARB = angiotensin receptor blocker
ARMD = age related macular degeneration
AS = ankylosing spondylitis
ASD = atrial septal defect
AST = aspartate transaminase
AUDIT = alcohol use disorders identification test
AVSD = atrioventricular septal defect
β-blockers = beta blockers
β-hCG = β human chorionic gonadotropin
B12 = vitamin B12
BCC = basal cell carcinoma
BCG = bacillus Calmette-Guérin
BD = twice daily
BM = blood sugar level
BMD = bone mineral density
BMI = body mass index
BNF = British National Formulary
BNP = B-type natriuretic peptide
BP = blood pressure
BPH = benign prostatic hypertrophy
bpm = beats per minute
BPO = benzoyl peroxide
BPPV = benign paroxysmal positional vertigo
BRCA = breast cancer
BTS = British Thoracic Society
Ca^{2+} = calcium
CAMHS = child and adolescent mental health services
CBT = cognitive behavioural therapy
CCB = calcium channel blocker
CCF = congestive cardiac failure
CCG = clinical commissioning group
CEA = carcinoembryonic antigen
CES = cauda equina syndrome
CF = cystic fibrosis
CHA_2DS_2-VASc = clinical prediction calculator for estimating risk of stroke in patients with AF
CHC = combined hormonal contraception
Chol = cholesterol
CI = contraindication(s)
CK = creatinine kinase
CKD = chronic kidney disease
CKS = Clinical Knowledge Summaries (NICE)
CMV = cytomegaloviurs
CN = cranial nerve
COC/COCP = combined oral contraceptive pill
COPD = chronic obstructive pulmonary disease
CPAP = continuous positive airway pressure
CRB65 = confusion, respiratory rate, BP, age – assessment tool for community acquired pneumonia
CRP = C reactive protein
CSA = clinical skills assessment
CSF = cerebrospinal fluid
CT = computed tomography
CT CAP = CT chest abdomen and pelvis
CT KUB = CT kidney ureters and bladder
Cu-IUD = copper coil
CV = cardiovascular
CVA = cerebrovascular accident (stroke)
CVD = cardiovascular disease
CXR = chest X-ray
DAFNE = dose adjustment for normal eating
DAU = day assessment unit
DBP = diastolic blood pressure
DC = direct current

DESMOND = diabetes education and self-management for ongoing and newly diagnosed
DEXA = dual energy X-ray absorptiometry
DH = drug history
DHEAS = dehydroepiandrosterone sulfate
DKA = diabetic ketoacidosis
DM = diabetes mellitus
DMSA = dimercaptosuccinic acid scintigraphy scan
DN = district nurse
DNA = did not attend (i.e. missed appointment)
DNACPR = do not attempt cardiopulmonary resuscitation
DPP4 = dipeptidyl peptidase 4
DRE = digital rectal exam
DSM-IV = Diagnostic and Statistical Manual of Mental Disorders, 4th Edition
DV = domestic violence
DVLA = Driver and Vehicle Licensing Agency
DVT = deep vein thrombosis
EBV = Epstein-Barr virus
ECG = electrocardiography
ECHO = echocardiogram
ECP = emergency contraceptive pill
ED = erectile dysfunction
EE = ethinyl estradiol
EEG = electroencephalography
eGFR = estimated glomerular filtration rate
eGFRcysC = glomerular filtration rate (eGFR) by standardised cystatin C
ELSCS = emergency lower segment caesarian section
ENT = ear nose and throat
EPAU = early pregnancy assessment unit
ESM = ejection systolic murmur
ESR = erythrocyte sedimentation rate
F = female
f/up = follow up
FB = foreign body
FBC = full blood count
FBG = fasting blood glucose
FEV1 = forced expiratory volume in 1 second
FH = family history
FHR = foetal heart rate
FOB = faecal occult blood
FODMAPs = fermentable oligosaccharides, disaccharides, monosaccharides and polyols.
FRAX = fracture risk assessment tool
FSH = follicle stimulating hormone
fT4 = free thyroxine
FVC = forced vital capacity
g = grams
G = gravida

G2P2 = gravida 2, parity 2
GAD = general anxiety disorder
GCS = Glasgow Coma Scale
GCSE = general certificate of secondary education
GFR = glomerular filtration rate
GGT = gamma-glutamyltransferase
GI = gastrointestinal
GI = glycaemic index
GLP = glucagon-like peptide
GnRH = gonadotropin-releasing hormone
GORD = gastro-oesophageal reflux disease
GP = general practitioner
GSV = great saphenous vein
GTN = glyceryl trinitrate
GUM = genitourinary medicine
H2/H2RA = H2 receptor antagonists
HAS-BLED – score for major bleeding risk
HbA1c = Glycated haemoglobin
HbeAg/Ab = hepatitis B e antigen/antibody
HBsAg = hepatitis B surface antigen
HBV DNA = hepatitis B virus deoxyribonucleic acid
HCA = health care assistant
HCU = homocystinuria
HCV RNA = hepatitis C virus ribonucleic acid
HF = heart failure
HFE = haemochromatosis gene
Hib = haemophilus influenza type B (vaccine)
HIV – human immunodeficiency virus
HLA B27 = human leukocyte antigen B27
HOCM = hypertrophic obstructive cardiomyopathy
HONK = hyperosmolar non-ketotic acidosis
HPV = human papilloma virus
HR = heart rate
HRT = hormone replacement therapy
HS = heart sounds
HTN = hypertension
IBD = inflammatory bowel disease
IBS = inflammatory bowel syndrome
ICD-10 = International Classification of Diseases 10th Revision
ICE = ideas, concerns and expectations
ICH = intracranial haemorrhage
ICP = intracranial pressure
ICS = inhaled corticosteroids
ID = intellectual disability
Ig = immunoglobulin
IgG = immunoglobulin G
IgM = immunoglobulin M
IHD = ischaemic heart disease
IM = intramuscular
IMB = intermenstrual bleeding

IPSS = International Prostate Symptom Score
IQ = intelligence quotient
ISMN = isosorbide mononitrate
IT = information technology
ITU = intensive treatment unit
IUD = intrauterine device (copper coil)
IUS = intrauterine system (e.g. Mirena)
IV = intravenous
IVDU = intravenous drug use
IVF = in vitro fertilisation
JVP = jugular venous pressure
K = potassium
LA = local anaesthetic
LABA = long acting beta agonist
LAM = lactation amenorrhea method
LAMA = long acting muscarinic antagonist
LARC = long acting reversible contraception
LD = learning disability
LDH = lactate dehydrogenase
LFT = liver function test
LH = luteinising hormone
LIF = left iliac fossa
LMP = last menstrual period
LMWH = low molecular weight heparin
LOC = loss of consciousness
LRTI = lower respiratory tract infection
LTOT = long term oxygen therapy
LUTS = lower urinary tract symptoms
LV = left ventricular
LVD = left ventricular dysfunction
LVH = left ventricular hypertrophy
M = male
m = metre
M/R = modified release
MAU = maternity assessment unit
MCADD = medium chain acyl-CoA dehydrogenase deficiency
mcg = micrograms
MCUG = micturating cystourethrogram
MDT = multidisciplinary team
MEN2 = multiple endocrine neoplasia type 2
MenC = meningitis C (vaccine)
mg = milligrams
MI = myocardial infarction
mL = millilitres
MMR = measles mumps and rubella
MRC = Medical Research Council
MRI = magnetic resonance imaging
MS = multiple sclerosis
MSK = musculoskeletal
MSU = mid-stream urine
MUSE = medicated urethral system for erections
N&V = nausea and vomiting

Na = sodium
NAD = no abnormality detected
NAFLD = non-alcoholic fatty liver disease
NASH = non-alcoholic steatohepatitis
NHS = National Health Service
NICE = National Institute for Health and Care Excellence
NIH – CPSI = National Institutes of Health Chronic Prostatitis Symptom Index
NKDA = no known drug allergies
NOACs = novel oral anticoagulants
NOGG = national osteoporosis guidance group
NOK = next of kin
NSAID = non-steroidal anti-inflammatory drug
NTD = neural tube defect
NVD = normal vaginal delivery
NYHA= New York Heart Association
OA = osteoarthritis
OAB = overactive bladder
obs = clinical observations (temperature, pulse, BP etc)
OCP = oral contraceptive pill
OD = once daily
Ofsted = office for standards in children's education, children's services and skills
OGTT = oral glucose tolerance test
OM = once in the morning
ON = once at night
OOH = out of hours GP
OSA = obstructive sleep apnoea
OTC = over the counter
OCP = oral contraceptive pill
OGTT = oral glucose tolerance test
OOH = out of hours GP
OSA = obstructive sleep apnoea
OTC = over the counter
P = parity
PA = personal assistant
PAPP-A = pregnancy-associated plasma protein A
Para = parity
PC = presenting complaint
PCB = post-coital bleeding
PCKD = polycystic kidney disease
PCOS = polycystic ovarian syndrome
PCR = protein creatinine ratio
PCV = pneumococcal conjugate vaccine
PE = pulmonary embolus
PEF = peak expiratory flow
PERLA = pupils equal and react to light and accommodation
PET = positron emission tomography
PF = plantar fasciitis
PGP = pelvic girdle pain

PID = pelvic inflammatory disease
PIL = patient information leaflet
PMB = post-menopausal bleeding
PMH = past medical history
PMR = polymyalgia rheumatic
PN = practice nurse
PND = paroxysmal nocturnal dyspnoea
POP = progesterone only contraception pill
PPI = proton pump inhibitors
PR = per rectum (rectal examination)
PRN = as required
PSA = prostate specific antigen
PSV = public service vehicle licence
PT = prothrombin time
PTH = parathyroid hormone
PUD = peptic ulcer disease
PV = per vaginam (vaginal examination)
PVD = peripheral vascular disease
QDS = four times daily
QOL = quality of life
QRISK2 = algorithm for cardiovascular disease
RACPC = rapid access chest pain clinic
RAST = radioallergosorbent test
RBG = random blood glucose
RCGP = Royal College of General Practitioners
RCO = Royal College of Ophthalmologists
RFs = risk factors
RhD = rhesus D
RLQ = right lower quadrant
RNIB = Royal National Institute of Blind People
ROM = range of movement
RPOC = retained products of conception
RR = respiratory rate
RUQ = right upper quadrant
Rx = treatment
s/c = subcutaneous
SABA = short acting beta agonist
SADQ = severity of alcohol dependence questionnaire
Sats = oxygen saturation
SBP = systolic blood pressure
SCC = squamous cell carcinoma
SDH = subdural haematoma
SFH = symphysis fundal height
SH = social history
SHBG = sex hormone binding globulin
SLR = straight leg raise
SMART = self management and recovery training
SNHL = sensorineural hearing loss
SNRI = serotonin-norepinephrine reuptake inhibitors

SNT = soft, non-tender
SOB = shortness of breath
SOBOE = short of breath on exertion
SOCRATES = site, onset, character, radiation, associated factors, time, exacerbating/relieving factors, severity (pain history)
SOL = space occupying lesion
SPD = symphysis pubis dysfunction
SSRI = selective serotonin reuptake inhibitor
STI = sexually transmitted infection
SUI = stress urinary incontinence
SVC = superior vena cava
SVT = supraventricular tachycardia
T1DM = type 1 diabetes/diabetics
T2DM = type 2 diabetes/diabetics
T4 = thyroxine level
TAH = total abdominal hysterectomy
TCA = tricyclic antidepressant
TCI = to come in
TDS = three times daily
TENS = transcutaneous electrical nerve stimulation
TFT = thyroid function test
TIA = transient ischaemic attack
TIBC = total iron binding capacity
TP = tumour protein
Trg = triglyceride
TSH = thyroid stimulating hormone
TURP = transurethral resection of the prostate
TVUSS = transvaginal ultrasound
U&E = urea and electrolytes and eGFR
UC = ulcerative colitis
UI = urinary incontinence
UKMEC = UK medical eligibility criteria for contraceptive use
UMN = upper motor neurone
UO = urinary output
UPSI = unprotected sexual intercourse
URTI = upper respiratory tract infection
USS = ultrasound scan
UTI = urinary tract infection
VA = visual acuity
VEGF = vascular endothelial growth factor
vs = versus
VTE = venous thromboembolism
VZIG = varicella zoster immunoglobulin
VZV = varicella zoster virus
WCC = white cell count
WHO = World Health Organization

Disclaimer

The information or guidance contained in this book is intended for use by medical professionals (specifically General Practitioners or General Practitioner Trainees) only and is provided strictly as a supplement to the reader's own judgement, their knowledge of the patient's medical history, relevant manufacturers' instructions and the appropriate best practice guidelines. The guidance we refer to within this book is specifically for General Practitioners based in the UK, and international readers should refer to local guidance and advice. Because of the rapid advances in medical science, any information or advice on dosages, procedures or diagnoses should be independently verified. The reader should take into account that the information within this book is only part of any guidance mentioned and is strongly urged to consult the full text of up to date guidance. The text is not to replace specialist advice. The reader is strongly urged to consult the relevant national drug formulary and the drug companies' and device or material manufacturers' printed instructions, and their websites, before administering or utilising any of the drugs, devices or materials mentioned in this book. This book does not indicate whether a particular treatment is appropriate or suitable for a particular individual. Ultimately, it is the sole responsibility of the medical professional to make his or her own professional judgements, so as to advise and treat patients appropriately. We do not accept any liability or responsibility for any form of loss or any decision made by the reader.

CHAPTER 2 OVERVIEW
Healthy People

	Cases in this chapter	Within the RCGP curriculum: Healthy People, Promoting Health and Preventing Disease RCGP Curriculum Online March 2016[1]	Learning points in the chapter include:
1	Immunisation Refusal	'Be able to explain the benefits and risks of child immunisation and vaccination in order to reassure parents effectively'	MMR refusal, other reasons for immunisation refusal and legal considerations. Immunisation schedules and conditions immunisations protect against
2	Cervical Screening	'Promote self-care and empower patients and their families whenever appropriate' 'Explain to the patient and/or their relatives the evidence about a screening programme …'	Cervical cytology procedure, results and counselling Other NHS screening programmes
3	Inappropriate Use of Services	'Understand approaches to behavioural change and their relevance to health promotion and self-care'	Educating families with regards to how to use local services
4	High Cholesterol	'Assess a healthy individual patient's risk factors' 'Understand the concept of risk and be able to communicate risk effectively to patients and their families'	Cardiovascular risk scores Statin discussion
5	Wants to Lose Weight	'Consider how to minimise the impact of the patient's symptoms on his or her well-being by taking into account the patient's personality, family, daily life and physical and social surroundings'	The importance of understanding the patient to help guide behaviour change See also The Motivational Interview in the Introduction
Extra notes	Immunisation Schedule	'Be able to explain the benefits and risks of child immunisation and vaccination in order to reassure parents effectively'	Current immunisation schedule Live attenuated vaccines
	Immunisation/ Vaccine Preventable Diseases	'Be able to explain the benefits and risks of child immunisation and vaccination in order to reassure parents effectively'	Symptoms, complications and mortality rates
	Cervical Screening Programme	'Understand the ethical aspects of prevention, presymptomatic diagnostics, asymptomatic therapy and factors that influence lifestyles'	Who should be screened
	Other NHS Screening Programmes	'Promote health through a health promotion or disease prevention programme'	Bowel cancer, breast cancer, diabetic retinopathy, AAA, newborn and antenatal screening
	Diet and Exercise Advice	'Promote health through a health promotion or disease prevention programme'	NICE Guideline. CG181. Cardiovascular disease: risk assessment and reduction, including lipid modification. July 2014
	Statins	'Assess a healthy individual patient's risk factors'	Primary and secondary prevention

1. http://www.rcgp.org.uk/training-exams/gp-curriculum-overview/online-curriculum.aspx

CHAPTER 2 REFERENCES

Immunisation Refusal
1. http://www.nhs.uk/Conditions/vaccinations/Pages/mmrvaccine.aspx September 2016
2. Harmsen et al. Why parents refuse childhood vaccination: a qualitative study using online focus groups. *BMC Public Health* 2013; **13**: 1183. http://bmcpublichealth.biomedcentral.com/articles/10.1186/1471-2458-13-1183
3. http://www.nhs.uk/Conditions/Consent-to-treatment/Pages/Children-under-16.aspx. Sep 2016

Cervical Screening
1. http://patient.info/doctor/cervical-screening-cervical-smear-test-pro
2. Cervical cancer screening. http://www.cancerresearchuk.org/about-cancer/type/cervical-cancer/about/cervical-cancer-screening. Jun 2016
3. Human papillomavirus (HPV) and cervical cancer. Fact sheet. Updated June 2016. http://www.who.int/mediacentre/factsheets/fs380/en/
4. NICE. http://cks.nice.org.uk/cervical-screening#!scenario:1. Revised February 2015.

High Cholesterol
1. NICE Guidelines. CG181. Cardiovascular disease: risk assessment and reduction, including lipid modification. July 2014.

Wants to Lose Weight
1. NICE Guidelines. CG189. Obesity: identification, assessment and management. Nov 2014.

Extra notes

Immunisation Schedule
1. http://www.nhs.uk/Conditions/vaccinations/Pages/vaccination-schedule-age-checklist.aspx. Jun 2016
2. https://www.gov.uk/government/uploads/system/uploads/attachment_data/file/532787/PHE_Complete_Immunisation_Schedule_SUMMER2016.pdf. Contains public sector information licensed under the Open Government Licence v3.0.

Conditions Immunisations Protect Against
3. http://www.nhs.uk/conditions/Pages/hub.aspx. Jun 2016
4. http://www.who.int
5. http://www.cdc.gov/.

Cervical Screening
6. Cervical cancer screening. http://www.cancerresearchuk.org/about-cancer/type/cervical-cancer/about/cervical-cancer-screening. Jun 2016

Other Screening Programmes
7. http://patient.info/doctor/screening-programmes-in-the-uk
8. https://www.gov.uk/guidance/fetal-anomaly-screening-programme-overview. Contains public sector information licensed by the Open Government Licence v3.0.

Diet and Exercise
9. NICE Guidelines. CG181. Cardiovascular disease: risk assessment and reduction, including lipid modification. July 2014.
10. https://www.gov.uk/government/uploads/system/uploads/attachment_data/file/489796/CMO_alcohol_guidelines.pdf. Contains public sector information licensed by the Open Government Licence v3.0.

Statins
11. NICE Guidelines. CG181. Cardiovascular disease: risk assessment and reduction, including lipid modification. July 2014.
12. NICE technology appraisal guidance 132. Ezetimibe for the treatment of primary (heterozygous-familial and non-familial) hypercholesterolaemia. 2008.

Healthy People

Doctor's Notes

Patient   Bhakti Shukla   12 months   F
PMH   No information
Medications   No current medications
Allergies   No information
Consultations Last appointment with practice nurse 2 weeks ago.

'Attended for 12 month vaccinations. Hib/MenC, PCV, Meningitis B given.

Mum refused MMR. Asked to book in with doctor for discussion.'

Investigations No information
Household

Name	Age	Sex
Laksha Shukla	32 years	F
Aaditya Shukla	32 years	M
Samir Shukla	6 years	M
Chaman Shukla	5 years	F
Sabrang Shukla	3 years	F
Talika Shukla	60 years	F

Example Consultation — Immunisation Refusal

Open □ — What would you like to talk about today? Thank you for taking the time to see me. You have concerns about the MMR vaccine? Can you tell me more about what has been going through your mind about this vaccination? Let's discuss it today so you have all the information you need to help you decide.

Sense □ — I can see you want to ensure you are making the best decision for your children.

History □ — First, can you please tell me more about your family and their health? I see Bhakti has had her other vaccinations. Did she have any problems with them?

Risk □ — Does Bhakti have any allergies? Is she otherwise fit and well?

ICE □ — What do you know about the vaccination? Do you know what the letters MMR stand for? Correct. Would you like me to explain more about those diseases? Okay, we will go through that. How much do you know already? Was there any other information you were hoping to gain today? Was there anything else you were hoping for? Is there anything else that worries you apart from autism?

Experience □ — What is your experience of autism? So you fear this condition in your children?

Curious □ — How do you feel about vaccinations in general? What does Bhakti's father think?

Summary □ — So, generally, you are all for vaccination but you remember a lot of bad press about the MMR vaccination in the news, in particular about a link between the MMR vaccine and autism. It is important to you that your children have the best education and, having seen another child with autism, you hope to protect your children as best you can. You would like some more information about the MMR vaccination.

Explanation □ — The MMR vaccine is designed to protect against Measles, Mumps and Rubella. You're right, there was a scare about the MMR vaccination a few years back. This followed a piece of research which was published in 1998. However, this piece of research did have many flaws and subsequent research has discredited the initial research. In short, there has been a lot of research into the possible link between autism and the MMR vaccination, and no link has been found. After reviewing all the available information, the World Health Organization recommends that the MMR vaccine is given. Is there anything I have said that doesn't make sense so far?

Explanation □ — Measles is a virus which causes cold-like symptoms, high fever and a rash. It is often a mild illness but can have serious complications such as pneumonia, deafness, blindness and inflammation of the brain called encephalitis. Thankfully the death rate is low but there are about 1–2 deaths per 1000 cases. Mumps is a viral infection which affects the salivary glands of the cheeks. It usually gets better on its own but can affect the testicles and ovaries which, rarely, affects fertility. It, too, can cause deafness and can also cause meningitis. Rubella is another virus which causes high fever, a rash and cold-like symptoms. The main worry with rubella is for women who are pregnant catching it, as it can cause problems with the baby's development.

Options □ — As a parent you have the right to refuse vaccinations, but I hope I have reassured you that the MMR vaccination is safe and that it is there to protect against some serious infections. I recommend the vaccination to protect against these diseases as, after reading the studies myself, I am confident there is no link to autism.

Empathy □ — I understand it can be scary to make decisions which may put our children at risk.

Empower □ — Would you like some information to take away which you can read in your own time? You can discuss it with your husband. What are your thoughts at this time?

Future □ — Let me know when you've made a decision and we can arrange an appointment if you wish Bhakti to have the vaccination.

Safety net □ — If you have any concerns or wish to discuss anything further, please give me a call.

Patient's Story

Immunisation Refusal

Doctor's notes	Bhakti Shukla. 12 months. No information in medical history. Last appointment with practice nurse 2 weeks ago.
	'Attended for 12 month vaccinations. Hib/MenC, PCV, Meningitis B given.
	Mum refused MMR. Asked to book in with doctor for discussion.'
How to act	Concerned
PC	*'Hi Doctor, your nurse asked me to come and see you. I don't want Bhakti to have the MMR vaccination. I've heard it can cause autism.'*
History	Your name is Laksha Shukla. You are 32 years old and live with your husband, mother-in law and four children: Samir, Chaman, Sabrang and Bhakti.
	Generally, you are all for vaccinations. You grew up in India and saw the damage polio can do. You moved to the UK when you were 12 years old. You remember reading about the MMR vaccination causing autism so you don't want Bhakti to have this. Bhakti is developing well, and she has recently started walking. She has been well up until now and you have no concerns about her health.
Social	You are a full-time mum. Your husband feels Bhakti should have the vaccination but thought you should get some more information first to put your mind at ease. You have Hindu faith.
ICE	You believe there is a link between the MMR vaccination and autism. You would prefer Bhakti not to have the vaccination. You aren't sure what diseases the MMR vaccine protects against, but you suspect they aren't as bad as autism. You expect the doctor to be able to give you information about the link between the MMR vaccination and autism. You would also like to know more about measles, mumps and rubella. There is a boy in your oldest child's class who has autism and he has real difficulties at school. He struggles to learn and you hope your children have a good education.

Learning Points

Immunisation Refusal

The immunisation schedule is included in the extra notes, along with some information about the recent changes and some further points.

MMR and autism?[1]

The scare regarding the MMR vaccine and autism came about in 1998 after a study was published in the *Lancet*. The study claimed that the MMR vaccine had been linked to regression (loss of skills), autistic spectrum disorders, inflammation of the small intestine (enterocolitis) and that children with autism had higher levels of measles antibodies in their bloodstream. Since this study the claims have been widely discredited in follow-up studies looking into these claims. There were some flaws in the original study which could have led to bias. Based on the subsequent trials there is no reason to suspect that the MMR vaccine is linked to autism, and therefore the MMR is recommended by the World Health Organization as it is more effective than giving the separate vaccines for measles, mumps and rubella. Interestingly, the rates of autism continued to increase in Japan even after the vaccine had been withdrawn, adding further evidence of no causal link.

Other reasons for vaccination refusal

There is a multitude of reasons for parents refusing vaccination. Consider the following and how you would discuss these with the parents. One study[2] found the following were often cited:

- Perceptions about the child's body and immune system – too young for immune system to cope with immunisation or child already protected by breast feeding.
- Perceived risks of disease. The belief of a low risk of catching the illness, the belief that conditions can be easily treated and the belief the diseases are not serious.
- Vaccine efficacy. The belief that the vaccines don't work.
- Side effects.
- Perceived advantages of experiencing the disease.
- Prior negative experience with vaccination.

Legal considerations[3]

If one person with parental responsibility consents to treatment but another refuses, the healthcare professional can give treatment based on the consent given by one adult with parental responsibility or if there is great dispute, the case can be referred to the courts for a decision on the child's behalf.

Doctor's Notes

Patient	Chloe Atherton　　25 years　　F
PMH	Tonsillitis aged 22 years.
	Viral respiratory tract infection aged 14 years.
	Urinary tract infection aged 4 years.
Medications	Rigevidon
Allergies	No information
Consultations	Last appointment with practice nurse 3 weeks ago. Cervical smear taken.
Investigations	Recent Cervical Cytology Result:
	Mild dyskaryosis, high risk HPV detected. A colposcopy referral has been made.
Household	No household contacts.

Example Consultation — Cervical Screening

Open — Firstly let me reassure you that the test result has not found cancer. Before we discuss it in more detail, may I ask you a few background questions to ensure I understand what has happened so far? This will help me interpret your result.

History — What led to you having the test done? Are you otherwise well? Any problems with your periods or bleeding pattern? Do you smoke? Do you work? Regarding your women's health, when was your last period? Have you any abnormal bleeding? Have you ever been pregnant? Do you have a sexual partner? Do you have any abnormal vaginal discharge? Have you ever had a sexually transmitted infection?

Risk — Any bleeding between periods or after sex? Have you had any pain? Have you ever had a smear test before? Is there any family history of cervical cancer or women's problems? I'd like to reassure you this is not connected to the ovary.

ICE — You have mentioned that you are worried about cancer. Is there anything else that has been concerning you? Were you hoping I would do anything in particular today?

Summary — So you have no worrying symptoms, but received a letter telling you that your smear was abnormal and that you have been referred to the hospital. You are worried that you have cancer and whether this could be related to your aunt's cancer. You are concerned about the colposcopy test and whether it will be painful.

Experience — What do you know about smear tests already? Have you known anyone who has had it done? Or had problems with the cervix?

Explanation — The cervix is the neck of your womb. I can see from your record that you have mild dyskaryosis. This means that when the cells from your cervix were looked at under a microscope the middle of the cells looked a little abnormal. In your case, the changes are only mild. Often, in cases like yours, the cells will go back to normal all on their own. However, we know that cervical cancer is caused by the HPV virus, so in cases with changes we test for the presence of the virus. If found, which it is in a large percentage of the population and it was in your case, we offer a further test called colposcopy to look at the cervix in more detail. Smear tests look for changes in the cervix which, if left, may develop into cancer. So having an abnormal test rarely indicates cancer, but early changes. We then monitor the cervix or treat it to prevent cancer. Is there anything I have said which you are unclear about or that I haven't explained well enough? Would you like to know about colposcopy?

Explanation — Colposcopy is a procedure where a doctor looks at the cervix under a microscope directly. You will be asked to undress from the waist down and usually sit in a special chair which supports your legs. A speculum is put into the vagina so the cervix can be seen, like when you had the smear test. The doctor will usually put a special stain on the cervix which shows any abnormal cells. If any are found, the doctor will often take a biopsy or offer to treat the cells there and then by removing them after giving a local anaesthetic. If this happens, the doctor will explain this to you. Like a smear test, it can be uncomfortable but you shouldn't experience much pain. Any questions?

Options — How do you feel about the colposcopy now? Do you feel you will go?

Empathy — I understand getting abnormal results is scary, especially if there is a possibility of cancer. But hopefully there are just some abnormal cells which can be taken away.

Empower — Would you like to take some information away to read in your own time?

Future — We will get a letter from the hospital after your appointment but I would be happy to see you after the appointment if you'd like to discuss what happened.

Safety net — In the meantime, if you do have any bleeding not during your period or pain please let me know. Please don't hesitate to contact me if you have questions.

Patient's Story

Cervical Screening

Doctor's notes Chloe Atherton, 25 years. PMH: Tonsillitis aged 22 years. Viral respiratory tract infection aged 14 years. Urinary tract infection aged 4 years. Medication: Rigevidon

How to act Concerned.

Investigations Recent Cervical Cytology Result:

Mild dyskaryosis, high risk HPV detected. A colposcopy referral has been made.

PC *'Hi Doctor, I've recently had my smear done but the results have come back abnormal. Do I have cancer?'*

History You attended for your first cervical cytology test 3 weeks ago following receiving an invitation after your 25th birthday. You were unsure about going for the test but discussed it with a friend who is older than you and she said the test was fine, so you booked in. The nurse doing the test explained that if the results were abnormal you would be referred to the hospital for more tests. You are worried about this. Before the test you had no symptoms; no intermenstrual bleeding, no post-coital bleeding and no dyspareunia. There is no family history of cervical cancer but your aunt died of ovarian cancer and you thought this could be related. You take the oral contraceptive pill so feel pregnancy is unlikely; you always remember to take it. Last Menstrual Period 1 week ago.

Social You work as a barmaid and waitress. You have a boyfriend. You have been together 3 years. He knows about the result and how worried you are, so has offered to go to the hospital with you.

You don't smoke and only drink alcohol at weekends.

ICE You think you may have cervical cancer. You are concerned about the colposcopy test as you don't know what this will involve. You hope the doctor will be able to reassure you that you don't have cancer and explain the colposcopy test to you. You fear it will be painful.

Learning Points

Cervical Screening

Details of the cervical screening programme can be found in the 'extra notes' section.

Cervical cytology procedure[1]
- Liquid-based cytology is the preferred technique for collecting cervical cells.
- This uses a brush and pot of liquid. The brush is used to collect the sample then the head of the brush is snapped off and put into the pot. Therefore, the term 'smear test' is now outdated but often is still used by patients and healthcare workers.
- Ideally the test should be done around day 14 of the woman's cycle. Lubricant jelly and spermicide gels should be avoided 24 hours before.
- **If the history is concerning (e.g. PCB) or the cervix looks abnormal or ulcerated, do not take the smear but refer urgently to colposcopy.**

Results
- 1 in 20 results show abnormal cells.[2] Most of these will return to normal without treatment. Therefore, if abnormal cells are detected, HPV testing is done.
- There are 100 different types of human papilloma virus (HPV) but two are considered high risk for cervical cancer: HPV-16 and HPV-18. These cause 70% of cervical cancers.[3]

Result	Management[4]
Normal	Return to normal recall
Inadequate	Repeat test
Borderline or Mild Dyskaryosis	Test for high risk HPV: • Negative – return to normal recall • Positive – colposcopy examination/assessment
Moderate or Severe Dyskaryosis	Colposcopy examination/assessment

Important counselling points
- The screening test is a test for abnormal cells and not cancer cells. The purpose of the test is to detect abnormal cells before they become cancerous. Therefore, an abnormal result does not usually indicate cancer.
- Colposcopy is a procedure to look at the cervix in more detail. It is similar to having a smear in that a speculum is inserted to make the cervix visible, but then the doctor will look at the cervix using a microscope called a colposcope. The colposcope itself doesn't enter the body. The doctor will usually put a special stain on the cervix to show up any abnormal areas.
- If abnormal areas are found, biopsies may be taken or the doctor may decide to treat the cells there and then. If that is the case, the doctor will explain what they would like to do. Any removal of tissue is usually done with local anaesthetic.

Doctor's Notes

Patient   Sara Azmeh   28 years   F
PMH   No information
Medications   No current medications
Allergies   No information
Consultations No recent consultations
Investigations No information
Household   Yusuf Azmeh   29 years   M
                  Lilah Azmeh   7 years   F
                  Najm Azmeh   5 years   M
                  Akram Azmeh   4 years   M
                  Rasha Azmeh   6 months   F

During a recent 'Unplanned Admissions Review' your practice has noted that this family have been attending A&E and out-of-hours services regularly. You have sent a letter to the parents to ask them to come in to discuss the health of the family and the services available.

7 A&E attendances in 2 months with viral URTI symptoms between four children.

1 A&E attendance with eczema (Akram).

1 A&E attendance with vomiting (Rasha).

1 out-of-hours attendance due to running out of salbutamol inhaler (Lilah).

1 attendance to out of hours with hay fever symptoms (Yusuf).

No admissions required, discharged back to GP care after each attendance.

Example Consultation — Inappropriate Use of Services

Open ☐ — Thank you for coming. We hoped to discuss your family's health problems, and offer help and support. As you have recently joined our practice, could you tell me more about your family? Welcome to Nottingham. How are you settling in? What were your experiences in Syria? I'm sorry to hear what your family has been through.

Impact ☐ — How have you coped with the stress of the move? We are here to help your family.

History ☐ — Are you well physically and mentally? And your husband? Have you made friends? Did you work in Syria? Giving yourselves time to settle in is important, but do you have any plans? Ah, best of luck with your future studies. Are your children in school? Tell me about each member of your family; how they are coping and their health.

Sense ☐ — I sense you are particularly worried about breathing problems in the children.

Curious ☐ — Have you had any bad experiences with asthma or chest infections?

ICE ☐ — How do you feel the children are at present? Do you have any particular worries about yourself, your husband or your children? Have you had any thoughts about what could help? Was there anything you were hoping I would do today?

Experience ☐ — Do you know where you can get help from if someone in the family is poorly?

Summary ☐ — To summarise, your family have moved away from where you felt in great danger and it has been hard for you all. You feel exhausted and miss your loved ones, your husband has the stress of trying to find work and your children have been quiet. You feel this is from the shock of what they have experienced. You worry about Lilah's asthma, Akram's eczema and don't know where to get Rasha weighed. You would like some information about healthcare in England. Let's make a plan together.

Empathy ☐ — I cannot imagine what you have been through but I am glad you now feel safe.

Explanation ☐ — In the UK there are lots of different ways to seek help. For problems like hay fever or colds, you can go to a pharmacy where there are medications which you can buy. The pharmacists are experienced in giving advice for these problems so they are often a good first point of call. You may be able to sign up to 'Pharmacy First' which enables you to get free prescriptions for some things like paracetamol for the children. At the practice we can offer emergency appointments if your family are unwell. Please phone our receptionist who will provide you with an appointment. We also have doctors and nurses at the practice who help to manage long-term conditions like asthma or eczema. When the practice is closed and your problem cannot wait, you can phone 111. This includes evenings, night-time and weekends. They will provide advice or arrange an appointment with another GP. If someone is very poorly or has been in a bad accident, this is when you should go to A&E or call 999 on the telephone. This is a lot to take in. Any questions so far? It must be difficult when things are so different in a new country.

Options ☐ — Would it help if I booked Akram in to assess his eczema and also see Lilah for her asthma? I'd also like to refer you to our health visitor service. Health visitors look after families with children under 5 years old and can advise you on minor problems and do health checks like weighing children. You can just turn up with Rasha to the health visitor's clinic once a week to get Rasha weighed. The health visitor can also put you in touch with other services like Sure Start which supports mums and runs mum and baby groups. Does any of that sound helpful? If you continue to worry about your children, we could arrange counselling for them.

Empower ☐ — Would you like me to give you an information sheet with the practice information? Helpful website addresses include NHS choices and patient.co.uk.

Future ☐ — Shall I book those appointments for you? I look forward to meeting your family.

Safety net ☐ — If you are ever worried about a health problem, don't hesitate to give us a call.

Healthy People – 3

Patient's Story

Inappropriate Use of Services

Doctor's notes Sara Azmeh, 28 years. PMH: No information.

During a recent 'Unplanned Admissions Review' your practice has noted that this family have been attending A&E and out-of-hours services regularly. You have sent a letter to the parents to ask them to come in to discuss the health of the family and the services available.

Household			
	Yusuf Azmeh	29 years	M
	Lilah Azmeh	7 years	F
	Najm Azmeh	5 years	M
	Akram Azmeh	4 years	M
	Rasha Azmeh	6 months	F

How to act Confused.

PC *'Hello Doctor, you have asked me to come in to discuss this letter I have received.'*

History You, your husband and four children moved to the UK 4 months ago. You are Syrian asylum seekers. You are unsure how the healthcare system works in the UK. You love your children dearly and get frightened when they are unwell. You and your husband are both well. Over recent years you have had very little access to healthcare in Syria and worry about Lilah's asthma which isn't well controlled. You have had an inhaler from the practice which helps but she keeps running out. You also have trouble managing Akram's eczema; although you know it isn't life threatening, it often becomes sore and stops him sleeping. You are aware that you have been to A&E quite a lot but are unsure what else you should do when the practice is closed or if you can't get through on the phone. After you had been to hospital a couple of times they told you to ring 111 next time, so you did when you required the extra inhaler for Lilah and they helped your husband when he had problems with his nose.

Social Your asylum request is being processed at present but you are very hopeful that it will be granted. Your husband used to work in local government in Syria. Since having children you have been a full-time mum but do hope to train as a nurse in the future. You have met a nice elderly lady who is your neighbour and has been helping to look after the children if you need to run errands. You hope your children can start school soon and your husband will find work.

In Syria you were very frightened and your family walked for days to safety. You feel exhausted but you are thankful that you are safe. You cry when you think of home. You left your elderly relatives who were not able to travel. You lost contact with your parents but believe they are safe as they were with you until you crossed the border. The children have become very quiet since you left. You imagine they are shocked but you give them lots of love and tell them they will be okay now.

ICE You feel that if the children are poorly you should take them to A&E where they can see a doctor and will be safe. You are concerned about Lilah's asthma and Akram's eczema. You also wonder where you should get Rasha weighed. You expect the doctor to tell you off for going to A&E too much but you worry about your children and didn't know what else to do. You hope that the doctor may help your children's chronic problems but you do not feel you should tell the doctor what to do. You knew a few babies in Syria who died of chest infections as they didn't get seen by a doctor quick enough so you worry if any of the children start coughing.

Healthy People – 3

Learning Points   Inappropriate Use of Services

Avoiding unplanned admissions and directing appropriate use of services can be quite difficult. It is important that patients are given as much information as possible to allow them to make the right decisions regarding their health.

Make sure you are aware of what is available in your area:
- How do you access your health visitor/midwife/community nurses/community mental health services? How can patients access these in an emergency or out of hours?
- Does your practice offer extended opening hours or is there a NHS walk-in centre nearby?
- Do your patients know about the 111 helpline?
- Is 'Pharmacy First' available in your area? (Scheme running in certain areas to allow patients to receive prescription medicines for some conditions without the patient seeing a GP.)

Chronic conditions
In patients with chronic health problems such as asthma, COPD and heart failure, it is good practice to develop a care plan or action plan with the patient. For example, an asthma action plan would be based on symptoms and peak expiratory flow rate and include when the patient should go to see a GP or phone an ambulance. Likewise, does the COPD sufferer have clear instructions about when to start antibiotics or steroids? These care plans can be effective in reducing hospital attendances by empowering the patients to manage their condition themselves and giving them good advice about which signs and symptoms need routine, urgent or emergency attention.

Doctor's Notes

Patient	Vincent Riley 60 years M
PMH	Hypertension
	Ex-smoker
Medications	Amlodipine 10 mg daily
Allergies	No allergies
Consultations	Nurse appointment for bloods and blood pressure.
	Letter to patient. 'Dear Mr Riley. Thank you for having your blood tests for your medication review. I would be grateful if you could please make an appointment with the doctor to discuss your cholesterol. Best wishes. Dr Emily Blount.'
Investigations	BP 130/80
	Height 185 cm
	Weight 70 kg
	BMI 20.4
	Cholesterol/HDL ratio 4.7
	Q risk 15.8%
Household	No household members registered.

Example Consultation — High Cholesterol

Open ☐	Thank you for coming. Is there anything else that you would like to talk about?
History ☐	Your cholesterol is a little high but what we need to do about this depends on your general health. I'm interested to know more about you. How do you feel your health is? You have an active lifestyle … How often a week are you doing exercise? When did you stop smoking? How much alcohol do you drink? Who is in your life?
Flags ☐	Do you ever become breathless or have any chest or leg pains?
Sense ☐	I sense you feel this is a waste of time but if there is anything we can do to protect you from having angina, a heart attack or stroke, I want to offer help. Are you interested in discussing ways to prevent problems down the line?
Risk ☐	Do you have a family history of angina or heart disease in relatives when they were under 60 years old?
ICE ☐	Since reading the letter we sent you, have you been concerned? Has anything else gone through your mind? Do you have an idea about what I may talk about today?
Curious ☐	I'm interested … Tell me more about how you have come across statins?
Impact ☐	It sounds as if you are healthy but is there anything more you can try, do you think, to improve your diet? Do you avoid saturated fats in your food?
O/E ☐	Can I feel your pulse and listen to your heart for a check-up please? Great, that sounds normal.
Summary ☐	To summarise, you feel well and your blood pressure is well controlled. Your cholesterol is slightly high. Your friends have had bad experiences with statins.
Empower ☐	I want to ensure you have the information you need to make an informed decision.
Impression ☐	We put all this information into a medical calculator. It is not perfect but it is based on research so we can share with you, if you wish, your predicted risk of having a heart attack or a stroke in the next 10 years. Are you interested in knowing your risk? We take into account if your vessels may have been affected by cigarettes or require blood pressure treatment. Your risk is predicted to be 15.8%. This means that if there were 100 people just like you, about 16 of them would have a heart attack or stroke in the next 10 years. This is not extremely high but we want to do everything we can to bring that down. Your cholesterol was 4.7, which is not bad. However, research advises that if your risk if greater than 10%, you may benefit from a statin treatment. What are your thoughts?
Empathy ☐	I appreciate I am being pessimistic when talking about events like heart attacks and strokes which is not what you want to hear when you do all you can for your health. I appreciate this is a big decision as it involves taking a tablet every day.
Experience ☐	What do you know about statins? Do you know how they work?
Explanation ☐	Statins lower cholesterol, but they seem to have extra benefit above what we would expect from just lowering cholesterol. Because you already lead a healthy lifestyle and have stopped smoking, the only other thing we can change to reduce your risk is lower your cholesterol. Guidance suggests we start atorvastatin 20 mg, taken at night. Like all tablets there are potential side effects of statins which can include feeling unwell with stomach and muscle aches. Rarely, statins can cause muscle breakdown. Statins can also affect the liver; however, we monitor this and if this occurs we stop the statin. Many people feel well on statins and they usually do lower cholesterol. Whether you choose to take the statin or not will depend on your own perception of the risk versus the downsides of taking a tablet every day.
Options ☐	What do you think? You are always welcome to come to discuss this again and we will continue to invite you for an annual health check. Are you interested in reading material to take home? Do you have any questions?
Future ☐	I respect your decision. Thank you for taking the time to listen to me today. If you ever want to talk again, please don't hesitate to make another appointment.

Healthy People – 4

Patient's Story

High Cholesterol

Doctor's notes	Vincent Riley, 60 years. PMH: Hypertension and ex-smoker.
	Medications: Amlodipine 10 mg daily.
	Consultations: Nurse appointment for bloods and blood pressure. Letter to patient. 'Dear Mr Riley. Thank you for having your blood tests for your medication review. I would be grateful if you could please make an appointment with the doctor to discuss your cholesterol. Best wishes. Dr Emily Blount.'
	Investigations: BP: 130/80, Height: 185 cm, Weight: 70 kg, BMI: 20.4, Cholesterol/HDL ratio: 4.7, Q risk: 15.8%.
How to act	Apprehensive about why the doctor has called you in today.
PC	*'I had a letter asking me to come in to talk about cholesterol treatment.'*
History	You feel very well. Apart from well-controlled high blood pressure you have no other medical history.
Social	You are a semi-professional golfer but are starting to spend more time helping around the clubhouse. You remain active, usually playing a few rounds a week and you also enjoy running and cycling. You eat a healthy diet. You are divorced and have a new female partner since last year. Things are going well and you are very happy. You used to smoke until the age of 48 years, on average 10 cigarettes a day. You drink 1–2 beers a couple of nights a week. You have three children with your ex-wife and they live in different parts of the world.
ICE	You are not concerned about your health. You feel very fit and active.
	You ask the doctor: *'Is this a box-ticking exercise, Doc?'*
	You have heard about statins. Several of your friends have tried them and felt awful on them. You are interested to hear what the doctor has to say but you do not accept any cholesterol treatment.
Examination	HS normal and HR regular 64 bpm. No stigmata of hyperlipidaemia.

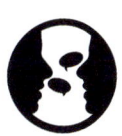

Learning Points

High Cholesterol

Notes from NICE guidelines [CG181]. Cardiovascular disease: risk assessment and reduction, including lipid modification. July 2014

Who should we screen using a CVD risk score (e.g. QRISK2)?[1]
>40 years – 84 years without pre-existing CVD.

Excluding type 1 diabetics and those with inherited disorders of lipid metabolism.

Excluding eGFR <60 ml/min/1.73 m² and/or albuminuria – see CKD guidance.

'Consider people aged 85 or older to be at increased risk of CVD because of age alone, particularly people who smoke or have raised blood pressure. For people 85 years or older consider atorvastatin 20 mg as statins may be of benefit in reducing the risk of **non-fatal** myocardial infarction.'[1]

CVD risk scores will underestimate risk in people with ...
'HIV, serious mental health conditions, immunosuppressants, antipsychotics and corticosteroids and autoimmune and systemic inflammatory disorders ... Those taking antihypertensive or lipid modification therapy or who have recently stopped smoking and a triglyceride concentration > 4.5.'[1]

Management
'Treat comorbidities and secondary causes of dyslipidaemia:'[1]

Address smoking, alcohol, obesity and hypertension.

Investigations: lipid screen (non-fasting), HbA1c, eGFR and renal function, ALT and TSH.[1]

Screening for familial hypercholesterolaemia
Ask about 'the likelihood of a familial lipid disorder rather than the use of strict lipid cut-off values alone and consider if: a total cholesterol concentration more than 7.5 mmol/litre and a family history of premature coronary heart disease ...

Refer if the total cholesterol concentration is >9.0 mmol/litre or a non-HDL cholesterol concentration of >7.5 mmol/litre even in the absence of a first-degree family history of premature coronary heart disease.'[1]

For information about managing raised cholesterol and triglycerides – see Extra Notes.

Doctor's Notes

Patient	Kirsten Cameron
Age	40 years
PMH	Gastro-oesophageal reflux disease
	Gallstones
	Depression
	BMI 40
	3 × NVD
	Tonsillitis
	Mild OA knees
	Menorrhagia
Medications	No current medications
Allergies	No information
Consultations	Recent consultations for OA knees and directed to physiotherapy.
Investigations	X-ray knees – mild OA.
Household	Richard Cameron 46 years
	Winnie Cameron 7 years
	Grace Cameron 6 years
	Thomas Cameron 4 years

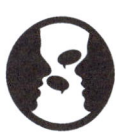

Example Consultation — Wants to Lose Weight

Open ☐ — Tell me more about what has led to you coming here today? What has triggered you coming this week in particular? There can be emotional or social stress that can all lead to weight gain. Are either of these factors something you can relate to?

History ☐ — It's helpful to know more about you and the stressors in your life so we can plan around them. Tell me about past problems with your health. And now? What have you tried? With a job and three children, what exercise do you manage to do at the moment? Do you smoke? How much alcohol do you drink? Who else in your life might support you?

Sense ☐ — I'm hearing from you that this has now become a priority, is that correct?

Impact ☐ — What impact has this problem had on your life? Anything else?

Curious ☐ — You say it gets you down, what do you mean? What triggers feeling this way?

Empathy ☐ — It sounds like being overweight has affected your confidence, which was perhaps already low following the depression.

ICE ☐ — What is your goal? What do you think will be the challenges to you achieving that? Do you have any ideas or wishes about how you would like to achieve this? What did you think I would suggest today? I can see it is important we tailor our plan to your busy life otherwise we are swimming against the tide.

Empower ☐ — Usually we need to put several things, as well as medication, in place to help. What other steps could be squeezed into your schedule if your husband and friend support you? Are there any health professionals you might find helpful?

Impression ☐ — It sounds as if you have seriously taken the doctor's advice about losing weight to help your knees – and you now feel this has become a priority for your mental and physical well-being. This problem has contributed to your pain, feeling down and low confidence with your partner. Can you think of any other problems it has led to?

Experience ☐ — What problems might it also cause in your future?

Explanation ☐ — You are right; the health of vessels supplying the heart and brain can be at risk.

Risk ☐ — I would like to do some tests to make sure there is no medical issue contributing to your weight gain. I would like to test your ovulation hormones and thyroid. Also, can we do a health check of your cholesterol, sugar level, kidney function and BP?

Summary ☐ — To summarise, your knee pain and your friend's encouragement have led you to think about the impact your weight has had on your life. It is important for you to gain some control back, as your big fears are that your depression may return and further knee pain. You have a good relationship with your husband but you feel sad that you do not have a sexual relationship. You worried that I may say you should eat less and exercise more or join a programme, which is not practical advice for your circumstances, and you enjoy food and cooking. You believe your husband and friend will support you and can offer the flexibility you need, time-wise. Your goal is to run up that hill and meanwhile you plan to enjoy learning some new healthy recipes. Have I got it?

Options ☐ — There is a tablet called orlistat which reduces fat absorption. Your bowels become loose and it may give you tummy upset as you pass more fat in the stool. Is this something you would like to try? Can you make an appointment with the nurse for the blood tests and BP check at exactly 9 am and before your breakfast please?

Future ☐ — We will check your weight again in 3 months' time and you may continue this tablet if you have lost 5% of your current weight. It can also help to use calorie counting apps on your phone to keep track of what you're eating, and some women find exercise videos, which they can do at their convenience at home, helpful.

Safety net ☐ — If your mood does drop, or you are concerned about anything, please return.

Healthy People – 5

Patient's Story

Wants to Lose Weight

Doctor's notes Kirsten Cameron, 40 years. PMH: Gastro-oesophageal reflux disease, gallstones, depression, 3 × NVD, tonsillitis, mild OA knees, menorrhagia. BMI 40. Medications: Nil. Recent consultations for OA knees and directed to physiotherapy. Investigations. X-ray knees – mild OA.

How to act Quiet and embarrassed.

PC *'Doctor, I would like help to lose weight please.'*

History Your knees are becoming increasingly painful. Originally you were worried about arthritis but, following an X-ray, the doctor explained that treatment for osteoarthritis is either anti-inflammatories, injections or exercises. You were told they are not bad enough for surgery but have been advised to lose weight. You do not have time to do the physio exercises or lose weight. You have three small children at home. You do the school run after work. You have had multiple health problems, but currently only your knees are bothering you. Your depression resolved about a year ago but you don't have any confidence. It is obvious that your husband does not find you attractive as he has no interest in having sex. *'It gets me down.'* You remain good companions. He would be supportive of you losing weight and would help with the children if you asked. It has just become routine that you run the home. Reading women's magazines gets you down. You used to be a size 12 and, over the past decade, you have gradually gained weight; especially when you were depressed and you used to binge eat. You spoke to your friend and she told you to see the GP. Your friend said she would help with the kids or go on a walk with you at night. There's a lovely view from the top of the hill near your house and you have laughed with your friend that in a year you will run up it. You also know you comfort eat. You would like to get into healthy eating and might start searching for new recipes on websites. You enjoy cooking.

Social Your husband is an undertaker. You are a milliner. You do not smoke. You rarely drink alcohol as money is tight and you save where you can.

ICE You are aware that you are at risk of heart attacks and increasing knee pain. You know that you have to eat less and exercise more; easier said than done.

You are tired at the end of the day. Your big fear is your depression returning. You felt at rock bottom at the time and it impacted on enjoying life with your children. Then you felt guilty that you were missing out on their precious years. (Your mood is generally okay at present.) You would like the doctor to provide a weight loss tablet rather than tell you to go to an exercise class which you have never been able to commit to. You would like practical solutions for your personal circumstances and feel other doctors have just told you to join Weight Watchers or go to classes. If the doctor explores options with you, you will agree to increase your exercise but you cannot commit to an exercise programme as you need to be at work or home.

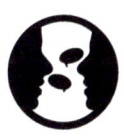

Learning Points

Wants to Lose Weight

Notes from NICE guidelines [CG189]. Obesity: identification, assessment and management. Nov 2014.

'Tailor the components of the planned weight management programme to the person's preferences, initial fitness, health status and lifestyle.'[1]

'The main requirement of a dietary approach to weight loss is that total energy intake should be less than energy expenditure.'[1]

Asian family origin — Consider lower threshold for intervention.

Children — 'Clinical intervention should be considered for children with a BMI at or above the 91st centile ... Encourage parents (or carers) to take main responsibility for lifestyle changes in children ...'[1]

Multicomponent interventions include behaviour change strategies for activity and eating behaviours.

Examination — BP, waist circumference.

Investigations — Lipid and HbA1c

Orlistat — 'Only after dietary, exercise and behavioural approaches have been started and evaluated ... a BMI of 28 kg/m² or more with associated risk factors or a BMI of 30 kg/m² or more.'[1]

'Continue orlistat therapy beyond 3 months only if the person has lost at least 5% of their initial body weight. Must review at 12 months. Diabetics will be slower to reach target.'[1]

Exercise — 'Encourage adults to do at least 30 minutes of moderate or greater intensity physical activity on 5 or more days a week. However, higher amounts may be needed to prevent obesity without dietary changes.'[1]

Diets — Suggest 'diets that have a 600 kcal/day deficit ...

Consider low-calorie diets (800–1600 kcal/day), but be aware these are less likely to be nutritionally complete.'[1]

Beware of free sugar content in fruit, juices and drinks.

Bariatric surgery

'Consider if:

BMI >40   OR

BMI >35 + comorbidities or BMI >30 + DM diagnosed in the last 10 years.'[1]

Consider a lower threshold in the Asian population.

'All appropriate non-surgical measures have been tried but the person has not achieved or maintained adequate, clinically beneficial weight loss ...

The person is generally fit for anaesthesia and surgery ...

The person commits to the need for long-term follow-up.'[1]

Extra Notes

Immunisation Schedule

Immunisation Schedule at the time of writing[1,2]

Age	Immunisation
8 weeks	- DTaP/IPV(polio)/Hib – diphtheria, tetanus, pertussis, polio and Haemophilus influenza type B - PCV (pneumococcal conjugate vaccine) - Rotavirus gastroenteritis, oral drops - Meningitis B
12 weeks	- DTaP/IPV(polio)/Hib – 2nd dose - Rotarix® – rotavirus gastroenteritis, oral drops
16 weeks	- DTaP/IPV(polio)/Hib – 3rd dose - PCV – 2nd dose - Meningitis B – 2nd dose
Between 12 and 13 months	- Hib/MenC = 4th dose of Hib and 1st dose of MenC - MMR – measles, mumps and rubella - PCV – 3rd dose - Meningitis B – 3rd dose
2–8 years (annual)	- Nasal flu spray
3 years 4 months	- Pre-school booster of DTaP/IPV (polio) - MMR – 2nd dose
11–14 years (girls)	- HPV – human papillomavirus types 16 and 18. Needs 2 injections, second given 6–24 months after the first
14 years	- Td/IPV (polio) – diphtheria, tetanus and polio booster - Men ACWY
Adults	- Men ACWY. If not received offer to students up to 25 years - Influenza and pneumococcal for those aged over 65 years and those in high-risk groups - Td/IPV(polio) – for those not fully immunised as a child - Influenza and DTaP/IPV(polio) for pregnant women - Shingles vaccine for adults either aged 70 or 78–79 years
High risk any age	- BCG – see http://www.nhs.uk/Conditions/vaccinations/Pages/bcg-tuberculosis-TB-vaccine.aspx - Hepatitis B vaccine for those with an increased risk of exposure, e.g. IVDU, healthcare workers. See http://www.nhs.uk/Conditions/vaccinations/Pages/hepatitis-b-vaccine.aspx

Live attenuated vaccines: MMR, chicken pox, rotavirus, yellow fever, oral polio, BCG, typhoid, Japanese encephalitis, rabies and cholera. They should not be given to immunosuppressed or pregnant patients.

Timing of vaccinations
See the Link Hub at CompleteCSA.co.uk for a link to timing and spacing of vaccines.

Healthy People

Extra Notes — Immunisation/Vaccine Preventable Diseases

Information collated from NHS Choices,[3] WHO,[4] Centers for Disease Control and Prevention[5]

Measles – cold-like symptoms, high temperature, white/grey spots inside cheeks, red/brown diffuse rash starting on head and neck then spreading to body. Serious complications: pneumonia, encephalitis, blindness, deafness. Death rate 0.1–0.2%.[5]

Mumps – painful swelling of the parotid glands. May cause testicular pain/swelling and can also affect ovaries. Serious complications: meningitis, fertility problems, deafness.

Rubella – red/pink rash of small spots with fever, viral symptoms and enlarged lymph nodes. Can cause complications in pregnancy (foetal abnormalities).

Diphtheria – high fever, thick grey/white coating back of throat with sore throat and breathing difficulties. Bacterial infection. Serious complications: myocarditis, problems with nervous system. 10% mortality rate despite treatment.[5]

Tetanus – wounds contaminated with soil or animal manure. High fever, muscle spasms and lockjaw. Bacterial infection (*Clostridium tetani*). Complications: PE, pneumonia. Suffocation or cardiac arrest may occur. 10–20% death rate.[5]

Pertussis – whooping cough. *Bordetella pertussis*. Persistent cough with secretions in airways, distinctive 'whoop' at end of cough. Complications: pneumonia, seizures, encephalopathy, apnoea, 1% death rate.[5]

Polio – viral infection, often asymptomatic but can cause paralysis which is life threatening. There is no cure. Although most cases pass without being noted, 1 in 200 with the condition have some degree of paralysis,[5] muscle atrophy, joint contractures and bony deformity such as twisted legs.

Haemophilus influenzae B – potentially serious bacterial infection. Can cause epiglottitis, meningitis, pericarditis, pneumonia, septicaemia, septic arthritis, cellulitis and osteomyelitis. Most serious complication is meningitis with a death rate of 1 in 20.[5]

Pneumococcal – bacterial. PCV protects against 13 types of *Streptococcus pneumoniae*. Typically causes respiratory tract infection (bronchitis, sinusitis) and otitis media but can cause invasive infection such as pneumonia, meningitis, septicaemia, osteomyelitis, and septic arthritis.

Rotavirus – virus causing gastroenteritis. Although rarely fatal, 1 in 5 present to their GP, and 1 in 10 cases in infants cause dehydration that requires hospitalisation.[3]

Meningitis B, C, ACWY – Protection against meningococcal groups B, C, A, W and Y. Causes meningitis and septicaemia. Complications include hearing damage, epilepsy, brain damage, limb amputation and death. Group W is most aggressive form. Symptoms: fever, headache, vomiting, muscle pains, cold hands and feet, non-blanching rash (petechial or purpuric).

Extra Notes

Cervical Screening Programme

Overview of Cervical Screening Programme[6]

All women between 25 and 64 years
- 25–49 years have 3-yearly recall
- 50–64 years have 5-yearly recall
- over 65 years are entitled to screening if they haven't been screened since they turned 50 years or if they have had recent abnormal results requiring follow-up.

Should screening be offered to younger women?
- In Scotland cervical screening begins at 20 years old.
- In England and Wales screening starts at 25 years. This is because:
  - Younger women are more likely to have abnormal cytology.
  - The abnormal cells are more likely to return to normal by themselves in younger women, making the development of cancer less likely.
  - Therefore, if the screening age was brought down this would be likely to result in an increase in unnecessary invasive tests/biopsies.

Who doesn't need cervical screening?
- Women with symptoms of cervical cancer should be referred directly via the suspected cancer pathway – cervical cytology should not be done (it is a screening test, not a diagnostic test).
- Unless under active follow-up for a previous abnormal result, pregnant women should wait until 3 months after delivery before having their routine cervical screening test.
- Women who have never been sexually active are at very low risk of cervical cancer so can choose not to be screened.
- Women who have had a total hysterectomy (i.e. cervix removed) do not require screening. However, in certain situations 'vault smears' are done – if this is required the patient's gynaecologist should arrange it.

Healthy People

Extra Notes

Other NHS Screening Programmes

What	Who	Comments
Bowel cancer	>55 years old	National bowel scope screening. This is a one-off test aimed at detecting polyps and removing them.
	60–74 years old	Home testing kits for faecal occult blood – 2 samples from each motion, 3 motions in total. Positive results referred for colonoscopy. Tested every 2 years.
	Information from https://www.gov.uk/guidance/bowel-cancer-screening-programme-overview. January 2015	
Breast cancer	Women 50–70 years (extending to 47–73 years)	3-yearly mammography.
	Information from https://www.gov.uk/guidance/breast-screening-programme-overview. June 2015	
Diabetic retinopathy	Annually (>12 years of age with diabetes)	Digital retinal photography
	Information from https://www.gov.uk/guidance/diabetic-eye-screening-programme-overview. January 2014	
Abdominal aortic aneurysm	Men aged 65 years	Ultrasound scan 3–5.4 cm wide – monitor >5.5 cm wide – offer surgery. Prevalence lower in women so currently not offered scan.
	Information from https://www.gov.uk/guidance/abdominal-aortic-aneurysm-screening-programme-overview. January 2015	
Newborn/Infant	All newborns – (hearing, bloodspot, physical examination)	Bloodspot now tests for: sickle cell, cystic fibrosis, hypothyroidism + 6 metabolic disorders (phenylketonuria, MCADD, maple syrup urine disease, isovaleric acidaemia, glutaric aciduria type 1 and HCU).
	Information from https://www.gov.uk/guidance/newborn-blood-spot-screening-programme-overview. Published January 2013	
Pregnancy	Pregnant women (foetal anomaly, infectious diseases, sickle cell/thalassaemia)	**Examination** – height, weight, fundal height, urine dip, BP **Blood tests** – blood-borne viruses, anaemia, rubella status, blood group, rhesus status, sickle cell, thalassaemia **Scans** – 12 weeks dating scan, 20-week anomaly scan **Down screening** – bloods 10–14 weeks. Best test is combined test (β-hCG, PAPP-A and nuchal translucency). Cut-off for further investigation is 1 in 150. Also Edwards' syndrome and Patau's syndrome now screened for.[8] Non-invasive pre-natal testing for Down Syndrome is being developed, which is based on maternal blood test, looking for foetal DNA within mother's blood. Promising but not considered diagnostic yet with ongoing trials.
	Information from https://www.gov.uk/guidance/infectious-diseases-in-pregnancy-screening-programme-overview. January 2015	

See reference[7] and weblinks above for more information.

Healthy People

Extra Notes

Diet and Exercise Advice – Summary

Information from NICE guidelines [CG181]. Cardiovascular disease: risk assessment and reduction, including lipid modification. July 2014.

Cardioprotective diet recommendations

Total fat intake <30% daily intake.[9]

Saturated fats <7% daily intake.[9]

Reduce/replace animal or saturated fats with mono-unsaturated or polyunsaturated fats.[9]

Olive oil is a healthy substitute for fat.

Choose wholegrain varieties of starchy food.[9]

'5 portions of fruit or vegetables a day'[9] (however, fruit may be high in sugar).

Fish twice a week (one portion of oily fish).[9]

'4 to 5 portions of unsalted nuts, seeds and legumes per week.'[9]

Exercise recommendations

'150 minutes of moderate intensity aerobic activity or … 75 minutes of vigorous intensity aerobic activity'[9] a week.

'Muscle-strengthening activities on 2 or more days a week that work all major muscle groups.'[9]

Encourage patients with a co-morbidity to 'exercise at their maximum safe capacity.'[9]

Alcohol consumption: Department of Health, January 2016[10]

Recommends maximum limit of **14 units** per week for **both men and women**. Those 14 units should be spread over 3 or more days.

Healthy People

Extra Notes

Statins

Information from NICE guidelines [CG181]. Cardiovascular disease: risk assessment and reduction, including lipid modification. July 2014[11]

Secondary prevention 80 mg atorvastatin and repeat lipid profile 3 months later

Primary prevention Offer lifestyle changes and retesting

Offer 20 mg atorvastatin if: ≥10% 10-year risk of developing CVD

>85 years

CKD

Consider in all T1DMs and offer if either:

>10 years of DM

>40 years

Established neuropathy

Other CVD risk factors

Advise of risks and adverse effects – an example explanation: *'Side effects include muscle pain or weakness, stomach problems or pain, and statins can affect the function of the liver. Rarely, they can cause muscle breakdown. (See BNF for full list.) If muscle pain or weakness develops seek help. Attend for another blood test to check the liver at 3 and 12 months. Avoid grapefruit juice when taking statins.'* Check no pre-existing generalised muscle pain and check CK level if present before starting. Remember to change simvastatin to atorvastatin if on amlodipine.

Measure liver transaminase enzymes at 'baseline, 3 moths and 12 months ... 12 months, but not again unless clinically indicated'.[11]

Follow-up for secondary prevention includes a lipid retest after 3/12. If >40% reduction (non-HDL) is not achieved, discuss compliance. Consider ezetimibe if target not achieved on full-dose statin.

Follow-up for primary prevention in CKD includes a lipid retest and consider increasing the statin dose (especially if 'judged to be at higher risk because of comorbidities').[11]

If eGFR <30 ml/min/1.73 m^2 discuss with a renal specialist first.

If intolerance of statins, consider stop/restart, 'reducing the dose ... or changing the statin to a lower intensity group.'[11] If there is muscle pain or weakness, check the CK.

Consider trying three different statins if possible and the patient is not at risk.

Triglycerides

>20 mmol/litre Refer urgently if not secondary to alcohol or poor glycaemic control[11]

10–20 mmol/litre Repeat day 5–14 then refer after considering secondary causes[11]

4.5–9.9 mmol/litre Optimise CV health and seek advice if >7.5 mmol/litre[11]

Ezetimibe monotherapy may be used in primary hypercholesterolaemia if the patient is intolerant of statins or if drug interactions prevent the use of statins.[12]

Seek specialist advice before considering **fenofibrates** (e.g. for hypertriglyceridaemia).

> **Lipid management**
> See the **Link Hub at CompleteCSA.co.uk** for a link to helpful information about lipid management.

Healthy People

CHAPTER 3 OVERVIEW
Genetics in Primary Care

	Cases in this chapter	Within the RCGP curriculum: Genetics in Primary Care RCGP Curriculum Online March 2016[1]	Learning points in the chapter
1	Down Syndrome	'Communicating genetic information'	Notes on Down Syndrome
2	Cystic Fibrosis	Giving information of 'genetic susceptibility in common conditions'	Lists of genetic disorders: autosomal recessive, X-linked and chromosomal
3	Familial Adenomatous Polyposis	'Taking and considering a genetic family history' 'Demonstrate comprehensive management for those patients with, or at risk of, genetic conditions'	Autosomal dominant disorders
4	Breast Cancer BRCA Gene	'Identify patients with, or at risk of, a genetic condition'	Notes on the genetics referral criteria for breast cancer
5	HOCM	Giving information of 'genetic susceptibility in common conditions'	Notes on HOCM

1. http://www.rcgp.org.uk/training-exams/gp-curriculum-overview/online-curriculum/applying-clinical-knowledge-section-1/3-02-genetics-in-primary-care.aspx

CHAPTER 3 REFERENCES

Down Syndrome
1. http://patient.info/health/downs-syndrome-leaflet
2. http://www.nhs.uk/Conditions/pregnancy-and-baby/pages/screening-amniocentesis-downs-syndrome.aspx
3. http://www.rapid.nhs.uk/guides-to-nipd-nipt/nipt-for-down-syndrome/

Breast Cancer
1. NICE Guidelines. CG164. Familial breast cancer: classification, care and managing breast cancer and related risks in people with a family history of breast cancer. June 2013.
2. http://www.nice.org.uk/guidance/cg164/ifp/chapter/about-this-information.

Doctor's Notes

Patient	Heather Mumford
Age	33 years
PMH	NVD aged 33 years
Medications	No current medications
Allergies	No information
Consultations	No recent consultations
Investigations	No recent investigations
Household	David Mumford, 35 years
	Emma Mumford, 2 weeks

Example Consultation — Down Syndrome

Open ☐ — I'm so sorry to hear that. How is Emma doing? And you? What have the hospital doctors said? How do you feel about this diagnosis? Were you given any warning?

Empathy ☐ — It is a huge worry when a new baby needs an operation.

History ☐ — This is the first time we've met. Please tell me more about you. Where is Emma now? Have you always been well? And during the pregnancy? Who are you close to? Do you feel you are receiving much support? What do you do for a living?

Empathy ☐ — It must be upsetting when others are not getting in touch.

Impact ☐ — Has this news changed you or your relationship? How is your bond with Emma?

Sense ☐ — I'm hearing from you that you have unanswered questions and lots on your mind.

Impression ☐ — Have you had a talk with a doctor about what this means? Shall we do that today?

ICE ☐ — When you walked through the door, was there anything else you were hoping we would discuss? I'll take note of everything you wish to talk about then we'll go through it. What other questions do you have? What else has been going through your mind? What worries you most? Anything else you're wondering?

Curious ☐ — What do mean when you say you feel guilty?

Summary ☐ — To summarise, you have bonded very well with Emma. Your immediate family are supportive. Your main concern is Emma's health and you are especially worried about the heart operation and any other medical problems Emma may develop. You feel guilty for thinking about the impact on your own life. You have questioned how independent Emma will be and whether she has the potential to live a long life. You would like to discuss how this has happened and whether it is likely to happen in a future pregnancy. Have I got it? Is there anything else you were hoping for today?

Empathy ☐ — It is natural to hope that you will have a healthy baby. If there are any problems, it is normal to consider how this will impact on your own life.

Experience ☐ — What is your understanding of Down Syndrome?

Explanation ☐ — At conception, genetic instructions are passed from parent to child within genes and chromosomes. To help understand the difference, if you imagine a book, all the words in a book are the genes. The genes are grouped into chapters, chromosomes. In Down Syndrome an extra chromosome is made during the transfer of genetic instructions, so you have not necessarily passed down a faulty gene. There is about a '10 times increased risk'[1] of having a baby with Down syndrome in another pregnancy. However, overall your risk may still be small. There is a new test which is more accurate for Down syndrome which you may think about at the time.

Future ☐ — What do you know about an AVSD? It means there is a hole in the muscle in the heart. Therefore, blood with and without oxygen is mixed up. Emma may also have other medical problems such as altered vision and hearing. There is an increased risk of problems later in life like diabetes. There may be tough times ahead and Emma may have more challenges than most. However, Emma may live happily until a fine old age and she has a loving family on her side. Regarding Emma's future independence, the range of learning difficulties is very variable, but we hope Emma will find her own path. Often personalities are naturally very warm, cheerful and gentle,[1] and so Emma may soon win the hearts of everyone she meets.

Empower ☐ — Shall we catch up again after you have had a chance to talk to your husband and absorb what we have talked about? Is there anything else you would like to talk about next time? Come and see me any time or after the appointment with the consultant. I look forward to meeting Emma. She'll be a delight I'm sure.

Patient's Story

Down Syndrome

Doctor's notes	Heather Mumford, 33 years. PMH: NVD 2 weeks ago. Medication: Nil.
How to act	Anxious. Upset.
PC	*'Doctor, Emma was born with Down syndrome.'*
History	You had a normal delivery 2 weeks ago following a normal pregnancy.
	Emma is doing okay and she is breast feeding nicely.
	After testing during pregnancy, you were told your risk of a baby with Down syndrome was low.
	Your husband, David, is at home with Emma.
	Both you and David have quickly become very fond of Emma.
	You have always been well. You take no medicines.
Social	You are an actuary. Your husband is a 35-year-old lawyer.
	You have never smoked, or taken drugs. You used to drink occasionally.
	You have a strong relationship. You have a couple of close friends who have been very supportive but most others have not been in touch and you have only received a couple of baby cards. Your parents died when you were a child but David's parents are supportive.
ICE	You are trying to read about Down syndrome but caring for Emma takes up your time. You are aware that in Down syndrome there are additional genes and another chromosome, although you are a little confused between genes and chromosomes.
	You are mainly concerned about Emma's future health.
	You've been told she has a heart condition called an AVSD and you have an appointment with a cardiologist next week to discuss an operation. You can't bear this thought.
	You stay awake wondering if Emma will have a normal life.
	If the doctor explores your thoughts, you confide in the doctor that you feel guilty when you think about what this means for you and David.
	By this you mean that you always presumed you would have successful and independent children and you took for granted that you would have a normal family life.
	You fear that only you and David will ever love Emma.
	You are hoping today that the doctor can explain what Down syndrome is, why this has happened and what this means for Emma and your family.
Questions	Have you or your husband passed down a faulty gene?
	Would a second child also have Down syndrome?
	Will Emma die young? What else is Emma at risk of?
	Can the doctor explain the AVSD again?

Genetics in Primary Care – 1

Learning Points   Down Syndrome

Genetics	Trisomy 21 (in most cases).
Risk	of having a baby with Down syndrome
	Aged 20 years = 1/1500. Aged 30 years = 1/800. Aged 40 years = 1/100[1]
Combined test	Fluid collection measurement at the neck + hormonal levels + mother's age
	11–14 weeks' gestation
	Screening for Down syndrome, Edwards' syndrome and Patau's syndrome[2]
Quadruple test	Around 14–20 weeks' gestation[2]
High risk result	If initial tests estimate a risk of >1/150, diagnostic testing will be offered.[2]
Chorionic villous sampling	Around 11–14 weeks' gestation[2]
Amniocentesis	Around 15 weeks' gestation[2]
NIPT	Non-invasive pre-natal testing: 'NIPT' to detect Down syndrome … Edwards' syndrome, Patau's syndrome and Turner's syndrome
	… NIPT analyses the cell-free DNA in the mother's blood'[3] rather than hormone levels.
	Advertised as >98% sensitivity
	It is also therefore a screening test and women should be counselled regarding the benefits and limitations.

The start of a new relationship
What was achieved within this consultation was predominantly support at a time of need, providing a confidante to share thoughts and fears. Normalising the mother's emotions was important to offer relief from feelings of guilt. This consultation provided an introduction to a connection and relationship with the GP which is likely to be ongoing as Emma grows.

The patient breaks bad news
A patient may walk through the door and they break their bad news, without a warning shot, and often the discharge letter hasn't reached you. Have a think about what you may say when you are taken aback. Some things will be upsetting or may even trigger emotions or feelings from your own experiences. Show your interest and concern; however, be careful how you react and avoid judgement. Be guided by the patient.

Making connections
In this case there is a clear resonance between the mum's experience of her own parents dying when she was a child and her fears about what will happen to Emma when she and her husband die. The skilled clinician notices these connections but chooses wisely and carefully about when (or indeed if) to share them with the patient. Today's consultation would have been too soon.

Doctor's Notes

Patient   Olivia Wales
Age   29 years
PMH   No information
Medications   No current medications
Allergies   No information
Consultations No recent consultations
Investigations No recent investigations
Household   No household members registered

Example Consultation — Cystic Fibrosis

Open ☐	Tell me about your niece's experience? How is your niece? Apart from genetic testing, what other thoughts have gone through your mind?
Impact ☐	How has your niece's diagnosis impacted on your family? And you, how has it impacted on you?
Sense ☐	I can see this is very important to you.
ICE ☐	What do you fear the most? Do you have any other questions? You were hoping we could arrange a genetic test for yourself – is that correct? Is there anything else that is important to you? What would it mean to you if you did have a gene that put you at increased risk of having a child with cystic fibrosis – how would this impact on your life?
History ☐	You have always been well, is that correct? Do you take any medicines? Do you work?
Curious ☐	Does your husband think you should have the test? Are you close to your sister? What does she think you should do?
Summary ☐	To summarise what you have said so far, your sister's daughter, Grace, has had multiple chest infections and requires medication to help maintain her nutrition. You have watched the amount of stress your sister has had to go through and this has made you question whether you would like children. You are upset by the arguments you have had with your husband. You feel the test may help you to make the choice whether to have a child.
Empathy ☐	It sounds as if you have watched your sister through many sad and difficult times when Grace has been admitted to hospital. That must be hard.
Experience ☐	What is your understanding of cystic fibrosis? What do you know about what causes cystic fibrosis?
Explanation ☐	In cystic fibrosis there is a build-up of mucus in the chest and difficulty absorbing all the nutrients from the diet because an organ next to the stomach, called the pancreas, is not producing the chemicals needed to break food down so it can be absorbed. Unfortunately, it can also cause fertility problems in later life.
Risk ☐	When a child is conceived, information from both parents is passed to the child. This information is coded in genes, one from each parent. Both parents need to pass on a faulty gene for a child to have cystic fibrosis. Everyone has a one in 21 chance of carrying the gene for cystic fibrosis. Your sister must have inherited one faulty gene from your parents, which she unfortunately passed on. You may or may not have a faulty gene. If we take the worst-case scenario and assume that you did inherit the faulty gene too, your chance of passing on the faulty gene would be 50%. However, your child would also need to inherit a faulty gene from your husband, who has the background risk of 1 in 21. So, based on this, your risk would be 1 in 42 of having a child with cystic fibrosis. However, we don't know that you have inherited the faulty gene; if either you or your husband doesn't have a faulty gene, there is almost no risk of having a child with cystic fibrosis.
Options ☐	How would you feel about speaking to a counsellor about this? I can write to the genetics team and explain what impact this has had and we can be guided by them. If you don't hear from them in the next 6 weeks, let me know. They may offer a consultation for you to discuss what options are available. Relationship counselling is another option if you think this may be helpful.
Future ☐	If you decide to start trying for a family, come and see me again and we can discuss this in further detail.

Genetics in Primary Care – 2

Patient's Story

Cystic Fibrosis

Doctor's notes Olivia Wales, 29 years. PMH: Nil. Medication: Nil.

How to act Polite and quiet.

PC *'My husband and I would like to start a family but my niece has cystic fibrosis. I'm wondering if there are any special tests we could have?'*

History You are well, take no medicines and have been happily married for two years.

Your sister gave birth to Grace 10 years ago and soon afterwards they were told that she has cystic fibrosis. Your sister decided not to have another child. There have been no other members of the family with this condition. This includes your sister's husband's family.

Your sister's spirit seems to have gone over the years. The more Grace attends hospital the more sadness your sister has to go through. You believe the stress of the situation led to the breakdown of your sister's marriage. You worry that your sister will be alone if Grace dies.

Social You are a teacher. You drink no alcohol and have never smoked.

ICE You have seen your niece have lots of chest physiotherapy and she has had multiple lung infections requiring hospital admissions. She has to take medicines to help absorb her food.

A charity is taking her to Disney World. You are aware that Grace may not live long.

What is your risk of having a baby with cystic fibrosis?

Is there a test you can have done to make sure you don't have the faulty gene?

You don't know if you want a child if there is a high risk of bringing a child into the world who has to go through Grace's experience. Your husband is desperate for children. He does not want you to have genetic testing. He believes your chances are low and you should just start trying. This has led to arguments within your relationship. You were very excited when Grace was first born but now, watching your sister's life, you don't think you ever want children. You have not told your husband this.

It was your sister's idea to have the genetic test.

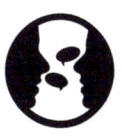

Genetics in Primary Care – 2

Learning Points

Cystic Fibrosis

We suggest you should be able to explain each condition in 1–2 sentences as well as being able to explain the probability of each condition being passed on to children.

Autosomal recessive disorders
Hereditary haemochromatosis
Sickle cell
Thalassaemia
Cystic fibrosis
Wilson's disease

X-linked recessive
Haemophilia A (factor VIII)
Haemophilia B (factor IX)
Becker muscular dystrophy
Duchenne muscular dystrophy

X-linked dominant
Fragile × syndrome

Chromosomal disorders
Turner's syndrome
Klinefelter's syndrome
Down syndrome

Doctor's Notes

Patient	Shane Dickens
Age	23 years
PMH	Hay fever
	Hand injury aged 11 years
Medications	No current medications
Allergies	No allergies
Consultations	No recent consultations
Investigations	No recent investigations
Household	No household members registered

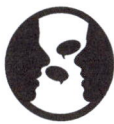

Example Consultation — Familial Adenomatous Polyposis

Open ☐	Tell me more about what's led to this. I'm sorry to hear that. How is Darren now?
Impact ☐	How has this affected you? What have you been thinking?
Sense ☐	I can see this has come as a shock and you are very worried.
Flags ☐	To help answer your questions I'd like to know more about you, please. Have you had any symptoms – such as changes in the bowel, weight loss or bleeding?
History ☐	Have you had any medical problems? Do you take any medicines? How much alcohol do you drink? Do you smoke or take drugs?
Risk ☐	I would like to explore your family history. Do you have any other brothers or sisters? Do you and Darren share a mum or a dad? Is your mum well? On your mum's side are there any medical conditions? Is your dad well? I'm sorry to hear that. Do you know if he suffered with the same condition? How about your dad's family? Do you know if Darren's mother or family have had bowel problems or young deaths in the family?
ICE ☐	You mentioned you can't stop thinking about this. What thoughts do you have? What do you think about when you think of Darren?
Sense ☐	You look sad. Is there anything else that keeps coming to mind? What do you fear most? Anything else? What did you think I may say today?
Empathy ☐	It must be really hard being such a distance away from your brother at this time.
Curious ☐	You mentioned your mum is worried. What have you talked about? And Darren?
Summary ☐	To summarise, Darren has been diagnosed with familial adenomatous polyposis. The news from the surgeon is not clear. You are struggling and feel sad that you have not always been close. Your mum has questioned whether your father and grandmother had the same condition. You would like to discuss this further. You have not had any symptoms and thought I may arrange a telescope test today.
Experience ☐	What do you know about familial adenomatous polyposis?
Impression ☐	Familial means it can run in families, adenomatous relates to the tissue in the gut and polyposis means little lumps, that can turn cancerous, forming from this tissue. This condition can occur randomly with no other family members affected, but usually parents and grandparents have this condition. Let's call it FAP.
Explanation ☐	We call the information which is passed from parent to child 'genes'. There are genes for every part of us. Genes come in pairs. We get one from our father and one from our mother. Which gene is stronger determines what we are like; for example, eye colour. Each parent also has two genes – from their mother and father. If one of their genes is faulty, there is therefore a 1 in 2 chance they have passed a faulty gene on to you. Anyone with this faulty gene will be affected by it. It is possible that your father and his mother had the problem as they both died young. But we don't know. This could have come from Darren's mum's side. If your father did have the gene for FAP, you have a 50% chance of having it. This is a serious condition and the only way to prevent death is to remove the bowel. It is difficult for me to comment on your brother's chances without having his information with me. If you have the test and it is negative, your risk of bowel cancer is the same as the risk for anyone in the population.
Options ☐	You mentioned arranging a telescope test but at this stage we could refer you to the genetics team. They may discuss having a genetic test. If we find you have the FAP gene, an operation will be stressful and challenging but potentially life-saving.
Future ☐	Do you know when you will return? I can arrange the referral today. When you return let's discuss how you are coping. In the meantime, look after your health by avoiding cigarettes and cannabis.
Empower ☐	Or do you wish to have time to think and talk again when you return?
Safety net ☐	If you ever see bleeding from the back passage, do not panic as most of the time this is harmless. However, always see a doctor to check it out.

Genetics in Primary Care – 3

Patient's Story

Familial Adenomatous Polyposis

Doctor's notes	Shane Dickens, 23 years. PMH: Hay fever and hand injury. Medications: Nil.
How to act	Concerned. Distracted in thought at times.
PC	*'My brother said I need a colonoscopy for familial adenomatous polyposis.'*
History	Darren is your half-brother. You share the same father. Darren lives in Australia.
	He has now told you that he had been bleeding from his bottom and thought this was due to haemorrhoids. He kept using haemorrhoid cream but it only got worse when he was opening his bowels and he started to lose weight.
	The doctor sent him for a colonoscopy and it has returned as cancer. Because he was young they did genetic tests and he has the gene for FAP.
	You are healthy. You have had no symptoms. You do not take medicines.
	Your bowels are normal. You have had no bleeding. Your weight is stable.
	You have no other siblings. Darren's mother's side of the family are well.
	Your mother and father were never married, and they separated two years after having you.
Maternal side:	Your mother, maternal grandparents and aunts are well.
Paternal side:	Your father drank a lot of alcohol and committed suicide when he was 39. You do not know his medical history.
	You never knew your father's mother. She died young.
	Your paternal grandfather has dementia.
	Your father had two sisters who are well. Their children are well.
Social	You have been travelling and finding work as you go in bars or in sports hire shops.
	Last year you completed a Geography degree.
	You have cut your travels short and you flew home once you were given this news.
	You plan to fly out next week to see your brother. You don't know when you will be back so you prefer not to arrange any hospital appointment at present.
	You are not in a relationship. You smoke cigarettes and smoke occasional cannabis.
	You drink alcohol socially but usually no more than 2 pints a night on average.
ICE	You have been reading about FAP and have some questions.
	You understand that you may need your bowel cut out like your brother.
	You are uncertain about Darren's prognosis as you were told 'the surgeons are not sure that they have got it all'.

1. You are confused by this and keep wondering if this means Darren will die.
2. *'Mum is worried it'll affect me too.'* She has been reading about the condition and is wondering whether your grandmother and father had the same problem.
   You want to know if this is likely to be the case. It may explain his suicide.
3. You feel anxious and are not sleeping well. You have started smoking more cannabis.

If the doctor is interested to know what has been on your mind, say, *'I can't stop thinking about Darren.'* If the doctor explores further, say, *'He's such a good guy'* and look to the floor, distracted in thought. If the doctor picks up on your cue you can say that you mean you have never been good at communicating with your brother and feel guilty that you did not reciprocate his interest in your life. You think about him often but he does not know this.

You expect the doctor will refer you for a telescope test into the bowel.

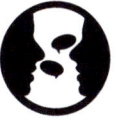

Genetics in Primary Care – 3

Learning Points — Autosomal Dominant Disorders

Familial adenomatous polyposis

Explanation	for patients ... *Familial means it can run in families, adenoma is the tissue in the large bowel and polyps are lumps in the bowel which can turn cancerous.*
Genetics	Refer for testing of the APC (adenomatous polyposis coli) gene, although some may be sporadic.
Symptoms	Asymptomatic, rectal bleeding or a change in bowels.
Complications	Obstruction, colorectal cancer or other tumours, e.g. thyroid, carcinoid, bone.
Monitoring	FBC, CEA, TFT, LFT, FOB, X-rays, advise dental monitoring and colonoscopy.

Polycystic kidney

Explanation	for patients ... *Poly means many, cysts are fluid filled sacs and kidneys make urine from body waste and water.*
Genetics	Autosomal dominant is most common
Features	Asymptomatic or there may be pain or haematuria
Complications	Recurrent infections, stones, hypertension, renal failure and need for dialysis
Investigations	U&E, BP, ACR and USS and seek renal advice
Monitoring	USS and U&E
Immunisations	Pneumococcus and influenza vaccine

HNPCC (hereditary non polyposis colon cancer)

Associations	Other cancers, e.g. ovary, prostate and stomach
Screening	Colonoscopy, endoscopy, cystoscopy and pelvic screening

Others which are or can be autosomal dominant

Ehlers-Danlos syndrome	Gilbert's disease
Hereditary haemorrhagic telangiectasia	Marfan's syndrome
Neurofibromatosis	Von Willebrand's disease
Familial hypercholesterolaemia	Huntington's disease
Prader-Willi syndrome	HOCM

There are more!

Doctor's Notes

Patient   Nicola Bennett
Age   42 years
PMH   3 × normal vaginal deliveries when aged 24, 26 and 30 years.
                   Focal migraine 18 years.
Medications   No current medications
Allergies   No information
Consultations No recent consultations
Investigations No recent investigations
Household   Duncan Bennett 46 years
                   Elizabeth Bennett 12 years
                   Benjamin Bennett 16 years
                   Arthur Bennett 18 years

Example Consultation — Breast Cancer BRCA Gene

Open ☐ — What has led to this decision? Tell me more about your mother's experience?

Curious ☐ — When you say you have built yourself up to this … in what way?

Impact ☐ — How has all of this impacted on your life? And on life day to day?

Sense ☐ — This has obviously played a large part in your life. It has taken courage to see me.

Risk ☐ — Has a member of the family already had a worrying gene identified? How old was your mother when she was diagnosed? I'm going to ask about factors which can affect your risk. I see you have had three children, the first when you were 24. Did you breastfeed? What contraception have you used? Did you smoke? Do you drink alcohol? That's all good news. Can you answer these questions about your mother? Do you have Jewish ancestors? Any other cancers in the family?

Flags ☐ — How often do you check your breasts? Have you noticed a lump or skin changes?

History ☐ — Tell me about your medical history. You mentioned not being able to concentrate … tell me more. Do you work? Is anyone else at home? How is your relationship?

ICE ☐ — What goes through your mind? Anything else? Or that you fear? What do your family think? How might a positive test for yourself affect your children?

O/E ☐ — Would you like me to examine your breasts today?

Summary ☐ — To summarise, you would like the genetic test after watching your mother go through breast cancer because you want to protect yourself and your children. Your sleep and concentration is affected. You have thought through potential scenarios and decided you would have a mastectomy. You hope, however, we can reassure you and therefore your children, but you are concerned about how a positive test may impact on them. Have I understood?

Empathy ☐ — This is important to you. You've had first-hand experience of the impact of cancer.

Impression ☐ — There have been studies looking into when we should do genetic testing. If your mother was over the age of 40 years, with no other cancers in the family, this is reassuring and genetic screening is not recommended. You have also decreased your risk of breast cancer by having three children quite young, all breastfed, and you used progesterone-only contraception. Your mother's hormone pattern was quite different and, combined with smoking, she was at increased risk.

Experience ☐ — What are your thoughts about what I have just said?

Explanation ☐ — You are correct we can never be certain of anyone's genes. We try to use the knowledge we have to base our recommendations on. Positive tests may impact on the mental well-being of families. It can be a very difficult decision.

Options ☐ — I'd like to help you reach a decision you are comfortable with. May I suggest that we meet again? If you still feel strongly I can write to the genetics team.

Future ☐ — I will download the public information NICE guidance leaflet which explains further what I have said today. In the meantime, as this has had such a huge impact on you, I will contact the genetics team to discuss your personal situation with them. We can then discuss what they suggest. How does this sound?

Empower ☐ — Whatever we decide, you will have lots on your mind. I am worried about how this is affecting you day to day. Have you had ideas on how we may be able to help with that? What about CBT? This is a therapy that helps you to work through how to manage powerful thoughts to avoid them impacting on your sleep, mood or concentration. I would recommend this. Have a think about it. We recommend that every woman checks her breasts and I will also print the breast awareness leaflet. Can we meet in a month?

Safety net ☐ — If you feel a lump or you have concerns or questions, don't hesitate to return.

Patient's Story

Breast Cancer BRCA Gene

Doctor's notes Nicola Bennett, 42 years.

PMH: 3 × normal vaginal deliveries aged 24, 26 and 30 years. Focal migraine 18 years. Medication: None.

How to act Determined and anxious.

PC *'Doctor, I would like to be referred for the genetic test for breast cancer please.'*

History You have always feared having breast cancer and it has taken a lot of courage to see the GP today. *'I've been building myself up to this.'* By this you mean you have had sleepless nights with a lack of concentration at work; however, this has not yet impacted on your ability to work effectively.

Your mother was diagnosed with breast cancer aged 45 years.

You are now aware that you are approaching this age.

Years ago you decided that you would not worry about this until your 40s.

This has recently been concerning you to the extent that you have played through in your mind all the possibilities which may occur.

Your mother had a mastectomy, chemotherapy and radiotherapy. She remained on tamoxifen but died 10 years later. The cancer had returned and had spread to her bones.

There are no other cancers in the family. Your mother smoked and she only had you aged 37 years. She never breastfed. Apart from three healthy children who were each breastfed for 1 year, and migraines in your teenage years, you have been healthy. You have used the copper coil as contraception since the birth of your third child. You used the progesterone-only contraception prior to this. You started your periods when you were 14 years old.

You are breast aware and check them every day in the shower.

Social You are a private physiotherapist. You are happily married and your eldest son is about to go to university. You were at university when your mother was diagnosed for the second time and remember feeling so far away at the time. The risk is beginning to feel real.

You drink alcohol rarely and have never smoked.

ICE You expect a referral to a geneticist.

You have considered in detail how you may react if the test is positive. You would want a mastectomy. You hope you will be able to cope better with bad news having gone through the possibilities in your mind. You fear how breast cancer may impact on your children. You don't want them to have to go through what you did, watching your mother.

You are hoping it will be negative so you can reassure your daughter. You will feel guilty if the test is positive and your daughter will have to go through this.

You have been worrying that either your children or your husband are getting fed up with you mentioning it.

If the doctor declines a referral, say:

'How can you say I am not at risk? I have the right to be referred.'

If the doctor declines, ask about a private referral. You have not read about the testing in detail, but you read about Angelina Jolie choosing a mastectomy.

If the doctor explores the extent of how this has impacted on your well-being and demonstrates an appreciation of this, you acknowledge and respect any advice. If the doctor provides an NHS referral, you are very happy.

Examination You decline an examination.

Genetics in Primary Care – 4

Learning Points

Breast Cancer BRCA Gene

Risk factors: Lifestyle: Alcohol and smoking. Overweight after the menopause
              Family history: Jewish ancestors and see below
              Hormonal: Early menarche, nulliparous or late pregnancies, OCP or HRT, limited/no breastfeeding

Breast screening 2016 aim = 47–73 years

1st invite is before 53 years. Then every 3 years

Genetics: 'A person who inherits a fault in a *BRCA1*, *BRCA2* or *TP53* gene is at high risk of developing breast cancer … Having a faulty gene is a risk factor, but does not automatically mean that you will develop breast cancer … All women who have a faulty *BRCA1*, *BRCA2* or *TP53* gene are at **high** risk … Women with a **high** risk have a 30% or greater chance of developing breast cancer in their lifetime.'[1,2]

Table showing the referral criteria. NICE[1]

Type of cancer in relative	Relatives affected	Age of relative at diagnosis
Female breast cancers only	1 first-degree relative	Under 40
	2 first-degree relatives	Any age
	1 first-degree and 1 second-degree relative	Any age
	3 first-degree or second-degree relatives	Any age
Male breast cancer	1 first-degree male relative	Any age
Bilateral breast cancer	1 first-degree relative	Under 50 at the diagnosis of the first cancer
Breast and ovarian cancer	1 first-degree or second-degree relative with breast cancer AND 1 first-degree or second-degree relative with ovarian cancer ONE SHOULD BE FIRST DEGREE	Any age

'Advice should be sought from the designated secondary care contact if any of the following are present in the family history in addition to breast cancers in relatives not fulfilling the above criteria: bilateral breast cancer, male breast cancer, ovarian cancer, Jewish ancestry, sarcoma in a relative younger than age 45 years, glioma or childhood adrenal cortical carcinomas, complicated patterns of multiple cancers at a young age, paternal history of breast cancer (two or more relatives on the father's side of the family). [2004]'[1]

Doctor's Notes

Patient   Jason Wright
Age   38 years
PMH   No medical history
Medications   No current medication
Allergies   No allergies
Consultations No recent consultations
Investigations No recent investigations
Household   No household members registered

Example Consultation — HOCM

Open ☐	I'm interested to know what has led to this decision.
Empathy ☐	I am so sorry. I understand why you feel the need to be investigated yourself.
Impact ☐	Since your brother's death how has this affected you? Do you feel different? Tell me about other members of the family? How are they doing?
History ☐	Have you noticed any (other) symptoms? And you have no medical problems? Tell me about you … do you work? Do you live with anyone?
Curious ☐	Can you confide in anyone else about how you have been feeling?
Flags ☐	Any pain or palpitations? And during exercise? Any fainting/collapsing episodes?
Risk ☐	Has any other member of the family died suddenly or had a heart condition?
Sense ☐	I feel this is now always on your mind.
ICE ☐	Have you any other fears that have been in your thoughts? You mentioned a referral to a cardiologist. Is there anything else you were hoping I would arrange today?
Summary ☐	To clarify what we've discussed so far, you fear you have inherited the same condition as your brother; you have been told this was cardiomyopathy. Since the diagnosis, you have noticed breathlessness at times and you feel you have changed; you have started distracting yourself with work but stopped doing sport. You fear most having to tell your family you have the same condition and feel we need to check your general health and send you to see a cardiologist. Have I understood you correctly?
O/E ☐	May I examine your heart, take your blood pressure and feel your pulse please?
Impression ☐	Today the examination of your heart is normal. Often if HOCM is present, a murmur will be heard. Thankfully this isn't the case in you. We will investigate; however, I don't think that your heart has caused your symptoms. It is very common that when we are very worried about something, we breathe differently and the fingers tingle.
Experience ☐	What is your understanding of your brother's condition?
Explanation ☐	HOCM is a condition that may not give symptoms but can cause SOB, collapses, chest pain or palpitations. The heart muscle is thickened but the vessels are not affected. We don't know what causes it. There is often a family link. In some cases, there is a 50% chance of inheriting the condition. Sudden death is rare but is believed to happen due to abnormal electrical activity causing the heart beat rhythm to change.
Options ☐	I will write today to the cardiology team. I imagine they will first perform a jelly scan of the heart, but I don't think you will hear from them this week. Therefore, we can do an ECG, which is a heart tracing, today. Would that be okay? I will ask the nurse to fit you in this morning.
Empower ☐	I hope you now feel reassured to return to your normal activity.
Future ☐	Shall I give you a ring with the ECG result? I wonder if bereavement counselling may help?
Safety net ☐	If you experience palpitations, pain or symptoms during exercise, let a doctor know.

Patient's Story

HOCM

Doctors notes	Jason Wright, 38 years. PMH: Nil. Medications: Nil
How to act	Concerned and anxious.
PC	*'I would like a referral to a cardiologist.'*
History	Your brother, Will, died a month ago when he was playing football.
	He played at a semi-professional level and collapsed during the match and died at the scene. Lots of people were watching; it was very distressing. The post-mortem diagnosed hypertrophic obstructive cardiomyopathy. You have been advised to 'get checked out'. You are also aware that this has happened to other footballers from news reports.
	Since then you have found that you are breathless.
	Your fingers tingle, usually in the evenings or in the car.
	You have no medical history. No other family history. No medicines.
	You are sad about your brother's death but have no symptoms of depression.
	You don't feel that you need any help with your grief.
Social	You are single.
	You have a busy work and social lifestyle. Never smoked. Alcohol 20 units/week.
	You have returned to work as a barman and you are very busy.
	You have no symptoms at work.
	You have been taking more on at work as a way of getting on with things.
	You have stopped playing football in fear the same will happen to you.
ICE	You were told that Will's heart got bigger.
	You then believe the vessel must have burst.
	You believe your heart is getting bigger.
	You fear having to tell your family you have the same condition.
	You just want to see a cardiologist this week before it's too late.
	You would like your cholesterol and blood pressure checked also.
Examination	Heart sounds normal. HR regular 70 bpm. BP 120/60.

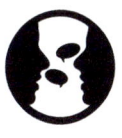

Genetics in Primary Care – 5

Learning Points

HOCM

Cause	Unknown
Genetics	Usually autosomal-dominant genetic condition.
Physiology	Hypertrophy of the undilated left ventricle with diastolic impairment.
Symptoms	If present (often asymptomatic): angina, dyspnoea, palpitations and syncope.
Examination	Raised JVP, murmur, AF.
Investigations	ECG, CXR, Echo and 24-hour tape.
Management	Control symptoms: heart failure, angina, and arrhythmias.
	Consider myectomy and septal ablation.
	Consider an implanted defibrillator to prevent sudden death.
Complications	May cause heart failure, AF, stroke or sudden death (usually from arrhythmia).

There are several aspects to this case. First, dealing with the patient's appropriate concern that he may have HOCM. There is a medical need to assess and refer him for investigation but also to reassure him if he shows no features of the illness at present. If time permits, there may be an opportunity to discuss the genetics of HOCM (autosomal-dominant inheritance) should the patient wish to know. The patient in the exam may directly ask you about this, so be prepared to explain patterns of inheritance in layperson's language or with use of diagrams. The patient's false belief that a vessel in his brother's heart had burst should also be sensitively addressed. Lastly, it is very important to acknowledge the devastating loss of his brother and offer support/bereavement counselling should he require it.

CHAPTER 4 OVERVIEW
Acutely Ill People

	Cases in this chapter	Within the RCGP curriculum: Care of Acutely Ill People RCGP Curriculum Online March 2016[1]	Learning points in the chapter include:
1	Abdominal Pain	'Recognise that an acute illness may be an acute exacerbation of a chronic disease'	Differential diagnosis of abdominal pain
2	Chest Pain of Recent Onset	'Know the main and common differential diagnoses …' 'Recognise the importance of knowing the protocols … acute illnesses' 'Know how … risk factors … influence the incidence and presentation of acute illnesses'	Differential diagnosis of chest pain. Chest Pain of Recent Onset NICE Guidance
3	SVT	'Recognise the signs of illnesses and conditions that require urgent intervention'	Assessment of palpitations
4	Angioedema	'Manage the difference between what you think is an appropriate medical course of action and the course of action desired by patients … carers' 'Know when it is safe and appropriate to manage a patient in the community'	Case involves negotiation with a parent. Resuscitation Council UK guidance
5	Hyperglycaemia	'Continuity of care for an individual patient undergoing an episode of acute illness can be maintained in all contexts'	Case involves offering continuity of care and follow-up after the acute treatment of hyperglycaemia. Ketones, HONK and lactic acidosis

1. http://www.rcgp.org.uk/training-exams/gp-curriculum-overview/online-curriculum/applying-clinical-knowledge-section-1/3-03-acutely-ill-people.aspx

CHAPTER 4 REFERENCES

Abdominal Pain
1. http://patient.info/doctor/acute-abdomen

Chest Pain of Recent Onset
1. NICE Guidelines. CG95. Chest Pain of Recent Onset. March 2010.

SVT
1. NICE http://cks.nice.org.uk/palpitations. Revised May 2015.

Angioedema and Anaphylaxis
1. http://www.nhs.uk/Conditions/Angioedema/Pages/Introduction.aspx. Jun 2016

Hyperglycaemia and DKA
1. http://www.diabetes.co.uk/diabetes_care/testing-for-ketones.html. Jun 2016

Doctor's Notes

Patient   Rosie Carpenter   40 years   F
PMH   Irritable bowel syndrome
Medications   Desogestrel
Allergies   No information
Consultations 1 month ago renewal of repeat contraception. No problems.
Investigations BP 116/62
                   BMI 31
Household   No household members registered

Example Consultation   Abdominal Pain

Sense ☐	I can see you are in a lot of pain. We do not have morphine here but as soon as we get to the bottom of what is causing your pain we will arrange urgent treatment.
Open ☐	Can you describe the pain? Please take me through your symptoms from when you first noticed something wasn't right. Anything else that you have noticed?
Flags ☐	Have you had a high temperature? Have you vomited? Did you see any blood or black when you vomited? What are your stools like? Have you noticed any blood or black colour in your stools? Have you been able to keep fluids down?
Risk ☐	Any history of tummy ulcers or gallstones? Have you noticed any symptoms of acid going up the gullet or pain after meals in the past months? When was your last period? Is there any chance you could be pregnant?
History ☐	Any problems passing urine? What medical problems have you had in the past? Do you take any medicines? Alcohol? Ibuprofen?
ICE ☐	Have you had thoughts about what could be causing this? What are you most worried it could be? Apart from morphine, is there anything else you thought I may suggest?
Curious ☐	Has a doctor given you morphine in the past?
O/E ☐	I'd like to examine you, take your temperature, breathing and heart rate, blood pressure in both arms and feel your stomach, as well as listen to your chest and heart if I may.
Summary ☐	So, for 24 hours you have had a pain which is severe. You have noticed stomach pains following eating. You vomited once and have had a fever. You fear this could be similar to the problem your father had when he died of a bleed in the stomach. I am sorry to hear that. Thankfully, I do not believe the same is happening to you.
Impression ☐	I believe you may have a gallbladder infection. The other possibility is a tummy ulcer but, due to the location of your pain and your fever, I believe you have a gallbladder infection. I don't think this is a rupture of your stomach or a blood vessel like your father because you have seen no blood and you do not drink alcohol which is likely to have led to his bleed.
Experience ☐	Are you aware of gallstones?
Explanation ☐	The gallbladder releases a liquid – I always compare it to Fairy Liquid – to help sort out the fat in our food. This liquid can turn into stones called gallstones which can then lead to a blockage. This blockage may cause intermittent pain, like the pain you have been experiencing after food. I think the pain you have been getting over the past few months is gallstones. The blockage from gallstones can also result in an infection.
Empathy ☐	It is extremely painful and makes you feel terribly unwell.
Options ☐	We need to get you to hospital.
Empower ☐	There is the possibility of an infection elsewhere, for example the pancreas. At the hospital they will do blood tests and possibly an ultrasound scan to confirm the diagnosis. Most cases of gallbladder infection get better with antibiotics, fluids and painkillers in hospital, but we need to get you to hospital without delay so you can start the antibiotics through your veins and get your pain under control.
Future ☐	If the diagnosis is confirmed I expect, once you are more comfortable, the doctors may talk to you about having your gallbladder removed at some point in the future.
Safety net ☐	We do not have any morphine in the practice. Would your husband be able to take you to hospital or would you prefer me to call an ambulance? Can we bring your husband in so I can explain the situation to him and see if he is happy to drive you? There is always the possibility you may become more unwell en route. If this happens your husband would have to stop the car and call 999. I will call the surgical team now so they can meet you at the other end. You will be going to the Surgical Admissions Unit. Please don't eat or drink anything until you've seen the surgical team.

Acutely Ill People – 1

Patient's Story

Abdominal Pain

Doctor's notes Rosie Carpenter, 40 years. PMH: Irritable bowel syndrome and BMI 31.

Medication: Desogestrel.

POP checked 1/12 ago and no problems.

How to act Keep putting pressure on the doctor. He/she needs to do something!

PC *'What's going on? I've never been in this much pain. I need morphine.'*

History The pain started yesterday and has gradually been getting worse. 10/10 severity.

It is in your upper stomach and radiating to the back and feels sharp.

It is worse after eating. You have had a fever.

You have no reflux symptoms and your bowels are normal.

You have been sick with the pain earlier this morning. You feel nauseous and unwell.

You have been getting pain in the upper abdomen over the past few months whenever you eat. You have not lost weight and have seen no melaena. You have no dysphagia.

You have no cardiac or respiratory symptoms.

You have no urinary symptoms. LMP was normal 2 weeks ago.

You have never had morphine but the paracetamol and ibuprofen you have taken have not helped.

Social You don't drink alcohol as your dad was an alcoholic. You don't smoke.

You work in publishing. You are married and live with your husband. You take no drugs.

ICE You fear this is an ulcer and that the ulcer may burst which you presume is what happened to your father when he died of a stomach haemorrhage. You expect the doctor to give you pain relief straight away and you want reassurance.

Examination Abdomen tender RUQ, Murphy's positive, normal bowel sounds.

No abdominal masses or organomegaly or ascites.

HR 114 regular, temperature 38.4°C BP 138/84 in both arms RR 18

HS normal and chest clear.

Your husband is in the waiting room. If the doctor advises going to hospital, your husband can drive you there as it is only around the corner.

Acutely Ill People – 1

Learning Points — Abdominal Pain

Differential diagnosis of abdominal pain[1]

Acute pancreatitis	Tender, distention, fever and tachycardic. Causes include gallstones, alcohol and raised cholesterol.
Peptic ulcer	Reflux symptoms (belching, heartburn, nausea) ± melaena.
Acute cholangitis	Charcot's triad (presents in <1/3) = fever, jaundice, RUQ pain (usually mild). Usually in older adults, e.g. secondary to a cancer obstructing the bile duct.
Cholecystitis	Murphy's sign (RUQ pain) or mass + fever or raised CRP/WCC ± vomiting, radiation to back, distention. Usually from gallstones. RFs = raised BMI/women/diabetes. Can be more severe in men.
Acute biliary colic	RUQ pain (with radiation to scapula) secondary to gallstones. Local tenderness but no fever.
Mesenteric ischaemia	Possible vascular history. Sudden onset. Systemically unwell. May appear SOB or vomit.
Appendicitis	Initial generalised pain before localising to RLQ + peritonitic.
Bowel obstruction	Vomiting + constipation + distended + not passing flatus. Peritonitic if perforated.
Renal colic	Severe loin to groin pain ± haematuria (macroscopic or microscopic).
Pyelonephritis	Urinary symptoms + loin pain + febrile + positive dipstick ± rigors.
Ectopic pregnancy	Lower abdominal pain (may radiate to shoulder) + β-hCG positive ± systemically unwell.
Ovarian cyst torsion	Severe pain radiating to iliac fossa or flank usually with nausea and vomiting.
Ovarian cyst rupture	May be peritonitic or haemodynamically unstable.
PID	Adnexal tenderness or cervical excitation + negative β-hCG ± history of STI. May be systemically unwell.
AAA rupture	Pain (abdominal or back) + haemodynamically unstable.
MI	Crushing central chest pain may radiate to arm or jaw (may present as abdominal pain) with SOB, nausea or vomiting and sweating. May be haemodynamically unstable.

Advice: β-hCG in any female (of reproductive age) despite recent LMP or contraception.

If for good reason (e.g. not had sexual intercourse for a year), history is 'taken in good faith'.

Most of the differential diagnoses listed require admission. Biliary colic and renal colic management will depend on the severity of the pain and your local access to scans. If there is no haematemesis/melaena and the patient is well, suspected peptic ulcer disease can be referred routinely for endoscopy via local protocols. Pyelonephritis can be treated in the community if the patient is afebrile and doesn't have significant pain but be aware of pyelonephritis complicating renal colic – this is a urological emergency! PID may be managed in the community if the patient is systemically well. If the patient is managed at home, provide careful safety netting advice and consider admission if there is no improvement in 48 hours.

This case is assessing your ability to manage a patient's demands and make a thorough assessment. It would be reasonable, if you felt the patient was very unwell, to check their observations first, explaining that you will return to ask them questions about the problem once you are happy they are not in immediate danger. Even if you are unsure of the cause, a febrile, tachycardic patient with abdominal pain warrants urgent further investigation.

Due to the regulation of controlled drugs, it is unusual for practices to keep morphine. If being pressured, as the patient is focused on morphine, address this then take the full history.

Acutely Ill People – 1

Doctor's Notes

Patient   Mary Jones   45 years   F

PMH   New patient questionnaire: Smoker. BMI 40.2. Three children.
                  No further information.

Medications   No information.

Allergies   No information

Consultations No information

Investigations No information.

Household   No household members registered

Example Consultation — Chest Pain of Recent Onset

Open ☐ — Please tell me more about the pain from when you first noticed it until now. When do you get the pain? Have you noticed any other symptoms?

Flags ☐ — Have you injured your neck? Do you have a headache? Any weakness or tingling in the arms? What are you doing when the pain comes on? Do you feel sick, sweaty or short of breath?

Risk ☐ — Do you suffer with raised BP or cholesterol? Has a family member under the age of 65 had a problem with their heart? Do you smoke?

History ☐ — Do you have any other medical conditions? Or take any medications?

ICE ☐ — What do you think is going on? Apart from giving you co-codamol, were you expecting me to do anything else today? Are there any other concerns you have?

Impact ☐ — Has this pain stopped you from doing anything?

Sense ☐ — I'm sorry that I have kept you waiting. I can see that you are in a rush; however, I am concerned about your pain.

O/E ☐ — May I examine your blood pressure in both arms, pulse and heart rate, take your temperature and listen to your heart please?

Summary ☐ — So you've had this pain a few times, initially when quite active, but this time it started whilst you were resting. It has now been present for 30 minutes in your chest and neck and you feel nauseous and sweaty. You believe it is due to your neck and hope I can provide co-codamol quickly as I have already kept you waiting.

Impression ☐ — I am concerned that this pain is coming from your heart (pause); this could be a heart attack.

Explanation ☐ — Your symptoms are typical of a pain from the heart even though you feel it in your neck. A heart attack is where a vessel to the heart becomes blocked and the lack of blood flow causes the pain.

Empathy ☐ — I appreciate this is very frightening and completely unexpected.

Options ☐ — I'd like to take you through to our treatment room where we can do a heart tracing called an ECG. I'm going to ask the receptionist to call an ambulance. I appreciate this sounds frightening, although if the pain is coming from your heart it is treatable. But we must not delay this treatment. I'd like to give you an aspirin tablet to help with the blood flow.

Empower ☐ — I appreciate you need to go to your son. However, I must tell you what is at risk here. You need to go to the hospital now otherwise your life could be in danger. I'm sorry. Do you have anyone our receptionist can call? Your husband? We will keep a close eye on you and have you seen by hospital staff straight away.

Future ☐ — At the hospital I expect they will do a blood test and they may take you to have a procedure which looks at the vessels to the heart. Do you have any questions?

Acutely Ill People – 2

Patient's Story

Chest Pain of Recent Onset

Doctor's notes Mary Jones, 45 years, New patient, BMI 40.2, Smoker, 3 children.

How to act You are in a rush. Tell the doctor this as he/she is running late.

You want to reassure the doctor it's just a pulled neck.

PC *'Doctor, I've got a pain in my neck.'*

History The pain in the upper left chest and neck has now been present for 30 minutes. You had not rushed here and this time it started 5 minutes after you arrived at the surgery.

It feels like something is pressing. You feel nauseous, sweaty and slightly SOB. You can't think of anything that takes it away. It just comes and goes but you think movement makes it worse as whenever you are doing something it comes on.

You also had the same pain 2 days ago when you were in the garden but it went away after 5–10 minutes when you rested.

You have had this pain a few times in the past two weeks.

For example, when running upstairs or watching television.

Your old GP gave you co-codamol for back pain so you would like this for your neck.

Your father died when you were a child due to his heart.

Social Mother of three. You have moved areas as your husband has been relocated. You have not found a job and used to work in a local tea room. Your husband works in the building supplies industry. You smoke 10 a day. You drink alcohol rarely.

ICE You believe you have pulled your neck. You have not made any connection with the heart. You would like a prescription for co-codamol and you will return another time if the doctor suggests anything else.

You can't go to hospital now. You have to go and watch your son in a school play.

You would just like the codeine. However, when the doctor explains the seriousness of the problem, you become upset and agree.

Examination HS normal, HR 124 regular, Sats 97% RR 18, BP 130/80 in both arms. 36.5°C.

No neck or cervical spine tenderness and full range of movement.

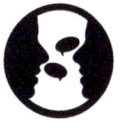

Learning Points

Chest Pain of Recent Onset

Beware: Cardiac pain at radiation sites + nausea/vomiting/sweating especially in women/elderly/diabetics.

Do they need to go to hospital today? Yes, if history of ACS within 72 hours. Otherwise RACPC.[1]

Emergency admission if current pain or pain within 12 hours + ECG abnormal/not available.

Yes, if pain resolved and signs of complications.

Do I need to call for an ambulance? Yes, if current chest pain[1] and consider in all possible ACS.

Always refer to full guidance.

Differential diagnosis

ACS: Pain >10 minutes or increasing frequency or onset with less activity or at rest.
Dissection: Sudden tearing pain radiating to the back between the scapulas.
Pericarditis: Sharp, relieved by sitting forward ± radiation, fever, cough and arthralgia.
Acute heart failure: Orthopnoea and breathlessness.
Arrhythmias: Associated with palpitations and syncope.
PE: SOB, tachycardia, hypoxia, ± haemoptysis ± leg swelling ± risk factors for VTE.
Pneumothorax: Risk factors include injury, tall male and COPD.
Pneumonia: SOB, fever, purulent sputum, cough ± pleuritic pain. Check the CRB65 score.
GORD/PUD: Belching, reflux and sharp/burning pain ± melaena.
MSK causes: From Tietze's, costochondritis or rib fracture. Recent activity, tender.
Anxiety: Tight chest, tingling in fingers, feeling of needing to breathe.
Referred thoracic pain: Back pain with possible back pain red flags.

When to give oxygen? Sats <94% and not at risk of carbon dioxide retention (aim for 94–98%).

Sats <88% and with COPD history (aim for 88–92%).

Acutely Ill People – 2

Doctor's Notes

Patient	Austin Winter	57 years	M
PMH	Radial fracture aged 34 years.		
	Lower respiratory tract infection aged 52 years.		
Medications	No current medications		
Allergies	No allergies		
Consultations	No information		
Investigations	BP 120/60	5 years ago	
Household	Elizabeth Winter	56 years	F

Example Consultation   SVT

Open ☐	How can I help? What do you mean by palpitations? Any other symptoms you have noticed? How do you feel in yourself?
Sense ☐	I can see you are distressed by what you are feeling. Can you tap the rhythm on the desk for me?
Flags ☐	Do you feel lightheaded? Any pain? Or breathless? Have you passed out ever?
History ☐	Do you have any medical conditions? Do you take any medicines or supplements? Tell me about your life at home and work please. Are you under stress at present?
Risk ☐	Regarding your general health, do you smoke or drink alcohol? Do you drink caffeine? In your family, is there any history of heart trouble or has anyone collapsed? Any sudden deaths? Have you noticed the palpitations during exercise?
ICE ☐	What do you think may be going on here? Is there anything you fear may be causing this? What did you think I might suggest before you left the surgery today?
Curious ☐	I'm wondering what made you think of angina? What do you know about angina?
Impact ☐	These episodes have been going on for a while. What has made you come now?
O/E ☐	I'd like to examine you. Would you mind taking off your shirt so I can listen to your heart and lungs, check your pulse and take your blood pressure? Then I would like to do a heart tracing. This involves some stickers on the chest. Is this okay?
Summary ☐	So, Mr Winter, your heart is beating fast but your blood pressure is fine. You have experienced this many times now and it can make you feel breathless. Due to your colleague's experience with the heart you wondered if you may have angina. You share the same stressful work as your colleague. You thought I may suggest aspirin and a cardiology referral, is that correct?
Impression ☐	You have a heart rhythm which is called supraventricular tachycardia or SVT for short. It is quite common but unsettling and can make you feel dreadful when it occurs. At this stage it is unclear what has caused this so we need to do some tests. I do not believe this is angina. Angina is usually a pain in the chest which is caused by the vessels being narrowed. You have rhythm disturbance caused by the electrical signals not vessels.
Experience ☐	We need to check the electrical signals in the heart, and the pathways that these signals travel along. There are drug or surgical treatments that will help. But first we need to try to slow the heart down. There are a few methods of doing this which may seem strange but they act on sensors in the body. First, we can try blowing into a syringe whilst lying down. If that doesn't work, we could try massaging the artery in your neck.
Empathy ☐	Okay, I appreciate a trip to the hospital is not what you were expecting today but your heart is still racing so we need to ask the hospital doctors to look at you.
Future ☐	I will call the medical team and let them know what's happening. I expect they will give you a drug called adenosine to slow down the heart. This may make you feel unwell but usually lasts just a couple of minutes. I expect a heart specialist may then talk to you about further tests.
Options ☐	How do you feel about going to hospital? We can call an ambulance or, because your blood pressure is fine, I am happy for your wife to take you if you are both comfortable with this.
Safety net ☐	If en route you have pain, feel lightheaded or more poorly, stop the car and call for an ambulance. May I check whether your wife is happy with this before you leave?

Acutely Ill People – 3

Patient's Story

SVT

Doctor's notes	Austin Winter, 57 years. PMH: Radial fracture aged 34 years. Lower respiratory tract infection aged 52 years. Medications: None.
How to act	Concerned.
PC	*'Doctor, I'm having palpitations. I'm having one now.'*
History	The palpitations are affecting your work.
	For the last 3 months, you have been aware of your heart beating quickly, a few times a week.
	This seems to have become more frequent.
	You don't feel dizzy but you can feel slightly breathless.
	You have no pain. You have no cardiovascular risk factors.
Social	You are a business advisor. You have a busy job but you do not feel stressed. Your wife and children are well.
	You do not smoke and rarely drink alcohol. You do drink a lot of coffee as you get up early and there is usually a coffee machine in the meetings.
ICE	You believe you have angina.
	Your colleague has just been diagnosed with angina and has been told he needs more exercise and less stress or he'll have a heart attack. You expect the doctor will tell you to start taking aspirin and refer you to a cardiologist.
Examination	HR 140 regular, HS normal, chest clear. BP 130/62. Apyrexial.
	ECG shows SVT

Your wife is in the waiting room.

Acutely Ill People – 3

Learning Points   SVT

Assessment of palpitations[1]

Does the patient need to go to hospital? Yes, if the SVT has not been controlled. No, if reverted.

The next common dilemma in an emergency consultation is: does the patient need an ambulance? Yes, if haemodynamically unstable.

If the patient is haemodynamically stable, this depends on the level of risk the doctor, patient and relative are comfortable to take which will be unique to each individual situation. Colleagues have different thresholds for calling an ambulance. It will also depend on the distance to A&E and your ambulance response time!

If this was AF with fast ventricular response or atrial flutter call 999 if haemodynamically unstable.

Otherwise treat any likely cause (infection), arrange blood tests and try a rate-limiting drug (beta-blocker or rate-limiting calcium channel blocker), e.g. bisoprolol, if no contraindications.

Metoprolol is shorter acting if the patient has side effects with the bisoprolol.

You would then also need to consider anticoagulation and, if new onset AF with no previous symptoms, possible cardioversion.

AF does not need a referral to cardiology. Atrial flutter is managed in a similar way but can be harder to treat and you may need advice.

Supraventricular tachycardia

SCENARIO: A patient returns from the cardiologist with a diagnosis of SVT.

'What does this mean, Doctor?'

A possible explanation may be …

'In the heart there is a pathway for electricity to flow. However, if there is a second pathway, the current can return and create a circuit which makes the heart beat too quickly. It depends where the extra pathway has formed. There may be days or months between episodes. Symptoms can include a feeling of a fast heart, feeling faint and chest pain.'

Note the SVT ECG may also show rate-related bundle branch block and inverted P waves.

Intermittent palpitations

SCENARIO: *'Doctor I've been having palpitations. It's not there at present.'*

Risk factors: Stress, caffeine, alcohol, recreational drugs.

Red flags: Family history of sudden collapse or death or heart conditions in the young. Symptoms with exercise.

Investigations: FBC, TFTs, ECG ± 24hr ECG or event monitor.

Differential diagnosis: Ectopic beats, SVT, AF, stress/anxiety or HOCM.

Acutely Ill People – 3

Doctor's Notes

Emergency walk-in patient

Patient	Joshua Middleton	11 years	M
PMH	Eczema		
Medications	Oilatum		
	Hydrocortisone		
Allergies	No information		
Consultations	Medication review. Eczema controlled. 1 year ago.		
Investigations	No information		
Household	Samantha Middleton	13 years	F
	David Middleton	46 years	M
	Angela Middleton	43 years	F

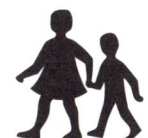

Example Consultation — Angioedema

Open — Hello Joshua, I'm Dr Blount. What happened? Is there anywhere else in your body that doesn't feel right? Angela, is there anything else you have noticed?

Flags — Joshua, does your breathing feel different? Does it feel swollen in your mouth?

Risk — Has this happened before?

O/E — Because this has happened so quickly, I would like to first have a closer look at you Joshua; at the rash and swelling … now your temperature in your ear … now this will squeeze your arm … now please put your finger in my gadget … may I look in your mouth please and listen to your chest? I can see the swelling around your eyes and the rash. You are okay Joshua but let's give you some medicine to get rid of this rash.

History — What time did this happen? When did the swelling around the eyes start? Has it got worse since you left the football pitch or stayed the same? How is your eczema? Angela, does Joshua have any other medical conditions? What medicines or creams is Joshua using? Any known allergies? Who is at home? Any pets?

ICE — Joshua, what do you think has caused this? Do you know why this might have happened? What did you think I may say today? What about you Angela: what has gone through your mind? It's helpful to know you have had training with EpiPens.

Impression — Joshua, you have had an allergic reaction, most likely to the peanuts.

Experience — Have you heard of the word allergy Joshua? What do you know about it?

Explanation — That's right Joshua. An allergy means your body doesn't like something. If you have an allergy you can have a rash or it can make your breathing difficult if you eat or touch the thing it doesn't like. Your friend cannot eat eggs. Lots of people have allergies. I would like you to see the allergy doctor at the hospital who will likely do tests to confirm the peanut allergy and may suggest other things you should avoid. For now, please avoid eating and touching all nuts until we know what is safe.

Empathy — The reaction on the face and skin must have been very frightening and it must be worrying you that it has not gone back to normal.

Options — Because Joshua's breathing has been normal and the swelling has not got worse since leaving the pitch and his observations are normal, I do not believe Joshua has had an anaphylactic reaction. Therefore, we could give Joshua an antihistamine and steroid tablets to take the swelling and rash down. I would expect these to work over the next few hours to a couple of days. The other option would be to go into hospital for a drip. I mention this option as, although I think it is unlikely, there is always a chance the swelling could get worse and affect the breathing. My suggestion, if you feel comfortable with this, is starting the tablets now, staying in the surgery for the next hour to make sure the swelling does not get worse, then if all is okay go home and complete the course of tablets, but with the plan that if anything gets worse or you are worried, then go to hospital. Or do you want to go there now?

Safety net — Okay, let's give you tablets. If in the meantime you feel unwell or different, or your tongue or breathing feels funny, please let me know. If, when you get home, any of these symptoms happen, call 999. If in the future you ever notice this happen again, call 999 straight away as it can happen quickly and affect the breathing.

Future — We will refer Joshua to an allergy specialist. EpiPens are prescribed initially by the specialist if they feel it is necessary. Because Joshua has not had an anaphylactic reaction they may say it is not necessary. I appreciate allergies can get worse the next time a reaction happens; however, we should be guided by their expertise as EpiPens can be dangerous. I will let them know in my referral letter that you have training to use EpiPens. Does that sound okay? Let's take you through to the treatment room and I'll keep popping in between patients to see you. If you are worried, just call for help.

Patient's Story

Angioedema

Doctor's notes — Emergency walk-in patient.

Joshua Middleton, 11 years. PMH: Eczema. Medications: Oilatum and hydrocortisone.

History

Mum — *'Joshua was eating peanuts and he immediately came out in a rash.'*

This has never happened before. Joshua is well and his eczema is controlled with emollients alone. He has no other allergies.

There is no family history.

Joshua — You were playing football and felt well.

Afterwards your friend gave you some peanuts. This was one hour ago now.

You can't remember if you've had peanuts before.

Within a minute you had come out in a rash and your eyes had started to swell. Since then there has been no change.

Your lips are slightly swollen but there is no tongue swelling and your breathing feels normal.

Social

Joshua — You are in the first year of secondary school.

You live with your parents and older sister.

ICE

Mum — You would like Joshua to have some medicine straight away.

You've heard of a child who died from a peanut reaction and this thought frightens you.

You would like to go home with an Epi-Pen but are happy to follow the doctor's advice.

You are a district nurse and have had Epi-Pen training.

Joshua — You feel scared and would like the swelling and rash to go away.

You don't know what this is.

Your friend has an allergy to eggs which means he can't have them.

Examination — Saturations 98% RR 18, HR 90 bpm regular and temperature 36.8°C. BP 106/60.

Widespread urticarial rash. Chest clear. Mouth and tongue normal. Mild lip swelling and mild swelling of the eyelids.

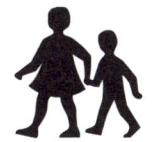

Acutely Ill People – 4

Learning Points

Angioedema and Anaphylaxis

Doctors are aware that anaphylaxis requires intramuscular adrenaline. However, the misuse of intramuscular adrenaline can be dangerous. When faced with a patient with swollen eyes and lips and a generalised urticarial rash, anaphylaxis is at the top of the differential diagnosis list.

Angioedema

Angioedema is a sign of a possible frightening medical emergency. Therefore, the above case of an acute IgE mediated reaction in the haemodynamically stable patient without respiratory compromise (which is not an uncommon scenario) may be approached differently by different GPs. GPs are likely to ask themselves:

Do I need to call an ambulance?

Do I need to give intramuscular adrenaline?

Should I give hydrocortisone and chlorphenamine (IM or slow IV) or oral treatment?

Anaphylaxis is a life-threatening risk to airway, breathing and circulation. Adrenaline is required if there are signs of risk to life.

The NHS website tells us angioedema 'sometimes occurs in combination with anaphylaxis …'[1], which reminds us that they are two separate diagnoses.

'Although most cases of angioedema get better without treatment after a few days, medication is often used …'[1]

'For cases of allergic and idiopathic angioedema, antihistamines and oral steroids can be used to relieve the swelling.'[1]

> **Anaphylaxis**
> See the **Link Hub at CompleteCSA.co.uk** for a useful link to anaphylaxis guidance from the Resuscitation Council (UK).
> Consider keeping a printout of this in your doctor's bag for reference in real-life emergencies.

Egg allergy is a contraindication to IM influenza/MMR/yellow fever/rabies vaccines.

Acutely Ill People – 4

Doctor's Notes

Patient	Mary Owen 35 years F
PMH	Type 1 diabetes
	Anxiety
	IBS
Medications	Insulin Glargine, NovoRapid, Citalopram and Buscopan.
Allergies	No information
Consultations	DNA letter from hospital diabetes clinic
Investigations	No information
Household	No household members registered

Example Consultation — Hyperglycaemia

Open — Oh dear. In what way unwell? When did you last feel your normal self? Okay, take it from that day and tell me what symptoms you noticed in sequence if you can. How is your general health usually?

Flags — How are your blood sugars at the moment? Do you have a ketone meter?

Risk — Any symptoms that may suggest infection, for example a cough, sore throat, diarrhoea, changes passing urine or tummy pain or abnormal vaginal discharge? Is it painful to pass urine? Are you racing to the toilet? Or passing a small or large amount each time? Any blood? Any rash, stiffness of the neck or discomfort looking at the light?

ICE — What do you think may have caused this? What is worrying you? What did you think I might suggest today?

History — Is the insulin regime appropriate for your lifestyle? Has everything been okay with taking your insulin recently? Do you have any other medical problems? How is your anxiety? How are your bowels at present? Do you work? Tell me more about work. Is anyone at home? Are you in a relationship? 'Not really?'

Curious — You say you have been forgetting to take the insulin. Why might this be? Why are you missing meals? You say you haven't got time to worry about work: is everything okay? I'm sorry your mother is not well.

Impact — Have you been struggling with your normal day? Are you feeling low?

O/E — I would like to check your BP, pulse, temperature, listen to your chest, feel your tummy and do a finger prick test for sugar and ketones. I think we also need a urine specimen from you, please, if you pop to the toilet whilst I make a plan.

Summary — To summarise, you have felt unwell for two days. You believe you have a urine infection, are frightened by your blood sugars being so high and thought I may make a suggestion of how to bring them down.

Empathy — It sounds like you are under stress physically and emotionally with a busy career, whilst taking care of your mother to whom you are very close.

Impression — Mary, I believe the raised blood sugar is likely due to a combination of stress, missing insulin doses and a urine infection. Urine infections are more likely after having sex and with raised sugars. I believe the diagnosis is a urine infection and diabetic ketoacidosis or DKA for short.

Experience — Have you heard of this?

Explanation — Because your body does not have a good supply of insulin to move all that sugar in your blood into your muscles to provide the muscles with energy, your muscle breaks down its protein to make ketones.

Options — You need to go to hospital for treatment through the veins otherwise you will be extremely unwell. Unfortunately, we cannot give this care at home. Is your mother a patient with us? What does she need? I can call your mother and suggest arranging emergency care through the Single Point of Access Team, whilst you are in hospital. I will phone the medical team at the hospital to let them know you need to come in. I will arrange for an ambulance to take you to hospital.

Future — At the hospital, I expect you will be given fluids, insulin and antibiotics.

Empower — When you are better, please return to see me to discuss your general health, support we could offer and changes to your insulin regime to better suit your lifestyle. We can also supply a ketone meter. I also recommend going to the toilet after sex to prevent water infections as this helps flush out the bacteria that may be pushed up to the bladder during sex. Does this make sense?

Safety net — If you feel unwell again, please don't hesitate to speak to a doctor.

Acutely Ill People – 5

Patient's Story

Hyperglycaemia

Doctor's notes	Mary Owen, 35 years. PMH: Type 1 diabetes, anxiety and IBS.
	Medications: Insulin Glargine, NovoRapid, Citalopram and Buscopan.
	Consultations: DNA letter from hospital diabetes clinic.
How to act	Look nauseated, slightly breathless and lacking in full concentration.
PC	*'I keep being sick. I feel really unwell.'*
History	Two days ago you started feeling unwell and tired and started to develop stomach pain.
	This morning you started vomiting with abdominal pain and a headache.
	You have no rash and no fever. You have no neck stiffness and no neurological symptoms. If the doctor asks you about your breathing, you do feel more breathless but have no other respiratory symptoms. Your blood sugar is 24.
	'I have been forgetting to take the insulin.'
	This is usually because you are *'always on the go'* and you have missed meals.
	You have no fever, but you have been passing urine more frequently over the past week. At first you thought you needed to go but then nothing came out and now you are passing much more urine, you have seen some blood and it is painful.
	Your bowels are currently normal. Your anxiety has been controlled recently.
	You have no other systemic symptoms. You do not have a ketone meter.
Social	You live alone. You are *'not really'* in a relationship. By this you mean you caught up with an old boyfriend and had sex 10 days ago. You used condoms.
	You work in advertising and have been successful in your career which can be stressful and you have suffered with the stress of meeting deadlines and presentations to clients in the past but *'I don't have time to worry about this now.'*
	You only drink minimal alcohol socially. You do not smoke.
	Your mother was diagnosed with leukaemia 3 months ago and she is currently having chemotherapy. You have been driving to see her after work and at the weekends, sometimes staying up with her through the night if she feels unwell.
	She isn't well at present but she made you come to the GP. You are very worried about your mum and will go back to see her after the consultation with the GP.
	You need to return to be with your mother. She has no one else. However, if the doctor explains why you need to go to hospital you will go. Your mother is a patient at the same GP practice. Can the doctors help? She needs someone to check in on her and make sure she has fluid and food tonight. She is very weak and in bed.
ICE	You are worried about your health and you are frightened that your blood sugars are so high. You believe you have a water infection after having sex.
	If the doctor's mention DKA, you have heard of it. You expect the doctor will tell you what to do with your insulin today to bring your sugars down.
Examination	HR 125 bpm, sats 97%, BP 115/70, RR 19, Temperature 37.4°C, abdomen soft, generally tender, no peritonism. Urine dipstick: Leucocytes ++, nitrite +++, protein +, blood ++, ketones ++++
	BM = 30 mmol/L. Blood ketones = 3.1 mmol/L. Clinically dehydrated.

Acutely Ill People – 5

Learning Points

Hyperglycaemia

The consultation

When asking if a patient has been compliant with medication, avoid sounding confrontational by asking: 'Are you taking your medicines correctly?' Instead ask: 'Has everything been okay with taking your medication in the way the doctor prescribed?' This is a much softer question and more likely to yield a truthful answer.

This case is challenging your skills at managing an emergency, practising holistically and your negotiation skills. Without a thorough social history and consideration of the patient's concerns, it is unlikely that the key information about the patient's mother will be retrieved. It is essential to address this concern and offer a solution to allow your patient to accept potentially lifesaving treatment.

Most areas have a 'crisis team' who can put emergency care in place (either at home or within a care home) for short-term care issues. It is very important to invite the patient back to discuss ways in which she can access help with her mother (both practically and financially) or at the very least signpost her to local carers' support groups. It is likely she will need long-term support to prevent her own health suffering.

Ketones From diabetes.co.uk.[1]

'<0.6 mmol/L	A normal blood ketone value.
0.6 – 1.5 mmol/L	Indicates that more ketones are being produced than normal, test again later to see if the value has lowered.
1.6 – 3.0 mmol/L	A high level of ketones and could present a risk of ketoacidosis.
	It is advisable to contact your healthcare team for advice.
>3.0 mmol/L	A dangerous level of ketones which will require immediate medical care.'[1]

HONK In type 2 diabetes.

Hyperglycaemic Hyperosmolar Nonketotic Coma.

This may present with extreme thirst, frequency, confusion and nausea, and may progress to coma if not treated promptly.

Lactic acidosis Diabetic patients may become acidotic especially if they are taking metformin.

CHAPTER 5 OVERVIEW
Children and Young People

	Cases in this chapter	Within the RCGP curriculum: Care of Children and Young People[1] RCGP Curriculum Online March 2016[1]	Learning points in the chapter
1	Baby Reflux	'Develop and apply the primary care consultation to bring about an effective doctor–patient–family relationship …'	Reflux management, cow's milk protein allergy, supplement replacement for breastfeeding mothers and lactose intolerance
2	Viral Illness	'Ensure that parents or carers … receive information and support to enable them to: Manage minor illnesses … Access appropriate services when necessary'	NICE Guidelines. CG160. Fever in under 5s: assessment and initial management. 2013
3	Head Injury	'Manage and appropriately treat common and rare but important paediatric conditions encountered in primary care'	Head injury assessment. NICE guidelines. CG176. Head injury: assessment and early management 2014
4	Recurrent UTI	'Receive information on medicines in a clear way …' 'Prescribe and advise appropriately about the use of medicines in children and young people, being competent at: Calculating drug doses …'	NICE guidelines. CG54. Urinary tract infection in under 16s: diagnosis and management. 2007
5	Nocturnal Enuresis	'Describe your role as a GP in dealing with enuresis, sleep disturbance'	Nocturnal enuresis management

1. http://www.rcgp.org.uk/training-exams/gp-curriculum-overview/online-curriculum/caring-for-the-whole-person/3-04-children-and-young-people.aspx

CHAPTER 5 REFERENCES

Baby Reflux
1. NICE http://cks.nice.org.uk/cows-milk-protein-allergy-in-children#!diagnosissub. Revised June 2015.
2. NICE. http://cks.nice.org.uk/cows-milk-protein-allergy-in-children#!diagnosissub/-617759 Revised June 2015.

Viral Illness
1. NICE Guidelines. CG160. Fever in under 5s: assessment and initial management. May 2013.

Head Injury
1. NICE Guidelines. CG176. Head injury. Assessment and early management. Jan 2014.
2. http://patient.info/doctor/head-injury
3. http://patient.info/health/head-injury-instructions
4. Scottish Intercollegiate Guidelines Network. Early management of patients with a head injury. May 2009. http://www.sign.ac.uk/pdf/sign110.pdf. Annex 11 page 76.

Recurrent UTI
1. NICE Guidelines. CG54. Urinary tract infection in under 16s: diagnosis and management. Aug 2007.
2. NICE Guidelines. CG160. Fever in under 5s: assessment and initial management. May 2013.

Nocturnal Enuresis
1. NICE Guidelines. (CG111). Bedwetting in under 19s. October 2010.

Doctor's Notes

Patient	Jacob Harris 9 weeks M
PMH	No information
Medications	No current medications
Allergies	No information
Consultations	8 week immunisations given.
	Health Visitor 1 week ago: Weighed 4.5 kg – growing along centile.
Investigations	No recent investigations
Household	Jasmine Harris 28 years F
	Paul Harris 29 years M

Example Consultation — Baby Reflux

Open ☐ — Oh dear, can you tell me more about his feeding pattern? What have you noticed? Is there anything else you have been concerned about? How is Jacob generally?

History ☐ — What milks has Jacob had so far? Has anything you have tried helped? How are his bowels? And skin?

Sense ☐ — I can hear how worried you are. Are you okay? Tell me more about yourself. Do you have support?

Risk ☐ — Any problems in your pregnancy, during or after birth? Did he have a dirty nappy within 24 hours?

Flags ☐ — Does he always vomit? Does the milk dribble out or would it hit the wall? Does he arch his back? Is he gaining weight nicely? Is the health visitor happy? Has his stool changed from black to yellow/brown? Any red or jelly in the stool? Do you ever see any lumps in the tummy? Is he producing lots of wet nappies?

Curious ☐ — What do you mean when you say something's not right?

Impact ☐ — Are you getting any sleep? Has this affected your mood at all?

ICE ☐ — What thoughts have crossed your mind as to what could be causing this? Is there anything you are worried about that we haven't mentioned? What thoughts did you have about what I may suggest today? Is there anything you were hoping for specifically? Tell me more about what your friend has said.

Summary ☐ — To summarise, Jacob is now 9 weeks and is arching his back, being sick and screaming a lot. He also makes a gurgling sound. You are worried that something is not right, cow's milk protein allergy is something you have wondered about and you would like me to see him and hope to be prescribed Neocate which your friend uses. Is this right?

Impression ☐ — All the symptoms you have described including the crying, arching of the back and vomiting are very common and in most cases due to reflux. It is reassuring that he seems to be gaining weight nicely.

Experience ☐ — Have you come across baby reflux?

Explanation ☐ — Some degree of reflux in babies is normal, as the muscular ring at the top of the stomach still needs to develop to stop milk coming out of the stomach. However, sometimes the reflux is severe and causes the baby distress; in these cases we offer treatment. The reason that I think an allergy is less likely is because the symptoms of arching the back, particularly on lying down, are common in reflux and there are no other symptoms to suggest an allergy, e.g. his bowels and skin are good and he is gaining weight. The Neocate your friend uses is given to babies with cow's milk allergy. However, the symptoms of reflux and milk allergy are similar so we'll keep this in mind.

Options ☐ — It sounds as if Jacob is distressed by his symptoms and I'd really like to see him before starting him on medication.

Future ☐ — If necessary, as a first step we could try mixing some Gaviscon sachets into his bottles. This usually works well but may cause constipation. Can you bring Jacob for an examination at 3 pm tomorrow?

Empower ☐ — In the meantime there are other simple things you can try, which include raising the head end of his Moses basket and holding him upright for 30 minutes after each feed.

Empathy ☐ — It can be very worrying and exhausting when a baby is not settled and crying, and the thought of them being in pain is also very distressing. However, babies with reflux often respond really well to treatment and frequently by 12 weeks the muscle ring has strengthened, allowing us to stop medication.

Safety net ☐ — If you have any concerns in the meantime, or you notice new symptoms, e.g. his skin is dry or he has fewer wet nappies, a temperature or a change in the bowels or you are worried, please give the surgery a call. If we are closed, it's 111 on the telephone.

Children and Young People – 1

Patient's Story

Baby Reflux

Doctor's notes	Jacob Harris, 9 weeks. 8-week immunisations given. Health Visitor 1 week ago: Weighed 4.5 kg – growing along centile.
How to act	Anxious.
PC	*'Hi Doctor, thanks for calling me back. Jacob keeps vomiting and he screams a lot. I'm sure he is in pain.'*
History	He is bottle fed now. You had to stop breastfeeding 4 weeks ago as you were worried you weren't producing enough milk as he always seemed hungry.
	He feeds every 4 hours and 5 oz (150 ml) each time. You feel he vomits more than other babies and cries after a feed, particularly if you lie him down in the crib. He'll often arch his back when crying.
	He opens his bowels every second day and it is yellow. He has plenty of wet nappies.
	No other symptoms. You've tried Comfort milk. It didn't work.
	You've tried anti-colic bottles too without success.
	You are exhausted. You hold the baby through the night as he's more settled when he's upright on your shoulder.
	You have been slightly tearful at times but on the whole have no symptoms of depression.
	Your pregnancy and the birth were fine. There have been no other complications.
	Jacob was born at term.
	'Something is not right.' By this you mean either he has a serious problem (you don't know what this could be) or you are doing something wrong. Sometimes at night he makes a gurgling sound in his throat if you try to put him down, which worries you.
Social	You have a supportive husband. You have a sister locally who helps when she can.
	You are a financial analyst. You plan to take 9 months of maternity leave.
	All the grandparents live a distance away. You have no additional support but do have some friends who have children.
ICE	You are worried he has cow's milk allergy (this is what your friend's baby has) or lactose intolerance. Jacob is gaining weight and the health visitor does not seem concerned.
	You are most worried that you are missing something serious.
	You hope the GP will see Jacob and then prescribe the Neocate, which your friend gives to her daughter. She says it's great. You don't think the GP will give it to you because it's expensive.

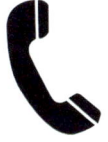

Children and Young People – 1

Learning Points — Baby Reflux

Reflux management

Change feeding regime or milk and check the baby is not overfeeding.

The recommended fluid intake for a baby over 1 week of age is 150 ml/kg/day. (1 oz = 30 ml.)

Stay Down or Comfort milk thickens in the stomach. Further options include Gaviscon sachets, omeprazole or ranitidine (off licence). Gaviscon can be mixed with feeds in bottle-fed babies or mixed with water and given immediately before feeds in breastfed infants.

Cow's milk protein allergy (CMPA)

Non IgE CMPA symptoms	Onset >2 hours. Symptoms include: Eczema, reflux, constipation and poor weight gain and others.[1]
IgE CMPA symptoms	Onset <2 hours.[2] Symptoms include: Swelling or breathing difficulties, rash, vomiting, diarrhoea and others.[1]
When to refer	If suspect IgE or severe reaction non-IgE CMPA. 'Consider referral to secondary or specialist care if there is: Faltering growth + ≥1 gastrointestinal symptom (see Table 1[2]) ≥1 acute systemic reactions. ≥1 severe delayed reactions. Significant atopic eczema and cross-reactive food allergies suspected. Persisting parental suspicion of food allergy ... Clinical suspicion of multiple food allergies.'[1] If uncertainty refer for IgE testing (RAST) or skin testing.
GP Management	If mild/moderate symptoms of non-IgE CMPA ... Seek a dietician's advice and eliminate CMP for 2–6 weeks and replace with extensively hydrolysed formulas, then reintroduce. ... Then eliminate again. If symptoms follow this pattern the diagnosis has been confirmed.[1] If there is no improvement seek advice[2] and consider an amino acid formula.
Child on solid foods	Ask a dietician for advice regarding sufficient calcium supplementation.
Breastfeeding mothers	Exclude all cow's milk from diet and give 1 g calcium and 10 mcg vitamin D daily.[1]
Extensively hydrolysed formula	Nutramigen LIPIL 1 up to 6/12 and Nutramigen LIPIL 2 from >6/12.
Soya	Specialist's advice only and for children >6 months (phytoestrogens).
Amino acid formula	Nutramigen AA / Neocate.
Reintroducing CMP – specialists	If reactions suggested IgE, severe non-IgE or even mild non-IgE symptoms; however, eczema is present at the time of reintroduction – follow specialist advice.
Reintroducing CMP – GPs	Reintroduce CMP at >9/12 of age and after at least 6/12 without symptoms. If symptoms return re-evaluate every 6 to 12 months.[2]

> See the **Link Hub at CompleteCSA.co.uk** for a link to the helpful **Milk Ladder**.

Lactose intolerance	Not an allergy. The lack of lactase prevents lactose breakdown. Can follow gastroenteritis. Investigations: Breath hydrogen test or stool-reducing substances. Lactose-free milk can be purchased OTC (e.g. SMA LF).

Children and Young People – 1

Doctor's Notes

Patient	Jayden Hall	13 months	M
PMH	No information		
Medications	No current medications		
Allergies	No information		
Consultations	Health Visitor drop-in session last month, growing well, no concerns		
Investigations	No recent investigations		
Household	Donna Hall	29 years	F
	Liam Hall	6 years	M
	Carly Hall	4 years	F

Example Consultation

Viral Illness

Open ☐ — Good morning, can I check who I am speaking to? Please could you confirm Jayden's date of birth and address? Great. How can I help? What is Jayden doing at the moment?

History ☐ — How long has Jayden been poorly? How high has his temperature been? Has it come down with paracetamol or ibuprofen? Has he been coughing? Does he have a runny nose? Any diarrhoea or vomiting? Does he seem in pain or distressed?

Risk ☐ — Has anyone he spends time with been poorly? Is he up to date with his vaccinations?

Flags ☐ — Is he eating and drinking okay? Has he been having wet nappies? Have you noticed a rash? Does he seem to be breathing more quickly than usual?

Sense ☐ — You seem to have a lot on your plate at the moment; is that right?

ICE ☐ — Have you had any thoughts about what may be wrong with Jayden and what might need to be done? How worried are you about Jayden at this moment?

Impression ☐ — From listening to the description of Jayden's symptoms, it sounds as if he has a viral infection but we should have a look at him, especially his ears, and listen to his chest.

Explanation ☐ — Usually when a child has a runny nose, cough and high temperature it is due to a viral infection, particularly if other people in the family have had similar symptoms. In these situations, antibiotics don't help as they won't treat a viral infection and can actually make children more poorly by causing side effects like diarrhoea.

Empathy ☐ — It must be really difficult having three poorly children at once.

Options ☐ — But it would be really helpful if you could bring Jayden down to the surgery so I can examine him here and check that he is okay. We try to reserve home visits for housebound patients so we have time to see more patients, like Jayden, at the surgery. I would be happy to see him at whatever time you are able to get down, this morning or this afternoon.

Empower ☐ — Could you ask a friend or relative to keep an eye on Liam and Carly while you bring Jayden to the surgery? Or get someone to come with you all to help? Thank you.

Future ☐ — I will see you both in a little while.

Safety net ☐ — Please give me a call if Jayden gets any worse in the meantime or, for example, if he becomes floppy, his breathing changes or develops new symptoms like a rash.

Children and Young People – 2

Patient's Story

Viral Illness

Doctor's notes	Jayden Hall, 13 months. PMH: No information
How to act	Harassed.
	Push the doctor for a home visit. Be delighted if they agree to visit.
	If the doctor is insistent that you come to the surgery and suggests options, reluctantly agree to come down. You could call your mum and ask her to babysit.
PC	*'Morning Doctor, I was wondering if you could visit. Jayden has a high temperature and is not well.'*
History	Jayden has had a high temperature on and off for 24 hours. You have an ear thermometer which has shown temperatures up to 38.6°C. You have given Jayden paracetamol which has brought his temperature down. Jayden was coughing all night and kept you awake. You are tired and stressed this morning as Jayden's two older siblings (Liam 6 years and Carly 4 years) are off school with colds, which they have had for a few days. Thankfully they seem to be on the mend. Jayden has a runny nose and is pulling at his ears. His appetite has reduced but he is still drinking well. He has had plenty of wet nappies. He has not been sick and doesn't have diarrhoea. Jayden is currently playing with his sister in the lounge. You would like a home visit as you feel Jayden needs looking at, but you feel it will be too much to bring all three children down to the surgery. You live within walking distance of the surgery.
	Jayden is up to date with his vaccinations and there were no concerns during the pregnancy or neonatal period. He is growing and developing normally.
Social	You are a single mum. You have a part-time cleaning job. This is fairly flexible and you work when your mother can babysit Jayden whilst the others are at school. Your mother lives nearby and you have some supportive friends. Jayden's dad sees him at the weekends.
ICE	You feel Jayden probably needs antibiotics for a chest infection but aren't overly concerned about him. You expect the doctor to visit to examine his chest and give you a prescription for antibiotics.

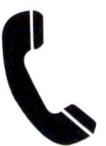

Children and Young People – 2

Learning Points

Viral Illness

Low Risk	• Normal skin tone, lips and tongue • Normal response to social cues • Smiling • Wakens quickly or remains awake • Not crying or strong normal cry • Moist mucous membranes • No Medium or High risk symptoms or signs

Medium Risk	• Pale skin tone reported by parent/carer
	• Abnormal response to social cues or not smiling
	• Prolonged stimulation required to awaken
	• Decreased activity
	• Nasal Flaring
	• Tachypnoea:
	  • RR > 50 breaths per minute, age 6–12 months
	  • RR > 40 breaths per minute, age >12 months
	• O_2 saturation ≤ 95% in air
	• Chest auscultation finds crackles
	• Tachycardia:
	  • >160 BPM, age <12 months
	  • >150 BPM, age 12–24 months
	  • >140 BPM, age 2–5 years
	• Capillary refill time ≥3 seconds
	• Dry mucous membranes
	• Poor feeding in infants or reduced urine output
	• Temperature ≥ 39°C and age between 3 and 6 months
	• Fever for > 5 days or more or rigors any time
	• Swelling in a limb or joint
	• Not weight bearing or avoidance of using a limb

High Risk	• Pale/mottled/ashen/blue skin tone, lips or tongue • Appears unwell to healthcare professional • No response to social cues • Unable to remain awake or does not wake when roused • Weak, high-pitched or continual cry • Grunting breaths • Tachypnoea: • RR >60 breaths per minute • Moderate or severe chest recession • Reduced skin turgor • Temperature ≥38°C; age <3 months • Non-blanching rash • Bulging fontanelle • Neck stiffness • Focal neurological signs • Focal seizures • Status epilepticus

Adapted from 'The Traffic Light System for Identifying Risk of Serious Illness.'
NICE guidelines. CG160. Fever in under 5s: assessment and initial management. May 2013.[1]

Children and Young People – 2

Doctor's Notes

Patient	Marcus Andrews	14 years	M
PMH	No information		
Medications	No current medications		
Allergies	No information		
Consultations	No recent consultations		
Investigations	No recent investigations		
Household	Tabitha Andrews	40 years	F
	Harry Andrews	42 years	M
	Katie Andrews	16 years	F

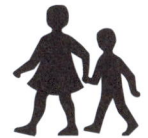

Example Consultation — Head Injury

Open ☐ — Please tell me more about what happened, Marcus? Mum, what did you see?

History ☐ — Where did you get hit? Does it still hurt? How do you feel now?

Risk ☐ — Do you know what you hit your head against?

Flags ☐ — Can you remember what happened in the moments before the tackle? Can you remember what happened straight after you were tackled? Do you think you lost consciousness, which means pass out? Have you been sick? Do you have a headache? Have you noticed a change in your vision? Are your arms and legs feeling and working okay? Can I just check that Marcus is usually fit and well? Is he on any medication? Has he had surgery or an injury to his head before? Did anything happen to Marcus that may have been a fit or seizure? Such as a collapse with shaking of his limbs?

Sense ☐ — Mum, I sense you are more concerned about the injury than Marcus is.

ICE ☐ — Is there anything specific you are worrying about? Marcus, is there anything you are worried about? Was there anything in particular you were hoping I would say or do? How do you feel about the match in a few days, Mum?

Summary ☐ — So you were running with the ball when you were tackled and hit the right side of your head against another player's knee. You remember what happened immediately before and after the tackle and you didn't lose consciousness. The impact hurt and made you feel dizzy. You felt sick once when you got back into the changing room but have been feeling okay since. You don't have any problems with your eyesight, arms or legs. Mum, you're concerned he may need a scan as he has been feeling sick and hoped I could arrange this. Marcus, you are concerned that you might not be able to play in your club match on Sunday, which would be very disappointing for you. Mum, after this head injury, you are concerned about the next match. Is there anything that I have missed?

Examination ☐ — Is it okay if I have a good look at your head? And I'd like to check your nose, ears, eyes and ask you to copy some movements to check the nerves in your head, arms and legs. Would that be okay? When you walked in, I saw you were walking normally: do you agree, Mum?

Impression ☐ — That is all reassuring. You have had a knock to the head but thankfully I don't think it is serious enough to need a head scan or for you to go to A&E.

Explanation ☐ — As you weren't knocked out, can remember what happened and haven't been sick, it is unlikely that there is any serious brain injury. There is no sign of a skull fracture.

Empathy ☐ — It must have been scary seeing Marcus get injured and it's only natural to want to make sure he is properly checked over. Marcus, I understand that the match is really important to you.

Empower ☐ — It's most likely that you'll recover completely by yourself over the next few days. If you have pain from your bump or a minor headache, you could try paracetamol or ibuprofen.

Future ☐ — With regards to your match, after a minor head injury it is advised that you don't return to sport for 7 days. I'm sorry if that means you'll miss your match.

Safety net ☐ — It's important to be vigilant for certain symptoms after a head injury. I'm going to give you a leaflet with advice about what to look out for. The sheet goes into detail but, briefly, things to look out for are drowsiness when Marcus would normally be wide awake, worsening headache, vomiting, seizures, bruising around the eyes or ears, bleeding from his ears, clear liquid from his nose or confusion. Please get in touch straight away if you have any concerns. When we are closed you can call 111 for advice or if you're really worried, go to A&E.

Children and Young People – 3

Patient's Story

Head Injury

Doctor's notes Marcus Andrews, 14 years. PMH: No information

How to act Attends with mum. Mum concerned and Marcus relaxed.

PC *'Hi Doctor, I was wondering if you could check Marcus over. He's taken a knock to his head in his school's rugby match.'*

History

Marcus: You are a keen rugby player, playing for both school and a local club. This morning during an inter-school rugby game, you hit your head against another player's knee during a tackle. You hit the right side of your head. It hurt a lot. You remember catching the ball and running forward with it. You remember the impact and remember seeing your mum run over – it was embarrassing! There was no bleeding. You felt a bit dizzy. Afterwards you felt sick but didn't vomit. You had a headache but this has gone now.

Mum: You had gone to watch the game so you saw what happened. As far as you are aware there was no loss of consciousness. Marcus looked a little dazed but recognised you immediately afterwards. You have checked for a cut and can't see one but there is a bit of a bump. The coach put an ice pack on Marcus's head. Marcus felt sick when he got back to the changing room so the coach advised you to go to your GP and hence the emergency appointment. No seizure symptoms. No PMH or DH.

ICE

Marcus: You want to know if you can play in your club's big cup match on Sunday – in 5 days' time. You are worried that you won't be allowed and you'll be really upset if you can't play. You think you are fine and expect to be sent home.

Mum: You are worried as he has been feeling sick. You think he might need a scan but didn't want to go to A&E without checking with your GP. You thought you might be seen quicker with a GP note. You don't want him to play in the cup match on Sunday and hope the GP will tell Marcus that he can't. The reason for this is that all the other boys are bigger than Marcus and you don't want Marcus to have another injury, especially when he will have bruising around his brain.

Social Lives with mum, dad and sister who is 16.

O/E Small 1 cm bruise but no swelling over right parietal region. No laceration. Nose and ears normal. No other bruising. Normal cranial and peripheral nerve examinations. GCS 15. Normal sensation and power in the arms and legs. Normal gait and coordination.

Children and Young People – 3

Learning Points

Head Injury

History should be focused on ruling in or out the following factors:

Criteria for transfer to hospital from community services (adults and children) NICE 2014:[1,2]

- Glasgow Coma Scale <15 at time of assessment.
- Any loss of consciousness as a result of the injury.
- Any focal neurological deficit since the injury.
- Any suspicion of a skull fracture or penetrating head injury.
- Amnesia for events before or after the injury.
- Persistent headache since the injury.
- Any vomiting episodes since the injury (clinical judgement should be used regarding the cause of vomiting in those aged 12 years or younger and the need for referral).
- Any seizure since the injury.
- Any previous brain surgery.
- A high-energy head injury. 'For example, pedestrian struck by motor vehicle, occupant ejected from motor vehicle, fall from a height of greater than 1 metre or more than 5 stairs, diving accident, high-speed motor vehicle collision, rollover motor accident, accident involving motorised recreational vehicles, bicycle collision, or any other potentially high-energy mechanism.'[1]
- Any history of bleeding or clotting disorders.
- Current anticoagulant therapy.
- Current drug or alcohol intoxication.
- Any safeguarding concerns (child with suspicious injury or vulnerable adult).
- Continuing concern by the professional about the diagnosis.

Consider referral if none of the above apply but there is:

- Irritability or altered behaviour, particularly in children under 5 years.
- Visible trauma to the head concerning the professional.
- No one to observe the injured person at home.
- Continuing concern by the injured person or their family/carer about the diagnosis.

Signs of basal skull fracture

Look for blood at the tympanic membrane (haemotympanum), bruising around the eyes or behind the ears and CSF in the ears or nose.

Patient.co.uk has a useful head injury instructions sheet. Main advice as per Example Consultation. Other points: advise patient not to be alone for 24 hours, keep in reach of phone and medical services. It is okay for parents to let children go to sleep; children are often tired after a head injury. Concerning drowsiness is when the person is unrousable. If a parent is very concerned about sleep, suggest waking the child after a couple of hours then let them go back to sleep.[3]

SIGN provides specific advice regarding return to sport. For minor head injuries they suggest a gradual return to sport but no sport (especially contact sport) for 7 days. For more serious injuries, i.e. those which caused amnesia or loss of consciousness, they recommend not returning to sports for 3 weeks.[4]

Doctor's Notes

Patient	Kalpesh Khan	6 years	M
PMH	\multicolumn{3}{l}{Urinary tract infection 6 weeks ago – *E. coli*, fully sensitive}	

Patient Kalpesh Khan 6 years M

PMH Urinary tract infection 6 weeks ago – *E. coli*, fully sensitive

Urinary tract infection 6 months ago – *E. coli*, fully sensitive

Medications No current medication

Past medication – 2 courses of trimethoprim

Allergies No information

Consultations Last appointment 2 days ago:

Attended with mum. Temperature 38.5°C, lower abdominal pain, dysuria, frequency and urgency.

Abdominal examination – suprapubic tenderness, abdomen soft, no masses.

Urine dip: protein +, blood +, leucocytes ++, nitrites ++.

MSU sent. Trimethoprim prescription given.

Investigations MSU result from 2 days ago – *E. coli*, resistant to amoxicillin and trimethoprim, sensitive to nitrofurantoin and cefalosporin

Household

Asaf Khan	43 years	M
Yasmin Khan	41 years	F
Ayub Khan	7 years	M
Raja Khan	3 years	M
Sabeen Khan	2 years	F

Example Consultation　　　　　　　　　　　　　Recurrent UTI

Open — I'm sorry to hear that Kalpesh is no better. Could you tell me what has been happening over the last couple of days? How is he now? What is he doing at present?

History — I see he has had two other urine infections in the past 6 months. In between his urine infections was he well? Has he had any other medical problems? Does he have any allergies you are aware of? Is there any family history of kidney problems?

Flags — Do you know if his urine stream is normal or reduced? What is his temperature at present? Is he complaining of tummy pain? Have you seen any blood? Has he vomited? Is he drinking well? When did he last pass urine? Does his urine smell? Is he complaining of back pain? Is he breathing normally? And is he drowsy or concentrating on the television at present?

Risk — Has he been growing and developing well? Were there any problems during your pregnancy? Has he had any tests at the hospital?

ICE — What is going through your mind about this? Have you had any thoughts about what you would like to happen next? Is anything particular worrying you?

Curious — What is your experience of septicaemia? I'm sorry to hear that.

Empathy — It must be worrying that Kalpesh has had these infections, especially after your experience with your father.

Impression — It seems that Kalpesh has another urine infection, but unfortunately this one isn't sensitive to the trimethoprim antibiotic, which explains why he hasn't got any better yet. The good news is that the laboratory has told us that another antibiotic should work.

Experience — Has another doctor talked to you about what tests we recommend with recurrent urine infections? Please tell me about what you have read.

Explanation — You are correct. Recurrent water infections in children aren't that common, and usually need investigation. However, they do usually respond to antibiotic medicines.

Options — Today I could either see Kalpesh in the surgery, if you feel he needs review, or send you a prescription for nitrofurantoin antibiotic which should kill the bacteria in his urine. Which would you prefer?

Future — As Kalpesh has now had three confirmed urinary infections, I would like to refer him to see a specialist. Would that be okay? It is likely that they will want to do some investigations such as an ultrasound scan to look at his kidneys and bladder. They may want to do some special tests which check that his bladder empties properly and that urine doesn't flow back up into the tubes towards the kidneys, as this is one cause of recurrent urine infection in children.

Safety net — I will do the prescription for nitrofurantoin. If Kalpesh gets any worse, please give us a ring straight away. I would expect him to start showing an improvement within 48 hours, so if he is no better please let me know. Should you become worried in the evening, night or weekend you can phone 111 for advice. If you think he is getting dry, perhaps due to vomiting, if he passes significantly less urine or you feel he is more unwell, don't hesitate to seek advice from a doctor straight away. I will get on with the referral to the specialist; you should receive an appointment letter within the next couple of weeks but please let the practice secretary know if this does not happen. Are you happy with the plan? To ensure I have been clear, can you tell me when you would ask for the help of a doctor? Thank you.

Children and Young People – 4

Patient's Story

Recurrent UTI

Doctor's notes	Kalpesh Khan, 6 years. PMH: 2 × UTIs – *E. coli*, fully sensitive in past 6 months and further UTI confirmed on MSU resistant to trimethoprim given.
How to act	Concerned.
PC	*'Hi Doctor, thanks for calling. I'm a bit worried about Kalpesh. He isn't responding to the antibiotics this time.'*
History	You attended the surgery 2 days ago when Kalpesh had symptoms of a urinary tract infection. You were given antibiotics by the doctor and told to phone back if he isn't improving. Unfortunately, this time he hasn't improved with trimethoprim. This is his third urinary tract infection in the last 6 months. Kalpesh was born at term following a normal pregnancy. He has been developing normally and is getting on well at school. He is otherwise fit and well (including since his last infection). Currently Kalpesh is lying on the sofa watching TV. He is still having a fever intermittently, has lower tummy pain and dysuria. His fever is 37.8°C at present after paracetamol and you plan to give him some ibuprofen. He is eating and drinking okay and passing urine every 2–3 hours. You have seen no blood and he has not complained of back pain. You have kept him off school for the last couple of days. There is no family history. He has no allergies.
ICE	You are worried that the antibiotics aren't working. You don't want Kalpesh to become really unwell, you are aware that infections can be serious, your father died of sepsis.
	'I just don't want this to become a septicaemia.'
	You have done some research and wonder if Kalpesh needs further tests. He has only had urine samples sent to date.
	'I've read about tests he may need.' Reading included an ultrasound scan and a kidney scan but this is all you understand.
	You would like to know what happens next. You are happy to accept antibiotics over the phone or an appointment at the surgery to check Kalpesh over. If given the option, and the doctor has clearly explained the problem and future plan, accept antibiotics over the phone. You would like Kalpesh to be referred.
Social	You are a married full-time mum and have three other children. They are all well. Kalpesh's father is a mechanic during the day and works as a taxi driver in the evenings so works long hours.

Children and Young People – 4

Learning Points

Recurrent UTI

NICE guidelines [CG54]. Urinary tract infection in under 16s: diagnosis and management. 2007

Most common signs and symptoms:
- Infants (0–3 months): Fever, vomiting, lethargy, irritability
  - Other: failure to thrive, poor feeding, jaundice, abdominal pain, haematuria and offensive urine.
- 3 months+ (preverbal): Fever
  - Other: abdominal pain, loin tenderness, vomiting, poor feeding, lethargy, irritability, haematuria, offensive urine, failure to thrive.
- 3 months+ (verbal): Frequency, dysuria
  - Dysfunctional voiding, changes in continence, abdominal pain, loin tenderness, fever, malaise, vomiting, haematuria, offensive urine, cloudy urine.

Child's age	Testing – clean catch ideally	Management – refer to full guidance[1] Also refer to NICE Guideline 'Feverish illness in children'[2]
<3 months	Send urine for culture	Admit to paediatrics
3 months – 3 years	Urgent microscopy and culture is the preferred method of diagnosis in this age group.	Child with specific UTI features: Start antibiotics Child with non-specific features: Urgent urine MC&S, if unavailable dipstick urine – nitrites positive then start antibiotics If well child, await MSU result
>3 years	Urine dip should be considered as it is as diagnostically useful as MSU in this age group.	+ve nitrite and leucocytes = treat +ve nitrite, -ve leucocytes = treat and send for culture -ve nitrite, +ve leucocytes = await MCS unless clinically UTI -ve nitrite and leucocytes = alternative diagnosis

Send an MSU if: Suspected upper UTI (Fever >38°C or loin pain), child <3 years, recurrent UTI, single positive for leucocytes or nitrites, no improvement after 48 hours (if sample not sent already)[1] child with intermediate to high risk serious illness,[2] or 'when clinical symptoms and dipstick do not correlate.'[1]

For antibiotic choice see your local antibiotic guidance and BNF.

Which investigations and should I refer?[1] depends on the type of UTI and the child's age.

Typical UTI (UTI): E. Coli which responds to treatment within 48 hours, no other features of AUTI or RUTI

Atypical UTI (AUTI): seriously ill[2], poor urine flow, abdominal or bladder mass, raised creatinine, non E. Coli species, not responding to treatment within 48 hours or septicaemia. Admission often required.

Recurrent UTI (RUTI): ≥ 2 UTIs (one must be upper) or ≥ 3 lower UTIs.

0–6 months: UTI: all require an USS within 6 weeks and if abnormal consider an MCUG
                     AUTI or RUTI: require urgent (during acute infection) USS*, DMSA + MCUG. Suggest refer**.

6 months–3 years: UTI: do not require investigation.
                     AUTI or RUTI: require USS (urgent for AUTI *, <6wk for RUTI) + DMSA ± MCUG. Suggest refer**.

Over 3 years: UTI: do not require investigation.
                     AUTI: urgent USS* only.
                     RUTI: USS within 6 weeks and DMSA 4–6 months after the infection. Suggest refer**.

*However in a non E. coli UTI but no other features of AUTI – USS within 6 weeks

**Referral to paediatrics/urology is likely to be required to access further investigations and interpretation; however, direct access to urgent USS may be available in your local area.

Children and Young People – 4

Doctor's Notes

Patient	Andrew Carr	7 years	M
PMH	No information		
Medications	No current medications		
Allergies	No information		
Consultations	No recent consultations		
Investigations	No recent investigations		
Household	Bernadette Carr	39 years	F
	Sarah Carr	9 years	F
	Kimberley Carr	4 years	F

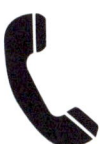

Example Consultation — Nocturnal Enuresis

Open ☐ — Can you tell me more about Andrew's bedwetting? Tell me more about Andrew. How's his health? Is there a pattern at all? Does he wet during the day?

Impact ☐ — How does he feel about it? How does this affect you?

History ☐ — Has he ever had dry nights? Is there a large amount of urine? Does it happen more than once a night? Does he wake afterwards? Does it happen at the same time? Have you tried anything already?

Risk ☐ — What are Andrew's bowel movements like? Does he have any accidents? Will he use the school toilets? Can you describe his fluid consumption through the day please?

Flags ☐ — Does he complain of pain when passing urine? Does he need to race to the toilet or has he been going more frequently? Has he been excessively thirsty or been passing more urine than usual? Has he lost any weight? Is he otherwise growing well? Have you ever had concerns about his development? Has school raised any concerns? Who's at home? Any problems at home? And at school? Does he drink tea or cola?

Sense ☐ — This has been going on a while; is there something that prompted you to phone today?

ICE ☐ — Have you had any thoughts about what could be causing it? Are you worried about anything in particular? Were you hoping that I would do anything specific today?

Summary ☐ — So, Andrew is dry during the day but has never been dry at night. He wets the bed 2–3 times a week. He is well and has no problems passing urine. He has some difficulties opening his bowels. He is developing well. Life has been stressful at home as Sarah's condition demands a lot of your time and Andrew was initially upset by the divorce but seems happy now. Both you and Andrew are concerned about the sleepover; he would love to go but fears wetting the bed. You were hoping that I would refer Andrew for further investigations, in particular to rule out diabetes.

Impression ☐ — Andrew has what we call 'primary nocturnal enuresis' as he has never been dry at night. Thankfully it doesn't sound like there are any major physical problems causing it. However, he may be constipated, which often makes the condition worse. At this stage there is plenty we can do without Andrew needing to go through hospital doors.

Explanation ☐ — Bedwetting at Andrew's age is still fairly common. Most cases resolve in time. First, you could try a star chart reward system. Children often like to help parents make this chart and it provides a great opportunity to discuss why it is important. Often children who wet the bed actually don't drink enough. Concentrated urine irritates the bladder, making it empty sooner. A child Andrew's age should drink around 1400 ml a day.[1]

Empower ☐ — Could you and Andrew complete a chart each day to show how much he has drunk? If he reaches 1400 ml you could reward him on the star chart. Recording when he passes urine and opens his bowels would also be helpful. Stars can also be given for helping change sheets or going to the toilet once he is wet as well as for dry nights. How does this sound? There is a very helpful website called ERIC which has information for parents, example charts, diaries and leaflets.

Options ☐ — You specifically wanted to check that Andrew does not have diabetes. We can do a blood test for this but, from what you have told me, diabetes seems unlikely. He is well, gaining weight and has no tummy pain. He has also had this problem for years. If a urine dipstick test does not show glucose, diabetes is very unlikely. What are your thoughts? It would be helpful if I could meet Andrew to see how he feels and examine him. He may need treatment for constipation, which may help with waterworks problems too. Another option is an alarm which goes off when the child passes urine. The school nurses are a good source of advice too. Medication can be used for occasions like sleepovers. Can we discuss this once I've seen Andrew?

Future ☐ — I have a slot tomorrow after school. How does that sound? Could you bring a urine sample in to test for infection and diabetes? I look forward to seeing you tomorrow.

Safety net ☐ — Please give me a call if Andrew appears unwell or you are concerned in the meantime.

Children and Young People – 5

Patient's Story

Nocturnal Enuresis

Doctor's notes	Andrew Carr, 7 years. PMH: No information.
How to act	Concerned.
PC	*'Hi Doctor, thanks for phoning back. I'm worried about Andrew; he is still wetting the bed.'*
History	Andrew has never been dry at night. He wets the bed 2–3 times a week. He has been dry during the day since he was 3 years old. He has been invited to a friend's sleepover party and Andrew is desperate to go but is very worried he will wet the bed. He is a shy boy and lacks confidence in social situations; you also worry an accident in front of friends would be disastrous for him. He is otherwise well. He drinks mostly water and squash. You have been stopping him drinking in the evening to try to prevent bedwetting. Overall, you think he probably has about 1 L to drink a day, perhaps a little less. You have two other children. Your eldest child, Sarah, has cerebral palsy so life is a bit hectic. You could really do without having to wash Andrew's sheets all the time. Andrew gets embarrassed by his bedwetting. He has at times hidden his wet pyjamas in the wardrobe. You have also found a stash of soiled underpants too. It seems Andrew hasn't been opening his bowels properly either. Andrew is a fussy eater and you struggle to get him to eat fruit and vegetables. He has not lost weight, is not excessively thirsty and doesn't complain of pain when passing urine.
ICE	You are worried there could be something seriously wrong. You've read that bedwetting can be a sign of diabetes. Your dad has diabetes so you thought this could be the cause. You would like Andrew to be referred to a paediatrician for investigations.
Social	You work part-time in a restaurant; it is difficult to work longer hours due to Sarah's condition. Unfortunately, your marriage to Andrew's father broke down a couple of years ago. Andrew sees his dad every other weekend. He also wets the bed there. He loves to see his dad. He is never tearful but is a quiet child. You think his mood is okay; he was upset during the divorce but he seems happy enough at school. He enjoys football and playing computer games with his sisters.

Children and Young People – 5

Learning Points

Nocturnal Enuresis

Bedwetting is considered normal in children under 5 years; however, do not exclude children from managing this condition based on age alone.[1]

It is prevalent in 1 in 7 five year olds and 1 in 20 ten year olds.

Primary nocturnal enuresis — Child has never been dry at night consistently.
Secondary nocturnal enuresis — Enuresis returns after >6 months of dry nights.

Risk factors:[1]

Primary	Secondary
Developmental delay	Stress/emotional upset
Neurological conditions, e.g. spina bifida, cerebral palsy	Urinary tract infection
Family history	Constipation
	Diabetes mellitus

Factors in history:[1]

- Large volume of urine in first few hours of night – typical bedwetting.
- Variable volume, more than once per night – possible overactive bladder (OAB).
- Bedwetting every night – more severe and less likely to resolve spontaneously.
- Daytime frequency, urgency, wetting, pain, poor stream (may suggest OAB/urological disease).
- Constipation – a common comorbidity that requires treatment. Soiling suggests impaction.
- Inadequate fluid intake – may mask underlying condition such as overactive bladder and prevents the bladder development to store urine.
- Behavioural, emotional and family problems may be a cause or consequence of wetting.

Practical tips:[1]

- Ensure there is access to a toilet and encourage regular use of the toilet including before bed.
- Ensure adequate hydration. See NICE guidance for targets per age range. Avoid caffeine.
- Put waterproof mattress and duvet covers on bed to help with cleaning.
- Waking or 'lifting' children at night to pass urine is not likely to promote long-term dryness.
- Reward systems (star chart) should be for achievable goals and not just dry nights. E.g. adequate hydration and going to the toilet before bedtime. Do not penalise or remove gained rewards.
- Ensure parents are aware it is not the child's fault.
- Alarms should be tried if the above fails. Alarms work best in conjunction with the reward system and should be assessed after 4 weeks; continue until minimum of 2 weeks of dry nights. Inform families that the alarms have a high success rate but can disrupt sleep and may need a parent to help wake the child; this requires commitment! The alarms help the child recognise the need to pass urine, then either hold on or get up to pass urine. Early signs of success may include smaller wet patches, waking to the alarm, the alarm going off later or fewer times.
- Desmopressin: offer to children >7 years and consider in ages 5–7 years for children who have failed with an alarm, an alarm was not appropriate or if rapid-onset or short-term relief of symptoms is required.
- Involve the school nurse or if not available seek advice from the enuresis nurse specialists.

Recurrence:

Rule out physical cause.
Consider using alarms again. Consider a combination of desmopressin and the alarm.[1]

ERIC
See the **Link Hub at CompleteCSA.co.uk** for a useful link to helpful information from The Children's Continence Charity.

CHAPTER 6 OVERVIEW

Older Adults

	Cases in this chapter	Within the RCGP curriculum: Care of Older Adults RCGP Curriculum Online March 2016[1]	Learning points in the chapter include:
1	Acute Kidney Injury	'Understand the management of the conditions and problems commonly associated with old age'	NICE Guidelines. CG169. Acute Kidney injury: Prevention, detection and management. August 2013
2	Chronic Kidney Disease	'Understand the special factors associated with drug treatment, e.g. the physiology of absorption, metabolism and excretion of drugs, the hazards posed by multiple prescribing, non-compliance and iatrogenic disease'	NICE Guidelines. CG182. Chronic kidney disease in adults: assessment and management. July 2014
3	Care Home	'Know the different forms of day-care and residential accommodation available and be able to advise patients about them'	Assessing capacity Funding a care home
4	Possible Dementia	'Understand the special features of psychiatric diseases in old age, including dementia'	The process of diagnosing dementia Resources for dementia
5	Distressed NOK	'Recognise your attitudes to the use of intensive or invasive tests and treatments and the use of limited healthcare resources in the care of the elderly'	Involving carers/relatives in care planning and end-of-life decisions

1. http://www.rcgp.org.uk/training-exams/gp-curriculum-overview/online-curriculum/caring-for-the-whole-person/3-05-older-adults.aspx

CHAPTER 6 REFERENCES

Acute Kidney Injury
1. NICE Guidelines. CG169. Acute Kidney injury: Prevention, detection and management. Aug 2013.
2. http://www.scottishpatientsafetyprogramme.scot.nhs.uk/programmes/primary-care/medicine-sick-day-rules-card. Polypharmacy Guidance. NHS. Scotland. Mar 2015.

Chronic Kidney Disease
1. NICE Guidelines. CG182. Chronic kidney disease in adults: assessment and management. Jul 2014.
2. NICE Guidelines. CG181. Cardiovascular disease: risk assessment and reduction, including lipid modification. Jul 2014.

Care Home
1. http://www.bma.org.uk/support-at-work/ethics/mental-capacity/mental-capacity-tool-kit
2. http://www.carehome.co.uk/fees/feeschart.cfm

Possible Dementia
1. NICE Guidelines. Dementia overview. Revised Dec 2015. http://pathways.nice.org.uk/pathways/dementia

Doctor's Notes

Patient Alexander Dickens 78 years M
PMH Chronic kidney disease, osteoarthritis and heart failure
Medications Paracetamol
Furosemide 20 mg
Spironolactone 50 mg
Indapamide 2.5 mg
Ramipril 5 mg
Bisoprolol 5 mg
Allergies No information
Consultations Last week seen by GP. Pitting oedema to knees. Sats 95%. Crepitations at lung bases. JVP 3 cm. Agreed to increase furosemide to 2 daily. BP 162/72. Ramipril increased from 2.5 mg to 5 mg.
Investigations Blood test 1 week ago: eGFR 51 ml/min/1.73 m^2, Creatinine 92 µmol/L,
Potassium 4.8 mmol/L and Sodium 143 mmol/L
Household Dorothy Dickens 74 years F

Message from biochemistry

eGFR 32 ml/min/1.73 m^2, Creatinine 196 µmol/L, Potassium 5.5 mmol/L and Sodium 142 mmol/L.

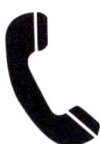

Example Consultation — Acute Kidney Injury

Open — Mr Dickens, I'm calling about your blood tests which show that your kidneys are struggling more than usual. I wanted to talk to you about what may be causing this so we can put them right again.

History — Tell me the story about what led the doctor to see you last week. What medication changes did you both make? How have you been since the doctor last saw you? Do you feel more tired at all? Are you passing urine normally? Who is at home with you? Is Mrs Dickens well?

Risk — It is likely that the cause is a combination of things: medicines; age, unfortunately. Do you have any problems with the flow of your urine or getting up at night? Good.

Flags — Any fevers, any pain passing urine or going more frequently? Any loose stools or vomiting recently? You started taking furosemide last week. What dose are you taking each day? And can I check which other medicines you take?

Curious — You mentioned your knee plays up. Do you ever take anything for that?

Impact — How active are you generally?

ICE — Is there anything that keeps worrying you? Anything else you have wondered? Is there anything else that you would like or would find helpful?

Summary — To summarise, you have been very worried that your breathing is getting worse, as it did 6 months ago, when you needed to go into hospital. You have been well on 80 mg furosemide previously. Your main concern now is balancing the kidneys with the breathing.

Impression — We call this acute kidney injury.

Experience — Have you had problems with your kidney blood tests before?

Explanation — I think what has caused it is a combination of factors that all impact on the kidney. The recent diarrhoea made the kidneys more dehydrated and increasing the ramipril and furosemide at the same time was just too much for the kidneys. The ibuprofen is also a contributor unfortunately.

Sense — You sound very disappointed.

Empathy — I appreciate it must be very disheartening going from one problem to another.

Options — Have you taken your medicines this morning? I would suggest you hold off taking them until I've seen you. Can you come in to see me at the end of morning surgery? I would like to examine you. We can recheck the blood tests when you come. When you arrive, can you please do a urine sample. We can look at your medicines, take your blood pressure, listen to your chest, look at your legs and knees and repeat your bloods. Does that sound okay? Your blood tests from today will be back in a few hours. We can then make a plan for if and when we involve hospital doctors.

Future — I wonder whether, to help monitor your breathing, we could involve the heart failure nurses?

Empower — You mentioned your weight has changed. Monitoring your weight is helpful to detect warning signs and guide your medications. I also have some information to give you which includes a card telling you what you can do when you feel unwell; it's called a medicines sick day rule card. How will you get to the surgery? Great. See you at midday.

Older Adults – 1

Patient's Story

Acute Kidney Injury

Doctor's notes Alexander Dickens, 78 years. PMH: Chronic kidney disease, osteoarthritis and heart failure.

Last week seen by GP. Pitting oedema to knees. Sats 95%. Crepitations at lung bases. JVP 3 cm. Agreed to increase furosemide to 2 daily. BP 162/72. Ramipril increased from 2.5 mg to 5 mg. Medication: Paracetamol, Furosemide 20 mg, Spironolactone 50 mg, Indapamide 2.5 mg, Ramipril 5 mg, Bisoprolol 5 mg. Blood test 1 week ago: eGFR 51 ml/min/1.73 m^2, Creatinine 92 µmol/L, Potassium 4.8 mmol/L and Sodium 143 mmol/L.

Message from biochemistry – eGFR 32 ml/min/1.73 m^2, Creatinine 196 µmol/L, Potassium 5.5 mmol/L and Sodium 142 mmol/L.

How to act You are surprised when the doctor calls.

PC *'Hello Doctor, what can I do for you? … I'm very well thank you.'*

History The doctor saw you last week. You were last in hospital 6 months ago when the fluid was on your lungs. This was frightening. Since then you have been *'not too bad'* but you started to feel the fluid coming back last week so called the doctor. You had noticed you were not moving around the house as easily with your breathing. When the doctor suggested taking 40 mg furosemide, initially it didn't seem to help so you increased it to 80 mg. They have given you 120 mg in hospital before, so you thought 80 mg would be fine. You can tell your fluid is going as your breathing is better and you have lost a little weight. You feel fine. Last week, however, your grandchild came around and you had a day with diarrhoea. You feel fine now. You are passing urine normally. You have no symptoms of a UTI. You have no fever. Your knee arthritis does 'play up'. If asked, tell the doctor you buy ibuprofen OTC for this. Otherwise you take only the prescribed medicines. You have not yet taken this morning's medication.

Social You live with your wife. Your son lives around the corner with your grandchildren.

You have a good circle of friends and don't let your medical conditions get you down.

You have noticed a general decline in your health over the last few years.

ICE You have never heard of the diagnosis 'acute kidney injury'.

You become very apologetic that you have changed the dose yourself without consulting the doctor and apologise to the doctor for causing an inconvenience to them.

'Oh dear Doctor, I am worried about my breathing … now my kidneys. I just can't win.'

You are hoping the doctor will examine you again. Your son could bring you in.

You would like reassurance that your chest is okay and to talk about your knees.

Learning Points

Acute Kidney Injury

Definition[1]
Serum creatinine rise of ≥26 micromol/litre within 48 hours.

≥50% rise in serum creatinine known or presumed to have occurred within the past 7 days.

A fall in UO to <0.5 ml/kg/hour for >6 hours in adults or >8 hours in children.

25% or greater fall in eGFR in children and young people within the past 7 days.

Risk factors for development of AKI[1]
- Age over 65 years
- Nephrotoxic drugs
- Previous AKI
- Chronic kidney disease
- Reliance on carer
- Hypovolaemia
- Sepsis or infection (e.g. urine)
- Vomiting
- Nephritis
- Heart failure
- Diabetes
- Liver disease
- Severe diarrhoea
- Oliguria (UO <0.5 ml/kg/hour)
- Iodinated contrast used in past week
- Urological obstruction
- Haematological malignancy
- Hypotension

Management Urinalysis, ±urgent USS, manage the cause, review nephrotoxic drugs and repeat bloods and consider admission for renal replacement therapy.[1]

Complications 'Hyperkalaemia, metabolic acidosis, symptoms or complications of uraemia (pericarditis, encephalopathy), fluid overload and pulmonary oedema.'[1]

Sick day rule card
The sick day rule card was originally developed by NHS Highland to advise patients which medicines to stop when they become unwell with either 'vomiting or diarrhoea (unless only minor), fever sweats or shaking'.[2] Medicines to stop include ACEIs, ARBs, NSAIDs, diuretics and metformin.[2]

Older Adults – 1

Doctor's Notes

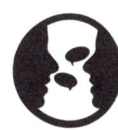

Patient Bob Riley   67 years   M
PMH   No information
Medications No current medications
Allergies   No information
Consultations Letter to patient 3 months ago – 'Please repeat your blood test in 2 weeks' time. Please also hand in another first morning urine sample.'

Letter to patient 2 months ago – 'Please repeat your blood test in 9 weeks' time.'

Investigations Blood results:

3 months ago	2 months ago	1 week ago
eGFR 40 ml/min/1.73 m^2	eGFR 42 ml/min/1.73 m^2	eGFR 41 ml/min/1.73 m^2
ACR = 10 mg/mmol	ACR = 11 mg/mmol	
Hb 146 g/L		
Na 137 mmol/L		
ALT 12 IU/L		
ALP 60 IU/L		
K 4.2 mmol/L		
PSA 0.8 ng/mL		
Cholesterol 3.3 mmol/L		
HbA1c 36.6 mmol/mol		

Household Phoebe Riley   66 years   F

Example Consultation — Chronic Kidney Disease

Sense ☐	I see you are worried and keen to know your results. To interpret these in the context of your health,
Curious ☐	I'm interested to know what led to these tests being taken. Were you feeling unwell in any way?
ICE ☐	Is there anything you are most concerned about? And what did you think they may show?
Impression ☐	The kidney blood tests have on both occasions been slightly low. The other tests are all normal. There is a name given to this result, chronic kidney disease.
Empathy ☐	I appreciate this sounds worrying, but 70% of people over 65 years have this diagnosis.
Experience ☐	Have you come across this diagnosis before?
Explanation ☐	There is often no cause but CKD can be caused by medical problems such as high blood pressure.
Risk ☐	What this means can depend on your medical history. Do you have any medical problems? Take any medicines including ibuprofen? Any family history of kidney problems? Have you ever smoked? Any problems passing urine, including needing to go at night, or again after you've just been or poor flow?
Flags ☐	Have you ever noticed any blood in your urine? Have you noticed any swelling around the ankles?
History ☐	Are you active? Did you work? Do you have family? How do you like to spend your time?
O/E ☐	I would like to take your blood pressure and dip the urine to check for blood please.
Summary ☐	So, to summarise, you have been very well, with no medical history or symptoms to report. You had the blood test for a routine health check and you were worried the abnormality may be from your cholesterol, which you are careful with, or your prostate. In fact it is only the kidney test which has shown a problem – the common finding of chronic kidney disease.
Options ☐	Now we have made the diagnosis, we need to protect your kidney vessels from raised blood pressure and cholesterol. I would like to recommend a cholesterol tablet. Although your cholesterol is good, research has shown that the tablet protects the vessels. The tablet is called atorvastatin 20 mg, which you take once a day. Have you heard of statins? There is the risk of side effects, e.g. muscle aches, but many people are fine on them. Rarely, there is a risk of muscle breakdown, so if your muscles did ache or you felt unwell then please tell your GP. This tablet can also affect the liver but we will be monitoring your blood tests. If your kidney tests changed quickly or fell to 30 we would ask the specialists to see you. The kidney test is currently at the level of 40. Normal is above 60. At present, because your urine test only showed a small amount of protein, we don't need to start any other tablets.
Empower ☐	To protect the health of the vessels, I suggest we monitor your blood pressure; it is currently slightly high but not at the level we need to give treatment. As much exercise as possible and decreasing your salt can be protective. If you decrease your salt by 6 g/day it can decrease your BP by 10! Might these be things you could do? You need to avoid taking certain tablets from the chemist, such as ibuprofen, which can make kidney function worse. Check first before you buy anything!
Future ☐	We should repeat your blood test and BP yearly.
Impact ☐	What might you tell your wife when you get home?
Safety net ☐	I don't expect that this diagnosis will cause you any symptoms. However, if you ever do notice anything new, for example ankle swelling or blood in the urine, please let me know.

Older Adults – 2

Patient's Story

Chronic Kidney Disease

Doctor's notes	Bob Riley, 67 years. PMH: None. Medications: None.
	Blood results 1 week ago: eGFR 41 ml/min/1.73 m^2
	Blood results 2 months ago: eGFR 42 ml/min/1.73 m^2, ACR = 11 mg/mmol
	Blood results 3 months ago: eGFR 40 ml/min/1.73 m^2
	Hb 146 g/L, Na 137 mmol/L, ALT 12 IU/L, ALP 60 IU/L, K 4.2 mmol/L, PSA 0.8 ng/mL, Cholesterol 3.3 mmol/L, HbA1c 36.6 mmol/mol, ACR 10 mg/mmol
How to act	Concerned. You would like to know what the result means as soon as the GP tells you the diagnosis.
PC	*'You wanted to see me for my blood test results. What's wrong?'*
History	You avoided meat before the tests and the urine was a first morning sample.
	You have been told to return to the GP because your blood test is 'abnormal'.
	You had the blood tests for a health check. You have no family history.
	You have no outflow obstruction symptoms including no nocturia.
Social	You live with your wife. You walk the dogs twice a day. This is your only exercise.
	You enjoy the taste of your food (you always add salt) but avoid sugary or fatty foods.
	You have never smoked. You drink alcohol occasionally. You take no medicines.
ICE	You presumed this was a problem with your cholesterol or prostate.
	You did not know what to expect.
Examination	BP is 137/82, urine dipstick is normal.

Older Adults – 2

Learning Points

Chronic Kidney Disease

'People with markers of kidney damage and those with a glomerular filtration rate (GFR) of less than 60 ml/min/1.73 m² on at least 2 occasions separated by a period of at least 90 days (with or without markers of kidney damage).'[1]

Markers – kidney damage	Albuminuria (ACR > 3 mg/mmol) or urinary sediment abnormalities[1]
	Electrolyte disorders, abnormal histology or renal imaging[1]
Risk factors	HTN, smoking, CVD, DM, proteinuria, AKI or haematuria, outflow obstruction nephrotoxic drugs (lithium/NSAIDs), vasculitis, systemic inflammatory disease, or a FH or African, African-Caribbean or Asian family origin.[1]
CKD investigations	Repeat the test after 2 weeks to exclude AKI.
	To make a diagnosis of CKD another test is required in 3 months.
	ACR must be a first urine of the day.
	Avoid meat 12 hours before the blood test.
	eGFRcysC test – if available can differentiate borderline CKD.
	'African-Caribbean or African family origin … multiply eGFR by 1.159.'[1]
CKD diagnosis	eGFR <45 OR ACR ≥3 (any eGFR) OR eGFR <60 and eGFRcysC unavailable.
Progressive CKD	Change in CKD category/12 months OR ↓eGFR 25% or 15 ml/min/1.73 m²/year.[1]
Classification	eGFR 45–59 = CKD3A. 30–45 = CKD3B, 15–29 = CKD4, eGFR <15 = CKD5
	ACR <3 = A1, ACR 3–30 = A2, ACR >30 = A3[1]
Further investigations	FBC (? Anaemia) and if eGFR <30, calcium, phosphate, PTH and vitamin D.
	Urine dip for haematuria. Use ACR (not dipstick) for protein measurement.
	Renal USS if eGFR <30, progressive CKD, haematuria, FH PCKD or obstruction.[1]
Management:	CVD lifestyle advice. No protein-free diet unless instructed by the renal team
	If possible, stop nephrotoxic drugs.
	No aspirin unless – CVD present and aspirin is required for secondary prevention.
BP aim	<140/90 OR in diabetics <130/80[1]
Atorvastatin 20 mg	If eGFR ≥ 30 and titrate if non-HDL cholesterol doesn't ↓by 40%.[2]
ACE inhibitor	Start if ACR (mg/mmol): ≥70 OR ≥ 30 + HTN OR ≥3 + DM *and* K <5 mmol/litre. Stop if change of eGFR ↓25% or creatinine ↑30% or K ≥6 mmol/litre.
Monitoring frequency	See Table 2 within reference[1]
Refer if	eGFR<30, ACR >70 (unless DM put on ACEi), ACR>30 + haematuria.
	Progressive CKD.
	Suspected renal artery stenosis or suspected inherited condition.
	≥4 antihypertensives[1]
Discuss with medics if	AKI, severe uraemia, fluid overload or hyperkalaemia.
Type 4 tubular acidosis	In a diabetic with CKD and raised potassium … test for a low bicarbonate.
	Manage BP and discuss with a specialist whether the Rx of furosemide (if oedematous) and fludrocortisone is appropriate.

Older Adults – 2

Doctor's Notes

Patient   Kathleen Wright   89 years   F
PMH   Atrial fibrillation
Medications   Apixaban
                  Bisoprolol
Allergies   No known drug allergies
Consultations A&E visit 4 weeks ago 'Laceration. Dressing, discharged.'
Investigations No recent investigations
Household   No household members registered

Example Consultation — Care Home

Open ☐	Hello Mrs Wright – I'm sorry to hear that. Tell me more about what's happened recently and that led to you coming here to discuss this with me today.
History ☐	When did your daughter come to visit? What did she say to you? I see you were at the hospital recently. What happened then?
Flags ☐	You stopped taking apixaban – tell me why that was.
Risk ☐	Tell me how you manage at home. Have you had any other falls? Can you manage the stairs? Where is the bathroom? How about cooking and shopping?
Sense ☐	I sense you are very clear that you want to stay at home, even though there are some challenges (e.g. with the stairs) and even if it might be risky.
ICE ☐	What are your own thoughts? Is there anything that worries you about staying at home? Was there anything in particular you were hoping I might be able to do today?
Impact ☐	You live alone – do you feel lonely there? Your daughter and her family are your only relatives – is this causing friction between you?
Curious ☐	Tell me how you felt when you looked around the care homes.
Summary ☐	To summarise, it has been getting harder lately at home, for example with stairs, and you had a fall when you couldn't get up. This prompted your daughter to visit and she thought you might be safer in a home where there are people to look after you.
O/E ☐	May I check your pulse and BP? May I ask you some questions to help me be sure you understand the choices? Tell me what you think are the risks of staying at home.
Empathy ☐	I understand your wish to stay at home and it must be difficult that it has caused friction with your daughter. I expect she cares about you and is worried for your safety.
Impression ☐	My impression is that you have what we call the capacity to make the decision to stay at home and that you do understand the risks. There may be things we can do to make it easier to stay home safely. I am a bit concerned you have stopped the apixaban and I would like you to book another appointment so we can discuss the pros and cons of this.
Experience ☐	Do you have friends who have help at home either from people or physical aids?
Options ☐	I would like your permission to arrange for an assessment to see if there are things that would make it easier to stay at home. For example, a stair lift or lift, a pendant alarm, mobility aids and rails. We could arrange a cleaner, or carers to assist you with meals. I appreciate you have had a bad experience with the previous cleaner but I wonder if help from others may keep you safe in your own home. We could also arrange an appointment with the falls prevention team. What are your thoughts?
Empower ☐	I would like to give you a leaflet to read about care at home and other options and about apixaban.*
Future ☐	May I ask our community nurse to visit you at home in a couple of weeks to see how you are doing? With your permission, I could speak to your daughter on the phone.
Safety net ☐	Please come back if you have any concerns or phone me and I can arrange a home visit.

*http://patient.info/health/preventing-stroke-when-you-have-atrial-fibrillation

Older Adults – 3

Patient's Story

Care Home

Doctor's notes Kathleen Wright, 89 years. Recent A&E attendance with laceration. PMH: Atrial fibrillation. Medications include apixaban and bisoprolol.

How to act Articulate but upset. Not confused, fully orientated.

PC *'I'm here under protest. My daughter booked the appointment. She thinks I should move to a care home and I don't agree.'*

History You are a retired school teacher (widowed 10 years ago) and live in the family home where you have lived for the last 50 years. It is far too big for you, Victorian with four floors. There are six bedrooms. You tend to live on the ground floor only and sometimes can't make it up the stairs to bed so at times you sleep on the sofa. A few weeks ago you had a bad fall and couldn't get up. You cut your arm and this didn't stop bleeding because of the apixaban. You went to hospital where they were very busy and just put a dressing on your arm and sent you home by taxi. You have stopped the apixaban in view of the bleeding as it is clearly causing problems.

Social Your only daughter Rachel is a busy GP who has her own family and lives 200 miles away. She came to visit recently (after the fall) and was very bossy, telling you that your house wasn't clean enough and that there was food well past its sell-by day in the fridge. She took you around several care homes, all of which were horrible and full of old people and she was asking if there was a place for you. You have a modest pension and could not afford care home fees from income. You sacked your cleaner because she stole money from you. A neighbour drives you to the shops once a week.

ICE You are a determined person and are clear that you wish to stay in your own home and die in your own bed. You fear that your daughter can manipulate the situation so that you have to give up your house and move to a home. You are worried that the doctor today will collude with your daughter, indeed that she may have already spoken to the doctor and been influential. You are worried you would have to sell the house to fund fees.

Ask the doctor *'Can she make me move to a care home?'*

'Is there any help for me to stay at home?'

Examination Pulse 100 AF. BP 130/90.

Older Adults – 3

Learning Points

Care Home

Assessing capacity

> **BMA's Mental Capacity Toolkit**
> See the **Link Hub at CompleteCSA.co.uk** for a useful link to the BMA's Mental Capacity Toolkit with series of very useful cards.

Information from the BMA's Mental Capacity Toolkit

Card 4 covers 'assessing capacity'. In brief:

- As part of your assessment of whether or not an individual can consent to treatment or care, you may need to assess whether or not they have capacity to make the decision or not.
- There are four aspects to consider and, if an individual fails any one of these, they are deemed not to have capacity to make a decision:
    - Understand information relevant to the decision.
    - Retain the information relevant to the decision.
    - Be able to weigh up or use the information.
    - Be able to communicate their view – in any way/by any means.[1]

You need to listen, where appropriate, to relatives or friends who may be able to provide useful additional information but must not be influenced by the views of the third party regarding the decision.

If you decide that someone lacks capacity, this should be based on your 'reasonable belief' and backed up by objective reasons.

The assessment of capacity relates to a specific decision at a specific time. If there is a change in the situation capacity should be reassessed.

Funding care home places

Total of savings and capital (e.g. property) <£23,250 – the local authority (LA) assists with fees[2]

Capital >£23,250 but savings less than this, the LA will pay for first 12 weeks[2]

Savings >£23,250, no help from LA[2]

Other financial help includes Pension credit, income support, and attendance allowance.

> **Funding care home places**
> See the **Link Hub at CompleteCSA.co.uk** for a useful link to advice for patients and relatives regarding care home fees.
>
> **Care options**
> See the **Link Hub at CompleteCSA.co.uk** for a useful link to advice for patients and families.

Older Adults – 3

Doctor's Notes

Patient	William Briggs	71 years	M
PMH	Hypertension		
	Is a carer – wife has MS		
Medications	Ramipril 5 mg daily		
Allergies	No known drug allergies		
Consultations	No recent consultations		
Investigations	Renal function and cholesterol normal 3 months ago		
Household	Hazel Briggs	71	F

Example Consultation — Possible Dementia

Open ☐	Hello Mr Briggs – you are most certainly not wasting my time or yours. Please tell me more about your concerns about your memory.
History ☐	Has this happened before? Has your wife or family noticed a problem?
Flags ☐	Have you ever found yourself in any danger or risk at home? For example, have you ever found saucepans boiling dry? Have you had any near misses when driving?
Risk ☐	Tell me how you manage at home. Do you have help in the house? How do you manage with Hazel? How about cooking and shopping?
Sense ☐	I sense you are very concerned about your memory and whether it might mean that you have a significant problem such as dementia or Alzheimer's disease.
ICE ☐	What are your own thoughts? Is there anything that worries you particularly? Was there anything specific you were hoping I might be able to do today?
Impact ☐	What other impact is this problem having on you day to day? Have you had thoughts about how it may impact on your life in the future? How is your mood?
Experience ☐	Have any of your friends or family had memory problems? Tell me more about their experience. Has your aunt been on your mind recently?
Summary ☐	To summarise, although you have been a bit forgetful for a while, recently there have been a few occasions when you have become aware of significant memory lapses which are quite out of character for you. You have been thinking about the impact of dementia and also how Hazel may cope. We should probably arrange a formal memory test, but first I would like to do a quick assessment of your memory myself.
O/E ☐	I would like to check your pulse and BP and do a short test of your memory – would that be okay? Thank you. There are six questions (1) What year is it? (2) What month is it? (3) Please remember this address – Peter White, 56 Commercial Street, Bedford. (4) About what time is it? (5) Count backwards from 20 to 1. (6) Say the months of the year in reverse. Repeat the address phrase.
Impression ☐	The short memory test suggests that there *might* be a problem with your memory. This is certainly not a diagnosis of dementia or Alzheimer's but it does mean that it might be useful to do some more tests.
Empathy ☐	I understand how worrying it must be, particularly when you were an accountant, to experience loss of memory and when you have Hazel to care for.
Options ☐	We should do more tests, then we could discuss referral to a memory clinic. If we find that you do have memory loss, some types may be helped by tablets. There is plenty of support available.
Empower ☐	I would like to give you a leaflet to read about memory problems and about driving.
Future ☐	We will arrange a blood test, urine test and ECG and a CXR to see if this sheds any more light on what is going on. You asked about driving and, so long as you feel safe, there is no reason to stop driving just now.
Safety net ☐	Please book an appointment with me in 2 weeks when we can discuss the test results.

Older Adults – 4

Patient's Story

Possible Dementia

Doctor's notes William Briggs, 71 years. PMH: Hypertension. Medication: Ramipril 5 mg

How to act Concerned, hesitant.

PC *'I'm sorry to bother you and I hope I'm not wasting your time, it's just I'm a bit worried about my memory.'*

History You are a retired accountant and are used to being organised and in control. You have noticed that you have become increasingly forgetful lately – losing your spectacles, keys etc. You put this down to normal absent-mindedness but a few things have made you more concerned. You have gone overdrawn at the bank and this has never happened before – you can't think how you could have been so careless. You phoned your son recently to check the date of your grandson (Freddie)'s birthday and your son said that you had in fact already sent a birthday card and cheque a week ago and then a further almost identical one arrived in the post today. He had been going to ring you to discuss. You have no recollection of buying or posting either of the cards or of writing the cheques, though when you looked in your cheque book the stubs were filled in in your handwriting so you must have done.

Your mood is fine.

Social You live with your wife, Hazel, who has had MS for years and is increasingly disabled. She is more or less housebound now. You have good neighbours. Your only son, Henry, lives with his wife and family about 100 miles away. You have two grandchildren, Freddie aged 16 and Rebecca aged 15. Since the village shop closed 10 years ago, you drive 5 miles to the supermarket 2–3 times a week.

ICE You are very worried that you are losing your memory and developing Alzheimer's. You are particularly worried about what this will mean for the care of Hazel. Will you have to go into a care home? What about Hazel? If you get a diagnosis of dementia, will you be able to drive?

You have no idea what the GP may suggest as you believe there is nothing that can be done for dementia.

Your aunt had dementia. You used to visit her in the care home and were saddened by how dependent she was and you have been thinking about how undignified the process of ageing can be. Your great fear, therefore, is needing to go into a home, your children seeing you lose your mind and having others attend to your personal hygiene.

Ask the doctor *'What's happening to me?'*

'Can this be reversed?'

'What will happen to Hazel?'

'Can I drive?'

Examination BP 130/90.

Memory test (e.g. 6 CIT) – you get about 70% correct and 30% wrong.

Older Adults – 4

Learning Points

Possible Dementia

Assessment of possible dementia

1. History, mental state, cognitive and physical examination. Medication review.

   Cognitive assessment includes: short- and long-term memory, orientation, attention and concentration, use of language. Cognitive testing suitable for GP consultations includes:
   - 6 CIT
   - GPCOG

   NICE also mentions two other screening tools which are suitable but less straightforward in GP[1]:
   - 7-minute screen – requires a set of picture cards
   - MMSE – is under copyright from Psychological Assessment Resources (PAR) and needs to be purchased from them.

2. Investigations

   FBC, ESR, U&E, Ca, LFT, Glucose, TFT, B12 and folate. Consider MSU (if acute confusion/delirium). ECG and CXR if appropriate.

3. Referral

   To specialist memory services.

Helpful articles and resources in geratology

> See the **Link Hub at CompleteCSA.co.uk** for useful links to very helpful articles on:
> - Unintentional weight loss in adults
> - Restless leg syndrome
> - Anticholinergic Burden Scale
> - Geratology PILs
> - Fact sheet about driving with dementia
> - PIL – Memory Loss and Dementia
>
> And dementia screening tools:
> - 6 CIT
> - GPCOG
> - 7-minute screen

Older Adults – 4

Doctor's Notes

Patient	Florence Matheson 89 years F	
PMH	Advanced Alzheimer's dementia	
	Do not attempt resuscitation	
	Daughter has power of attorney – health and financial decisions	
	Recurrent lower respiratory tract infections	
	Osteoarthritis – both knees	
	Pressure sore – sacral region	
	Dry skin	
Medications	Paracetamol 1 g QDS	
	Oilatum	
	Balneum cream	
Allergies	No known allergies	
Consultations	Yesterday	OOH note. Possible coffee ground vomiting during the night.
		Paramedics called and observations normal. For GP to review.
	Yesterday	Home visit by Locum GP. Eating and drinking. No further vomiting.
		Chest clear. Legs NAD.
		No melaena on PR examination. Abdomen soft non-tender.
		Carers' report – seems her normal self. Obs normal. Not distressed
		Message left on daughter, Kathleen Grimshaw's mobile.
Investigations	No recent investigations.	
Household	Nursing home resident.	

Telephone call – Kathleen Grimshaw would like an update from the doctor.

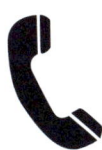

Example Consultation

Distressed NOK

Open ☐	Mrs Grimshaw, thank you for your call. I see the doctor tried to call you yesterday. What have you been told so far? How was your mother last night?
ICE ☐	You must have many questions. Please go ahead with any questions you have, I will take note of them and we will try to answer each one in turn. It is also helpful to know what your thoughts are … What has gone through your mind? What concerns you most? I see that you have power of attorney, which is very helpful. Were you hoping that we would make any specific decisions today?
History ☐	What do you know about your mother's health conditions? What problems has she had recently? Do you live locally? What support do you have? Siblings? A partner?
Curious ☐	What is your mother able to do? What changes have you seen in your mother over the last 6 months? What does she depend on others for? Has a doctor talked to your previously about your mum's health in general? Does she recognise you?
Summary ☐	May I summarise what we have said so far? Your mother is fully dependent on the carers due to advanced Alzheimer's disease. We are concerned that your mother may have had a bleed in the stomach. She has not had any further bleeding and there was no sign of blood when the doctor thoroughly examined her yesterday. However, the concern is that this may happen again and you called today to find out from the doctor why this may have happened and can it be fixed. You are afraid that your mother may be alone in the night. Therefore, you feel she should go to hospital.
Impression ☐	The carers saw what might have been blood in the vomit. Although this is only a possibility, the safest thing to do is make a plan for if this were the case.
Experience ☐	You were alarmed by the word haemorrhage. Have you come across this before?
Explanation ☐	Haemorrhage does mean a large bleed. The blood is likely to have come from the stomach. The reason may be due to acid building up causing an ulcer or even a tumour in the stomach which may have bled. There is the chance of this happening again and, if this happened, there may be a sudden significant amount of bleeding.
Empathy ☐	The thought of something happening to your mother is very distressing.
Sense ☐	I can hear that you are very worried about your mum. She is very frail and has been for some time now. What are your thoughts? Due to her Alzheimer's she is not strong and it sounds like she has been deteriorating over recent months. I do think she is approaching the end of her life as her body isn't working as it should. (Silence).
Options ☐	There are things that we can do at home, e.g. giving her a daily tablet, called omeprazole, to reduce the acid. We can also ask the nurses to do regular checks on your mum including through the night. But going through the emergency department is likely to cause your mother great distress. It is noisy, the lighting is different, people are different and I feel this would not be in your mother's best interests. The endoscopy procedure, to look inside the stomach, is invasive and your mother is frail. I would like to help your mother by preparing for a peaceful and comfortable end to her life as best we can, without going in an ambulance, through A&E and having tests which I do not believe will help. What are you thinking? You are welcome to think about this, come in and see me to discuss it again. However, as this can happen at any time, I would like to speak to the home about medicines that can be given quickly by the nurses if your mother became distressed and keep her where she can be peaceful. What would you like to do? May I make that plan and emphasise to the staff she needs regular monitoring?
Impact ☐	Losing your mother will have a great impact on you. I'm concerned about you also, especially as you do not have much support. Have you also spoken to your GP?
Future ☐	Please arrange to speak to me if you have further concerns or questions.

Older Adults – 5

Patient's Story

Distressed NOK

Doctor's notes Florence Matheson, 89 years. PMH: Advanced Alzheimer's disease, Possible coffee ground vomiting yesterday, ambulance called then GP visit. Multiple LRTIs, pressure sores and dry skin. Medication: Paracetamol, Oilatum and Balneum cream. DNA CPR.

Telephone call – Kathleen Grimshaw would like an update from the doctor.

How to act Anxious

PC *'I had a call from the doctor last night and missed it. I went to see my mother last night and they said they thought she had had a bleed. Can you tell me what's going on?'*

History You are Kathleen Grimshaw, the daughter of Florence. She lives in a care home.

You have power of attorney for your mother.

You see her every night after work. You have given up all your usual interests to care for your mother over the years. You are divorced and don't see your friends any more. You do not have siblings.

You have been informed that first the paramedic and then the doctor were called to see your mother, because of blood in her vomit. The word *'haemorrhage' was mentioned in the care folder* and you realise this is serious. You had an uncle who had a haemorrhage from his aorta.

If this happens again you would like her to go to hospital. You would like to know why this has happened, what treatment she will receive and if the problem can be fixed.

If the GP says the hospital would not treat your mother because of her age, become angry and find out what they would do if she was young.

If the doctor mentions an endoscopy, you would like your mother to have it.

However, if the doctor explains this is an invasive procedure, you do not make a decision but remain unsure.

'I don't want anything to happen to her.'

If the doctor agrees to call an ambulance and have your mother admitted, you are pleased. If, however, the doctor sensitively discusses the reasons why hospital care may not be in your mother's best interests, and takes time to listen to your views, you agree.

Last night your mother seemed peaceful. She was alert. You never really know if she recognises you or not, but she does not push you away.

Social Care home resident. Hoisted between chair and bed. Fully dependent on carers for all ADLs.

ICE You are worried that this will happen again and your mother will be vomiting blood through the night and the staff will not notice until the morning.

When you say you don't want anything to happen to her, you know that one day it will. You mean that you don't want her to die in a horrible way, vomiting blood. But you also still enjoy having a mother and it has been your fear throughout your life that your mother will one day be gone.

Ask the doctor *'Is this going to happen again?' 'What has caused this?' 'Can it be fixed?'*

'What would the hospital do?' 'Won't she be safer at hospital?'

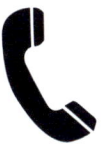

Learning Points

Distressed NOK

As a GP, using your clinical judgement, you try to act in what you believe are the best interests of the patient. However, relatives may not share your ideas. Respect their different opinions regarding what they believe is ethical. It is important to explore their opinions as there may be concerns that need addressing. It is also important to explore the emotional impact of the plan you propose. It may help to understand the relative's fear and bring your different viewpoints together so you are 'on the same page'. Remember that religious beliefs may be an important guide for the relative.

If, after presenting the options to the relative, they choose a plan that is not what you have recommended, as long as their decision is not putting the patient in danger, recognise that your own thoughts and beliefs are just your individual opinion so a paternalistic approach, blocking their request, may not be ethical. Negotiate a management plan which continues to deliver safe care.

Here is a repeat scenario of the above case, from the management options. However, in this situation the relative continued to push for hospital care.

Sense ☐   I can hear that you are very worried about your mum. She is very frail and has been for some time now. What are your thoughts? Due to her Alzheimer's she is not strong and it sounds like she has been deteriorating over recent months. Do you see any signs of happiness when you visit? What do you think your mother would want now? Do either you or your mother have a faith? I do think she is approaching the end of her life as the body isn't working as it should. (Silence) It sounds like you are very keen to ensure your mother receives the best care and you feel this would be safest in the hospital. It is important that I understand the reasons why you think hospital may be right for your mother, as this information can be helpful to hospital doctors. Even if your mother goes to hospital, I am concerned that she is approaching the end of her life and the doctors will not be able to reverse this. I hear that you would prefer your mother to be in hospital because you believe it would give her the best care. Can I also ask if there is anything else that worries you about her being in the care home rather than hospital? Some people worry about their loved one dying and what that might be like. Is that something that concerns you – that it might be frightening, perhaps? (Pause) Would it help if I were to talk with you about what happens when someone is nearing the end of their life and then dies?

Empathy ☐   For anyone – losing their mother can be the most frightening thought throughout life since childhood. (Silence)

Empathy ☐   How will it affect you personally? I'm concerned about you also. Especially as you do not have much support. Have you also spoken to your GP?

Options ☐   We have some options. The benefit of the hospital is that there are doctors and nurses to respond and react to your mother's needs. They would also make their own assessment of whether there is more they can do for your mother. My opinion is that I do not feel it is likely they would want to perform a procedure on your mother as she is so frail and I do not believe that this is in her best interests. I recommend keeping your mother here, where she is comfortable with the environment, to provide personalised end-of-life care. We can provide the same medicines as hospital doctors. Having medicines ready to manage any discomfort will enable us to provide excellent care for your mother's dignity and comfort. What do you think your mother would want? You would like her to go to hospital; is that still the case? OK, I will speak to the hospital doctors.

CHAPTER 7 OVERVIEW
Maternal Health

	Cases in this chapter	Within the RCGP curriculum: Maternal Health RCGP Curriculum Online March 2016[1]	Learning points in the chapter include:
1	New Pregnancy	'Recognise the prevalence of domestic violence and question sensitively where this may be an issue' 'Use screening strategies relevant to women'	Medications and supplements, risk assessments and screening in pregnancy
2	Antenatal Check	'Be familiar with and implement the key national guidelines that influence healthcare provision for women's problems'	Hyperemesis, hypertension in pregnancy and reduced foetal movements
3	Bleeding in Pregnancy	'Recognise and intervene immediately when patients present with [an] … obstetric emergency'	Bleeding in pregnancy and anti-D rhesus prophylaxis
4	Diabetes in Pregnancy	'Understand the impact of other illness.' 'Be able to advise on prevention strategies relevant to women … pre-pregnancy counselling, antenatal care'	Counselling pre-conception and risks of diabetes in pregnancy
5	Postnatal Check	'Know about the impact of culture and ethnicity on women's perceived role in society and their attendant health beliefs, and be able to tailor healthcare accordingly: for example, mental illness is kept "hidden" in some cultures because of the stigma attached to it'	Postnatal check, contraception and endometritis
Extra notes	Exposure to Chickenpox in Pregnancy		Varicella in pregnancy

1. http://www.rcgp.org.uk/training-exams/gp-curriculum-overview/online-curriculum/caring-for-the-whole-person/3-06-womens-health.aspx

CHAPTER 7 REFERENCES

New Pregnancy
1. NICE Guidelines. CG63. Diabetes in pregnancy. Management of diabetes and its complications from pre-conception to the postnatal period. Mar 2008.
2. NICE Guidelines. CG62. Antenatal care for uncomplicated pregnancies. Updated Mar 2016.
3. Obstetric Secondary Care Referral and Maternal Medical Risk Assessment (MMRA) Guideline. Oxford University Hospitals NHS Foundation Trust. September 2015. http://occg.oxnet.nhs.uk/General Practice/ClinicalGuidelines/Obstetrics/Maternal%20Risk%20Assessment.pdf
4. Alexander E.K., Marqusee E., Lawrence J., et al. Timing and magnitude of increases in levothyroxine requirements during pregnancy in women with hypothyroidism. *N Engl J Med* 2004; 351: 241–9. July 15, 2004. http://www.nejm.org/doi/full/10.1056/NEJMoa040079#t=abstract
5. NICE Guidelines. Hypertension in pregnancy: the management of hypertensive disorders during pregnancy. Aug 2010, updated Jan 2011.

Antenatal Check
1. NICE Guidelines. Hypertension in pregnancy: the management of hypertensive disorders during pregnancy. Aug 2010, updated Jan 2011.
2. White H., Threlfall H., et al. Maternity Assessment Unit Guideline. Oxford University Hospitals Foundation Trust. 28/4/16. Review date 28/4/19. http://ouh.oxnet.nhs.uk/Maternity/Maternity%20Guideline%20Documents/Maternity%20Assessment%20Unit/MAU%20Guideline,%20Full%20Guideline
3. NICE Guidelines. CG63. Diabetes in pregnancy Management of diabetes and its complications from pre-conception to the postnatal period. Mar 2008.
4. Reproduced from: Royal College of Obstetricians and Gynaecologists. *Reduced Fetal Movements*. Green-top Guideline number 57. London: RCOG; 2011 with the permission of the Royal College of Obstetricians and Gynaecologists.

Bleeding in Pregnancy
1. NICE Guidelines. CG154. Ectopic pregnancy and miscarriage: diagnosis and initial management. Dec 2012.
2. Reproduced from: Royal College of Obstetricians and Gynaecologists. *Use of Anti-D Immunoglobulin for Rh Prophylaxis*. Green-top Guideline number 22. London: RCOG; 2002 with the permission of the Royal College of Obstetricians and Gynaecologists.

Diabetes in Pregnancy
1. NICE Guidelines. CG63. Diabetes in pregnancy Management of diabetes and its complications from pre-conception to the postnatal period. Mar 2008.

Postnatal Check
1. FSRH Clinical Guidance. Postnatal Sexual and Reproductive Health. Sept 2009.
2. NICE Guidelines. CG63. Diabetes in pregnancy Management of diabetes and its complications from pre-conception to the postnatal period. Mar 2008.
3. NICE Guidelines. Hypertension in pregnancy: the management of hypertensive disorders during pregnancy. Aug 2010, updated Jan 2011.
4. Oxford University Hospital NHS Trust. Community Management for Hypertension. Information for community midwives and GPs. 2016

Exposure to Chickenpox in Pregnancy
1. Public Health England. Varicella: the green book, chapter 34. London: Public Health England; 2012. https://www.gov.uk/government/uploads/system/uploads/attachment_data/file/456562/Green_Book_Chapter_34_v3_0.pdf
2. Reproduced from: Royal College of Obstetricians and Gynaecologists. *Chickenpox in Pregnancy*. Green-top Guideline number 13. London: RCOG; 2015 with the permission of the Royal College of Obstetricians and Gynaecologists
3. Health Protection Agency. Guidance on viral rash in pregnancy: investigation, diagnosis and management of viral rash illness, or exposure to viral rash illness, in pregnancy. London: Health Protection Agency; 2011. https://www.gov.uk/government/uploads/system/uploads/attachment_data/file/322688/Viral_rash_in_pregnancy_guidance.pdf. Contains public sector information licenced under the Open Government Licence v3.0.

Maternal Health

Doctor's Notes

Patient	Jemma Black	32 years	F
PMH	Hypothyroidism		
Medications	Levothyroxine 75 micrograms daily		
Allergies	No information		
Consultations	No recent consultations		
Investigations	TFTs normal 1 year ago		
Household	No household contacts registered		

Example Consultation — New Pregnancy

Open ☐	That is big news, how do you feel about it?
Sense ☐	You sound delighted. Congratulations. May I ask, was it planned? Is this your first pregnancy? How are you feeling?
Flags ☐	Are you being sick? Any bleeding or pain? When was your LMP? How many days between your periods? Are you taking folic acid and vitamin D?
Risk ☐	Any history of depression? How is your relationship? Have you ever felt threatened or scared in your relationship? Any violence? Have you ever had a blood clot?
History ☐	I see you have an underactive thyroid and take thyroxine. Do you have any other medical problems? Do you smoke? How much alcohol do you drink? Do you take any drugs? What support do you have? What work do you do?
ICE ☐	Is there anything that's been on your mind or you've been wondering about? Or concerned about?
Examination ☐	Please may I check your blood pressure, weight and height and ask for a urine sample?
Impression ☐	You are about 5 weeks' pregnant but the 12-week scan will confirm that.
Options ☐	We should increase your levothyroxine to 100 micrograms, which is safe to do as the body requires a 30% higher dose in pregnancy. Let's also check your thyroid level and I will ask the specialist to see you. Another thing to talk about at this stage is screening for Down syndrome. Is this something you have thought about? The initial tests carry no risk. They include the blood test and the jelly scan which we do anyway. Unfortunately, this doesn't give us a definite answer, but this information can tell us whether you are at a higher or lower risk of having a baby with Down syndrome. If you were at higher risk, you would be offered further tests. These tests, however, do carry a risk of infection or miscarriage.
Curious ☐	You mentioned you spoke to your sister about the Down syndrome testing?
Empathy ☐	Some women feel they would want the tests as babies with Down syndrome can suffer with various medical conditions as well as have learning disabilities. Some women feel that they would prefer to end the pregnancy if Down syndrome was confirmed whereas others would continue. However, it can be a tricky decision whether to have the initial tests as, if the test result comes back suggesting we should offer further tests, the risk of having a miscarriage or infection from the tests can be higher than the risk of having a baby with Down syndrome. Does this make sense?
Empower ☐	You do not have to make a decision today and you are under no pressure. Perhaps you would like to talk this through with your husband.
Explanation ☐	To help the development of the baby, we recommend taking a folic acid and vitamin D tablet until 12 weeks of pregnancy. You can buy this from the pharmacy. Here is an information pack of all the foods you should avoid; for example, liver because it is full of vitamin A.
Future ☐	You can let your midwife know your decision. Please make an appointment to see the midwife in 4–5 weeks. I'll see you again after your dating scan.
Safety net ☐	If you experience any pain or bleeding or you are being sick and are struggling to keep fluids down then see a doctor. Can we keep an eye on your thyroid levels with a monthly blood test please?

Maternal Health – 1

Patient's Story

New Pregnancy

Doctor's notes	Mrs Jemma Black, 32 years. PMH: Hypothyroidism. Medication: levothyroxine 75 mcg.
How to act	You are excited.
PC	*'I'm pregnant. I don't know what I have to do next.'*
	LMP 5 weeks ago. Gravida 1 Para 0
History	You have been trying to conceive for 6 months.
	You have been taking folic acid but not vitamin D. No vomiting.
	You have hypothyroidism but are otherwise well.
	You have not vomited. No pain or bleeding.
Social	You are a dentist and live with your husband. Never smoked. No alcohol.
	You are in a happy relationship and have never experienced violence within your relationship.
ICE	You are unsure if you can continue your thyroid tablets.
	You don't know when to arrange the midwife appointment.
	If the doctor mentions Down syndrome screening, state: *'My sister told me there is a risk of miscarriage with the tests.'*
	If asked specifically about your sister, she had the initial screening and then had a miscarriage at 18 weeks, which was horrible. Once counselled, you would like the Down syndrome screening. You thought it was the initial tests that caused the risk of miscarriage.
Examination	BMI 22, BP 100/60, urine dipstick negative

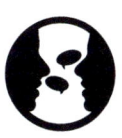

Maternal Health – 1

Learning Points

New Pregnancy

Medication and supplements

Folic acid 400 mcg or 5 mg daily if: epileptic Rx, sickle-cell disease, previous NTD, diabetic, folate deficiency, methotrexate/sulphasalazine Rx, BMI >30, malabsorption syndrome or methylene tetrahydrofolate reductase gene positive[1-3]

Vitamin D 10–25 mcg for all women[2,3]

Antidepressants Refer to perinatal psychiatry for advice if unable to stop medication.

Usually change to a TCA or fluoxetine (the only licenced SSRI).

Provide the woman with information to enable her to make an informed choice.

> **Teratology**
> See the **Link Hub at CompleteCSA.co.uk** for a useful link to teratology information for medicines taken in pregnancy.

Thyroxine Increase thyroxine by 30%[4] at the first visit then take monthly thyroid tests.

Risk assessments

BMI >30 5 mg folic acid, OGTT at 28 weeks and look for other VTE risk factors.[2,3]

>35 as above + increased pre-eclampsia surveillance. Consider aspirin if one other risk factor.[2,3]

>40 as above + refer to a consultant.[2,3]

Pre-eclampsia Aspirin 75 mg from 12 weeks for:

HTN or HTN in a previous pregnancy, CKD, autoimmune disease, or DM

Or ≥2 of: primigravida, >40 years, 10 years since last child, BMI >35, FH of pre-eclampsia (mum or sister) or multiple pregnancy.[3,5]

VTE Seek advice from the maternal medicine clinic to discuss LMWH if:

previous/FH VTE, thrombophilia, a comorbidity

or ≥3 of: BMI >30, age >35, parity >2, current smoker, varicose veins, systemic infection, immobility, current pre-eclampsia, multiple pregnancy or assisted conception.[3]

Anaemia If haemoglobin is <110 g/L at booking or <105 g/L at 28 weeks, iron supplementation should be considered.[2]

Diabetes If previous DM arrange OGTT, early glucose monitoring and refer to diabetes clinic.

OGTT at 28 weeks if a risk factor: BMI >30, previous baby >4.5 kg, FH diabetes (first-degree relative) or origin with a high prevalence.[1,3]

Screening

DS risk See Genetics chapter – Down syndrome for screening information.

Urine Urine dipstick to detect UTI which can lead to a miscarriage.

Mood Ask about mood and refer to perinatal mental health services if required.

Screen for domestic violence.

Maternal Health – 1

Doctor's Notes

Patient   Charlotte Bunton   31 years   F
PMH   NVD 2 years ago
Medications   No current medications
Allergies   No information
Consultations No recent consultations
Investigations No recent investigations
Household   Felix Bunton   2 years   M
                   Darius Bunton   33 years   M

Example Consultation — Antenatal Check

Open ☐	And how are you feeling? How many weeks are you now?
Impact ☐	Has your pregnancy caused you to feel unwell?
ICE ☐	Any worries at all? We can certainly do your check-up today. Was there anything you were hoping to discuss?
Flags ☐	Is baby moving well? Any swelling of the hands/feet? Headaches? Vision changes? Tummy pain?
Risk ☐	Any problems in the last pregnancy? Any drop in your mood? How is your relationship? Have you ever felt scared or unsafe at home? Any violence in the relationship? Have you ever had a blood clot?
Sense ☐	You seem very relaxed.
History ☐	And, medically, any other problems? Are you taking any medicines?
Curious ☐	It's the first time we've met; I'm interested to know more about you.
Summary ☐	So you are 32 weeks and no concerns at all. Your last pregnancy 2 years ago went smoothly. Is that correct?
O/E ☐	I'd like to examine you if I may: feel your tummy for the baby's lie and take the measurement. We can have a listen in to baby, check your weight and blood pressure. Is that okay? Do you have a urine sample?
Empathy ☐	Is sleeping starting to become difficult?
Impression ☐	All seems to be going very well.
Future ☐	Do you know when you are next planning to see the midwife?
Safety net ☐	Any problems then do let a doctor know. There are a few symptoms that you must tell either the doctor or midwife about; if you have any tummy pain, any bleeding, any headaches, vision changes or sudden swelling or decreased movements from baby. Any questions? Great, I'll see you at 38 weeks.

MATERNAL HEALTH – 2

Patient's Story

Antenatal Check

Doctor's notes	Charlotte Bunton, 31 years. PMH: NVD 2 years ago
How to act	Confident all is going well.
	You are here for your 32-week check.
PC	*'I've come for my routine review.'*
History	Gravida 2 Para 1 32/40
Social	You have a supportive husband. You are an engineer.
ICE	You are very clued up on your pregnancy and have no questions.
	You expect all will be well.
O/E	SFH 33 cm, foetal movement felt
	FHR 140, cephalic and 5/5 palpable
	Urine negative and BP 112/62
	Weight 62 kg, no oedema

Maternal Health – 2

Learning Points — Antenatal Check

When considering medication with pregnant patients, always discuss the advice in the BNF and refer to http://www.uktis.org/

Itching	Exclude obstetric cholestasis with LFTs and bile acids. Suggest calamine lotion.
Headache	Exclude pre-eclampsia. Consider paracetamol or codeine.
Hyperemesis	Examination: observations, hydration, abdomen and urine. Admit if ketones.
	The following are used: antihistamines (e.g. promethazine teoclate), prochlorperazine, cyclizine, metoclopramide, ondansetron, ginger and acupuncture.
HELLP syndrome	Haemolysis, elevated liver enzymes and low platelet count
Gestational hypertension	New HTN > 20 weeks without significant proteinuria[1]
Pre-eclampsia	New HTN (140/90 or >30/15 rise from booking) > 20 weeks with significant proteinuria (PCR> 30 mg/mmol or urine > 300 mg / 24 hours)[1]

	Symptoms	Headache, vision changes, pain below the ribs, vomiting or sudden oedema
	Examination	Proteinuria, liver tenderness, papilloedema, clonus, small for dates
	Tests	Urine and bloods: FBC, LFT including transaminases, LDH, U&E, urate and clotting
	Rx	Labetalol, methyldopa or nifedipine.
	Monitoring	BP and urine – at least twice weekly and weekly bloods

Examination findings, problems and action required

BP 140/90 – 150/100 and ≤ trace protein (and not high risk)	→ pre-eclampsia tests and DAU appointment[2]
BP >150/100 OR >140/90 and either high risk or protein +	→ same day MAU assessment[2]
Headaches/swelling but BP and urine normal	→ review in 1 week and safety netting advice
Abdominal pain	→ same day MAU assessment

SFH	from 24 weeks the gestation should equal SFH +/– 2 cm. If down by >2 cm → urgent scan.
	If up >2 cm consider polyhydramnios (movements may not be strong) and check for DM.
Foetal lie	From 34 weeks should be cephalic.
FHR	Not necessary if there is no concern present but usually performed for maternal satisfaction.
	Normal range is 110–160 bpm.
Weight	Aim <1 kg/week.
Glycosuria	Glucose trace → repeat (e.g. in 1 week) but usually no action required.
	'2+ or above on 1 occasion or 1+ or above on 2 or more occasions'[3] request an OGTT
Proteinuria	Send for MSU and PCR.
Reduced FM	→ MAU
	If unsure, lie on the left side for 2 hours and count foetal movements. If <10 → MAU
	Foetuses do have periods of sleep but these rarely last longer than 90 mins.[4]

Doctor's Notes

Patient   Debbie Paton   30 years   F
PMH   Miscarriage at 8 weeks
Medications   No current medications
Allergies   No information
Consultations No recent consultations
Investigations No recent investigations
Household   No household members registered

Example Consultation — Bleeding in Pregnancy

Open ☐	Oh dear. (Silence.)
Sense ☐	I can see you are very upset.
History ☐	When did you realise you were pregnant? (Encourages the history from the beginning.) What was the date of the first day of your last period?
Flags ☐	Do you feel lightheaded or unwell? Any severe pain?
Risk ☐	Have you had a heavy bleed? You have been pregnant before?
Impact ☐	What has been going through your mind since the bleeding?
ICE ☐	As you have experience of bleeding in pregnancy, do you know what happens next? Is there anything else you were wondering? Exercise is safe in the first trimester.
Curious ☐	I'm interested to know more about you. Do you have a partner? You mentioned your work?
Summary ☐	To summarise, you are having some spotting and lower discomfort 5 weeks into your second pregnancy. You previously had a miscarriage at 8 weeks. You are worried that netball could have triggered this bleeding. You are concerned about your fertility and hoping for further tests and a scan?
Empathy ☐	This must feel like a roller-coaster of emotions.
O/E ☐	I would like to examine you if I may; do another pregnancy test, take your blood pressure and pulse, feel your tummy, examine you internally to make sure you are not tender, as this may be a sign of an ectopic pregnancy, which is a pregnancy in the wrong place, then look at the neck of the womb, by inserting a speculum. Would this be okay? Would you like a chaperone?
Impression ☐	The neck of the womb is closed which is good. If the neck of the womb were open, a miscarriage would be inevitable. But as it is closed we can only wait and see. We call this a threatened miscarriage.
Empathy ☐	I appreciate it is an anxious time and frustrating when you have no control.
Explanation ☐	Although bleeding in pregnancy cannot be considered 'normal', it is very common, especially if it is light spotting without pain. It may be what we call an implantation bleed, which happens as the embryo settles into the womb. Many women in your situation will go on to have a normal pregnancy. However, unfortunately, about one in four pregnancies end in miscarriage. If this happens, then, even if you have two miscarriages, research has found this is usually just very bad luck. We can ask for genetic testing if you have three miscarriages but not two as this is very common. It is also very reassuring that you have fallen pregnant twice which means you do not need a fertility referral.
Empower ☐	You said work was stressful. Any opportunity to help your general well-being is important; regular exercise, eating and sleeping well and avoiding alcohol can all balance the stress, whether you are pregnant or trying for a baby.
Options ☐	I think we now need to keep a close eye on this pregnancy. Unfortunately, the pregnancy is too small for a scan: we don't see anything on a scan until 6 weeks. However, as you have had some pain, I am keen to do a couple of blood tests to measure the pregnancy hormone 48 hours apart which can be useful when determining if this is likely to be a pregnancy going to plan or whether this could be an ectopic pregnancy.
Future ☐	I will make an appointment at the EPAU clinic for your scan in 1 week's time. Please can you wait in reception and I will ask the phlebotomist to take your blood and please make a blood test appointment for around 48 hours later if possible. Is that okay?
Safety net ☐	If you have any increased pain or bleeding, any pain in your shoulder, feel lightheaded or unwell then you must see a doctor as he or she would then check this was not an ectopic pregnancy, but there is no sign of this today.

Patient's Story

Bleeding in Pregnancy

Doctor's notes Debbie Paton, 30 years, G2P0. PMH: Miscarriage at 8 weeks. Medications: None.

How to act Not tearful but upset.

PC *'I'm not sure if I'm having a miscarriage.'*

History You have felt your typical *'period drone'* for the past 2 days.

Then started spotting this morning.

No severe pains, mostly mild cramps.

You found out you were pregnant last week.

Since then, you have felt over the moon!

You lost your first pregnancy at 8 weeks.

Social You work in a bank. If asked about work, state: *'It is stressful.'*

You enjoy drinking alcohol but stopped once you knew you were pregnant.

You have a long-term partner. He wanted the pregnancy more than you at first but, after the first miscarriage, you realised it is what you want too.

ICE You worry if it is something that you have done.

'I played netball 2 days ago.'

You are worried there is something wrong and would like tests.

You expect the doctor will send you for a scan like last time.

You are also worried about conceiving again.

You have now been trying for over a year.

You are hoping for tests and a referral to fertility. Be pushy at first.

Examination Abdo SNT. Cervical os is closed. No adnexal tenderness.

BP 120/60. HR 72 bpm. Pregnancy test positive.

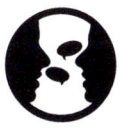

Maternal Health – 3

Learning Points

Bleeding in Pregnancy

EPAU for scan if >6 weeks and abdominal pain or bleeding
unknown gestation
previous ectopic or molar pregnancy   … remember to safety net!

Foetal heart activity would be expected from around 6 weeks.

Refer to same-day urgent gynaecology if there are symptoms/signs of an ectopic.

For a pregnancy of unknown location, EPAU may do serial β-hCGs (48 hours apart). The GP may do this if he/she feels confident to do so. If you are unsure, speak to your local EPAU for advice.

A viable uterine pregnancy should have an increased β-hCG of 63% in 48 hours.[1]

An ectopic may present with rectal/urinary symptoms
syncope or vague symptoms
shoulder pain

Bleeding and no pain <6 weeks Repeat the urine pregnancy test after 7 days.
Return if positive or symptoms continue.
Safety net for ectopic symptoms and pain.
A negative pregnancy test means the pregnancy has miscarried.
Consider an EPAU USS, if possible RPOC.

Examination required Abdomen
PV for adnexal tenderness or cervical excitation
  or sign of ectopic pregnancy
Cervical os
  for a threatened or complete (os closed) miscarriage
  or inevitable (os open) miscarriage
Observations to check if haemodynamically stable

Bleeding or pain >16 weeks Bleeding or moderate pain >16 weeks → MAU.
If severe bleeding 999 to delivery suite.
For mild pain consider SPD/PGP, constipation and rule out a UTI.
Consider all usual causes of abdominal pain.

Why give anti-D rhesus prophylaxis? A scenario to explain why …

Rhesus negative (antibody negative) mum-to-be → haemorrhage at birth → develops antibodies → haemolytic disease of baby 2.

Anti-D prophylaxis is offered to all Rhesus negative mums. However, recognising that the fetus may also be Rh D negative, some trusts now offer cell-free foetal DNA testing at 16 weeks. If this indicates the fetus is Rh D positive, Anti-D is offered at 28 weeks and delivery. If cell-free foetal DNA testing at 16 weeks indicates the fetus is Rh D negative, blood samples are taken at 28 weeks and delivery, but Anti-D is not offered.

Anti-D not required: if <12/40 and for a miscarriage or ectopic which is medically managed or threatened.[2]

MATERNAL HEALTH – 3

Doctor's Notes

Patient	Jayne Smith	37 years	F
PMH	Type 2 diabetes		
	Obesity – last BMI 35		
Medications	Metformin 1 g BD		
	Gliclazide 40 mg daily		
	Rigevidon		
Allergies	No information		
Consultations	No recent consultations		
Investigations	2 months ago HbA1c 51 mmol/mol		
Household	No household members registered		

Example Consultation

Diabetes in Pregnancy

Open — It's great that you are considering this in advance.

Experience — Are you aware of any risks of diabetes in pregnancy?

Sense — I can see you are keen to control your diabetes. We will look at your diabetes very carefully.

ICE — Is there anything that particularly frightens you? What have you been advised so far? Is there anything else you were wondering?

Curious — You seem to have a good understanding. Where has this information come from?

Explanation — Babies can be larger and therefore it's important to control your blood sugar as much as possible. Often babies need delivering a few weeks earlier. They do sometimes initially need help with their blood sugar after birth and some babies need help in the baby unit for a while. In later life, the children can have a higher risk of obesity or developing diabetes themselves. Being overweight can also put you at risk of pregnancy complications so you may need to take other medications such as aspirin when you do become pregnant.

Risk — Do you know what your last HbA1c was?

History — Are you otherwise well? When do you take your medicines? I'm interested to know more about you and your routine.

Impact — How does your diabetes impact on your life? Is there any time you struggle with your diabetes?

Summary — To summarise, you have had good control of your diabetes since diagnosis but your HbA1c has crept up and you are hoping for better control as you are planning a pregnancy. You are worried about risks to baby and are frightened about labour.

Empathy — I appreciate the risks can potentially be scary.

Impression — Being diligent about your health is likely to give a much better outcome for you and baby. You should be aiming for an HbA1c of <48 mmol/mol. This can be a challenge and we need to avoid hypos – a nickname for hypoglycaemic episodes – which means the blood sugar is too low, putting you at risk.

Explanation — When you do fall pregnant, blood sugars can be more erratic especially if vomiting.

Experience — Are you aware of the symptoms of a hypo?

Options — Do you have a blood glucose and ketone testing kit? You should start taking 5 mg folic acid, a higher dose than for non-diabetic women, and I will prescribe it for you. You also need extra vitamin D. Let's also arrange your diabetic eye check now. I will ask the secretary to arrange this. You will need more frequent eye checks in pregnancy. We should change your gliclazide to insulin. How do you feel about this? We then need to discuss the benefits of metformin. There is a special clinic which manages women with diabetes in pregnancy and I will refer you to this.

Empower — Continuing exercise will help control your blood sugar. You could see the dietician in case there are any other dietary changes you could make. Any extra weight loss you can achieve will both help you conceive and reduce risk in pregnancy.

Empathy — It is normal to feel anxious and concerned about labour. Is there anything specific which has been going through your mind? The team will be monitoring you and baby closely and discuss with you when they believe is the safest time to deliver baby. If you do feel that the worry and anxiety about labour is affecting you, come and see me and we can talk through your options. What are your thoughts?

Future — Shall we look at your blood readings again in a month, then consider insulin together? We should monitor your kidney function and check your chickenpox and rubella status when we take your bloods. Let's do this a couple of days before we meet next time so we can discuss your latest HbA1c then. Please bring a urine sample at the same time to check for protein.

Safety net — Until the HbA1c comes down, are you happy to continue contraception? That is a lot of information, do you have any questions?

Maternal Health – 4

Patient's Story

Diabetes in Pregnancy

Doctor's notes Jayne Smith, 37 years. PMH: type 2 diabetes, obesity. Last HbA1c 51 mmol/mol.
Medications: Metformin 1 g bd, Gliclazide 40 mg daily, Rigevidon.

How to act Very interested in your health

PC *'My husband and I would like to start a family.*
I just wanted some advice regarding my diabetes.'

History You have had diabetes for 2 years.

There is a strong history of type 2 diabetes in your family but you are aware your weight contributed to developing diabetes. The diagnosis provided motivation to make lifestyle changes needed to lose weight and get healthier. You are aware there is some way to go but are proud you have managed to get your BMI down from 46 to 35. You have changed your diet and taken up distance running.

You take great care but have recently been on holiday.

You expect your blood sugar may be worse than usual.

You eat well but often struggle to find time to exercise.

You have been reading a lot about diabetes and pregnancy.

You have a BM testing kit which you bought. You know the symptoms of a 'hypo'.

Social Dental nurse. Married 2 years ago. No alcohol and never smoked.

ICE You are unsure whether you should stay on your metformin.

You expect the GP will say start insulin and you are happy with this.

You are mostly worried about the risks to the baby after birth and in the future.

You are scared about the labour as you know babies with diabetic mums tend to be big.

You would like advice about preparing for pregnancy with DM.

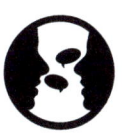

Maternal Health – 4

Learning Points   Diabetes in Pregnancy

OGTTs   'Diagnose gestational diabetes if the woman has either:

a fasting plasma glucose level of 5.6 mmol/litre or above or

a 2-hour plasma glucose level of 7.8 mmol/litre or above.'[1]

Counselling pre-conception[1]

Book an eye check and urine ACR before pregnancy. Eye checks recommended during pregnancy.[1]

Diet/exercise to aim for a healthy weight.

Folic acid 5 mg /day until 12 weeks.

Offer monthly HbA1c pre-pregnancy and a BM and ketone kit.

Pre-pregnancy and pregnancy HbA1c targets should be appropriate for the individual and an 'HbA1c level below 48 mmol/mol (6.5%)'[1] is recommended if possible and if hypoglycaemic risk is low.

Controlled blood sugars 'will reduce the risk of miscarriage, congenital malformation, stillbirth and neonatal death.'[1]

Offer a structured education programme.

'Women with diabetes may be advised to use metformin as an adjunct or alternative to insulin in the preconception period and during pregnancy, when the likely benefits from improved blood glucose control outweigh the potential for harm. All other oral blood glucose-lowering agents should be discontinued before pregnancy and insulin substituted. [2008]'[1]

Risks[1]

Increased risk of macrosomia and therefore birth complications.

The possibility of transient morbidity in the newborn and possible admission to the neonatal ITU.

The risk of obesity and diabetes in the child in later life.

Nausea and vomiting during pregnancy may affect blood sugar control.

Hypoglycaemia unawareness during pregnancy.

Metformin

Discuss the benefits of glycaemic control vs the potential for harm. Refer to http://www.uktis.org/

Diagnosed gestational diabetes

Refer to   'joint diabetes and antenatal clinic within 1 week [new 2015]'[1]

a dietitian.

'Offer immediate treatment with insulin, with or without metformin, as well as changes in diet and exercise, to women with gestational diabetes who have a fasting plasma glucose level of 7.0 mmol/litre or above at diagnosis. [new 2015]'[1]

Encourage foods with a low glycaemic index and regular daily exercise.

Targets   Do not use HbA1c routinely in the 2nd/3rd trimester.[1]

Without risking hypoglycaemia, if possible, aim for 'fasting: 5.3 mmol/litre and 1 hour after meals: 7.8 mmol/litre **or** 2 hours after meals: 6.4 mmol/litre. [new 2015]'[1]

Maternal Health – 4

Doctor's Notes

Patient	Jenny Eyre	26 years	F
PMH	Spontaneous vaginal delivery 6 weeks ago and 2 years ago.		
Medications	No current medications		
Allergies	No information		
Consultations	No recent consultations		
Investigations	No recent investigations		
Household	Olivia Eyre	6 weeks	F
	Logan Eyre	2 years	M
	Thomas Eyre	29 years	M

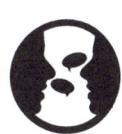

Example Consultation — Postnatal Check

Open ☐ — Congratulations. How are you doing? How is the little one?

Risk ☐ — What was your experience of pregnancy? And the birth? Any stitches? Any medical issues? And how is baby? How is feeding going? Any nipple or breast pain?

Empathy ☐ — Many women are tearful or feel low with the emotions and challenges of a new baby.

Flags ☐ — Emotionally, how have you been doing? What support do you have? Has your bleeding settled? Have you had any tummy pain? Fever? Or discharge? Do you know if your placenta was complete? Have you had intercourse yet? Have you had any thoughts about contraception going forward?

History ☐ — And you are otherwise well, no other medical problems? Who is at home?

Curious ☐ — I'm interested to know more about you. What support do you have?

ICE ☐ — Was there anything else you wanted to ask? Or weren't sure about? Is there anything you were hoping we would discuss today?

Summary ☐ — So just to summarise, all seems well; the only issue is bleeding.

Sense ☐ — You do not seem concerned by this.

O/E ☐ — I would like to take your blood pressure, heart rate and temperature, then examine you to ensure there is no sign of infection. By this stage your bleeding should have settled. May I feel your tummy? And I do think it would be helpful to feel your womb and take some swabs by doing a vaginal examination. Would this be okay? Would you like a chaperone?

Impression ☐ — You may have a minor infection of the womb called endometritis, which is common.

Experience ☐ — Have you come across this?

Explanation ☐ — Sometimes it is caused by remaining parts of the placenta being still inside the womb but it usually clears with antibiotics.

Options ☐ — I would recommend 1 week of a penicillin called co-amoxiclav, which is safe when breastfeeding. I would recommend treating, as we wouldn't want any infection to get worse and make you unwell. It is your choice so long as you are aware of the risks of not treating at this stage.

Future ☐ — If you prefer to monitor this we should meet again in a week …

Safety net ☐ — … or earlier if you noticed any tummy pain, fever, increased bleeding or discharge. Is this what you would like to do? Also if you find that your mood drops or if there are any problems with your breasts or new concerns do let me know.

Empower ☐ — With regards to the Mirena, you can book in for this at reception, but I would like to ensure your bleeding has settled before we do this. Would you like any other contraception such as the mini pill in the meantime? Okay, take care and do let me know if that bleeding continues, or there are any problems as we discussed. To ensure I have explained things clearly, could you please just tell me what symptoms you are looking out for that you would need to inform a doctor about? That's right. See you next week.

Patient's Story

Postnatal Check

Doctor's notes	Jenny Eyre, 26 years. PMH: SVD 6 weeks ago and 2 years ago. Medications: none.
How to act	You are feeling very well.
PC	*'I've come for my 6-week check.'*
History	All is well. You had a baby girl, Olivia, 6 weeks ago.
	G2P2
	Olivia had her check 2 days ago and she is great.
	You are breastfeeding.
	You have had no mood changes.
	You have full control of your bladder and bowels.
	You had no problems during the pregnancy or labour.
	You do still have some bleeding but no tummy pain. The lochia is still red and hasn't turned yellow yet but the amount is reducing. You were told that your placenta and membranes were intact. You did not require any stitches.
	You have not had intercourse yet due to the continued bleed and lack of opportunity!
	You decline further contraception at this stage as you intend to have a Mirena IUS fitted. You had one after your first pregnancy and got on well with it. You would rather use condoms and breastfeeding to prevent pregnancy whilst you wait for it to be fitted. You have never got on well with contraceptive pills.
ICE	You feel all is well. You have no concerns.
	You had bleeding at this stage with your son Logan, who is now 2, and it settled.
	You would prefer not to have antibiotics and give it one more week.
Social	You have a very supportive husband, and parents close by.
	You work in the research centre at the hospital.
Examination	BP 118/66 HR 62, 36.2°C
	Abdomen soft non-tender and no adnexal tenderness.
	Small amount of bloody discharge visible.

Learning Points — Postnatal Check

Postnatal contraception is not required until day 21.[1] Options:

LAM	If '<6 months postpartum, amenorrhoeic and fully breastfeeding, the lactational amenorrhoea method (LAM) is over 98% effective in preventing pregnancy'.[1]
COCP	May be used from day 21 if not breastfeeding. Additionally use condoms for 7 days.[1]
	If partially breastfeeding 'the benefits of CHC may outweigh the unknown risks'.[1]
POP	May be used from day 21. Additionally use condoms for 7 days.[1]
Injection	The progesterone injection can be given any time postpartum if not breastfeeding[1] and if breastfeeding (off licence) <6 weeks but ideally wait until day 21. Warn women about the risk of bleeding.[1]
Implanon	Can be inserted <21 days postpartum off licence (whether breastfeeding or not).[1]
IUD	Within 48 hours postpartum or from day 28. No additional contraception required.[1]
IUS	From day 28 + condoms for 7 days unless LAM.[1]
Endometritis	Consider if bleeding (which does not appear to be a period) at 6 weeks.
	Consider if abdominal pain or unusual discharge. Manage with antibiotics if systemically well.
	If after antibiotics and swabs it has not resolved, consider urgent USS for RPOC.

Check your local antibiotic guidance for advice on which antibiotics to use.

If features of low mood, be aware of the **Edinburgh Postnatal Depression Scale (EPDS)** but no need to memorise this.

If a fever develops within 14 days postpartum, discuss with obstetrics the need for IV antibiotics.

Sphincter control	1 month of pelvic floor exercises (for urethra, vagina and anus)
	Then refer to physio or bladder/bowel service.
Lochia:	Usually 3 stages: rubra (red blood), serosa (orange) and alba (yellow/white).
	Rubra usually settles by 4 days, serosa around 3 weeks and alba by 6 weeks. All may settle much more quickly.
	Sometimes rubra returns with a lot of physical activity but be aware of endometritis or RPOC if bleeding increases.

Postnatal management of gestational diabetes
Check a FBG at 6–13 weeks.[2]

Postnatal management of pre-eclampsia
In the postnatal period, measure the BP daily for the first 5 days, then every 1–2 days in the first 2 weeks following hospital discharge.[3,4] Weekly postnatal GP assessments are appropriate whilst gradually decreasing the antihypertensive treatment. Ask about headache and epigastric pain.[3]

Reduce the antihypertensive dose if the BP falls <130/80 and consider reducing treatment if the BP falls <140/90. Increase the dose if the BP is ≥ 150/100.[4]

Some women may be off all treatment by the 6-week check.

At the 6-week check a urine dipstick should be tested and if urine protein is ≥ +1, then a 3-month GP review should be arranged. At the 3-month review consider involving the renal team.[4]

Methyldopa should be changed to an alternative treatment following delivery, e.g. labetalol, nifedipine, enalapril, captopril, atenolol or metoprolol can all be used whilst breastfeeding.[4]

Maternal Health – 5

Extra Notes

Chickenpox in Pregnancy

Exposure to chickenpox in pregnancy

Step 1 Was there significant contact?

Contact in the same room for ≥15 minutes, face-to-face contact or contact in the setting of a large open ward.[1]

Step 2 Does she have immunity?

'If there is a definite past history of chickenpox, it is reasonable to assume that she is immune to varicella.'[2]

Step 3 If uncertain check VZV IgG (if the laboratory turnaround time is 24–48 hours).

'At least 80% of women tested will have VZV IgG and can be reassured.'[2]

Step 4 'If the pregnant woman is not immune to VZV and she has had a significant exposure to chickenpox or shingles, she should be offered VZIG as soon as possible or at the very latest within 10 days of the exposure. In the case of continuous household exposures, within 10 days of appearance of the rash in the index case.'[2,3]

'**Adverse effects of VZIG** include pain and erythema at the injection site. The risk of anaphylaxis is cited as less than 0.1%.'[2]

'Susceptible women who have had contact with chickenpox or shingles (regardless of whether or not they have received VZIG) should be asked to notify their doctor or midwife early if a rash develops.'[2]

'The incubation period is between 1 and 3 weeks and the disease is infectious 48 hours before the rash appears and continues to be infectious until the vesicles crust over.'[2]

When chickenpox rash develops in pregnancy

Risks   'pneumonia, hepatitis and encephalitis. Rarely … death'[2]

'Avoid contact with potentially susceptible individuals … until the lesions have crusted over.'[2]

'Symptomatic treatment and hygiene is advised to prevent secondary bacterial infection.'[2]

'**Oral aciclovir**	(off licence)
	for gestation ≥20/40 (and consider if <20/40)
	if presenting within 24 hours of the onset of the rash[2]
IV aciclovir	'to all pregnant women with severe chickenpox'[2]
VZIG	'has no therapeutic benefit once chickenpox has developed'[2]
Refer to hospital	if any complications OR
	'If the woman smokes cigarettes, has chronic lung disease, is immunosuppressed (including those who have taken systemic corticosteroids in the preceding 3 months) or is in the second half of pregnancy.'[2]

'If the pregnant woman develops varicella or shows serological conversion in the first 28 weeks of pregnancy, she has a small risk of FVS (Foetal Varicella Syndrome)'[2] which should be discussed.

Unknown rash in pregnancy – Also check parvovirus B19. Small risk of miscarriage and foetal hydrops.

Maternal Health

CHAPTER 8 OVERVIEW
Gynaecology

	Cases in this chapter	Within the RCGP curriculum: Women's Health RCGP Curriculum Online March 2016[1]	Learning points in the chapter include:
1	Menorrhagia	'Recognise common signs and symptoms of, and know how to manage, gynaecological disease'	NICE Guidance. Heavy Menstrual Bleeding: Assessment and Management. 2007 Dysfunctional Uterine Bleeding
2	PCOS	'Understand that as the sexual partners of some women are women, you must not make assumptions'	PCOS Metformin
3	PMB	'Intervene urgently with suspected malignancy'	CA125 test NICE Guidelines. Suspected Cancer: Recognition and Referral. 2015
4	Menopause and HRT	'Know how the social and biological features of the perimenopause and menopause period interact and affect health'	Menopause Premature menopause
5	Overactive Bladder	'Demonstrate knowledge of women's health problems, conditions and diseases'	Stress, urge and mixed incontinence
Extra Notes	Endometriosis	'Provide information to patients on possible local support services, referral services, networks and groups for women'	Endometriosis PMT
	Ovarian Cyst Management	'Data gathering and interpretation … the use of investigations and examination findings'	Oxfordshire guidance ovarian cyst management
	HRT Risks	'Be familiar with and implement the key national guidelines that influence healthcare provision for women's problems' 'Discuss the psychosocial component of women's health and the need, in some cases, to provide women patients with additional emotional and organisational support (e.g. in relation to … hormone replacement therapy …)'	Vascular risks Breast cancer risk Different preparations (oestrogen only/cyclical combined/continuous combined) Side effects Stopping HRT

1. http://www.rcgp.org.uk/training-exams/gp-curriculum-overview/online-curriculum/caring-for-the-whole-person/3-06-womens-health.aspx

CHAPTER 8 REFERENCES

Menorrhagia
1. NICE Guidelines. CG44. Heavy Menstrual Bleeding: assessment and management. 2007.
2. NICE Guidelines. NG12. Suspected Cancer – recognition and referral. 2015.
3. Mansour D. Safer prescribing of therapeutic norethisterone for women at risk of venous thromboembolism. *J Fam Plann Reprod Health Care*. 2012; 38(3): 148-9.

PCOS
1. NICE. http://cks.nice.org.uk/polycystic-ovary-syndrome#!scenariorecommendation. Revised Feb 2013.
2. http://www.advancedfertility.com/progesterone-withdrawal-test.htm

PMB/Suspected Gynaecological Cancer
1. NICE Guidelines. NG12. Suspected cancer: recognition and referral. June 2015.
2. Postmenopausal Bleeding – Patient Care Pathway. OXF234. Oxford University Hospitals NHS Foundation Trust. June 2014. http://occg.oxnet.nhs.uk/GeneralPractice/ClinicalGuidelines/Gynaecology/Post%20Menopausal%20Bleeding/PMB_pathway_V41.pdf

Menopause and HRT
1. http://www.fsrh.org/pdfs/ContraceptionOver40July10.pdf
2. NICE Guidelines. NG23. Menopause: diagnosis and management. Nov 2015.
3. https://www.evidence.nhs.uk/formulary/bnf/current/6-endocrine-system/64-sex-hormones/641-female-sex-hormones-and-their-modulators/6411-oestrogens-and-hrt/hormone-replacement-therapy
4. NICE. http://cks.nice.org.uk/menopause#!scenariorecommendation:2. Revised Oct 2015.

Overactive Bladder/Urinary Incontinence
1. NICE Guidelines. CG171. Urinary incontinence in women: management. Sep 2013.
2. 'The Guidelines Development Group defined "frail older women" as those with multiple comorbidities, functional impairments such as walking or dressing difficulties and any degree of cognitive impairment.'[1]
3. Gray S.L., et al. *JAMA Intern Med*. 2015; 175(3): 401–7.
4. http://www.oxfordshireccg.nhs.uk/wp-content/uploads/2015/01/Prescribing-Points-June-2015.pdf
5. NICE Guidelines. TA290. Mirabegron for treating symptoms of overactive bladder. Jun 2013.
6. 'At the time of publication (September 2013), desmopressin did not have a UK marketing authorisation for this indication. The prescriber should follow relevant professional guidance, taking full responsibility for the decision. Informed consent should be obtained and documented. See the General Medical Council's Good practice in prescribing and managing medicines and devices for further information.'[1]

Endometriosis
1. NICE. http://cks.nice.org.uk/endometriosis. Revised May 2014.

Ovarian Cysts
1. RCOG Guideline. Guideline No. 34. Ovarian cysts in post-menopausal women.
2. RCOG Guideline, Nov 2011 'Management of Suspected Ovarian Masses in Premenopausal Women'.
3. Oxford guidance. Price N., Traill Z., Goldstein M., et al. Management of ovarian cysts. Joint PCT/Radiology/Gynaecology/Gynae Oncology guidelines. Version 4. Dec 2012.

HRT
1. NICE Guidelines. NG23. Menopause: diagnosis and management. Nov 2015.
2. http://patient.info/doctor/hormone-replacement-therapy-including-benefits-and-risks
3. Kim H.K., Kang S.Y., Chung Y.J., et al. The recent review of the genitourinary syndrome of menopause. *J Menopausal Med*. 2015 Aug; 21(2): 65–71. doi: 10.6118/jmm.2015.21.2.65. Epub 2015 Aug 28.
4. Santen R.J. Vaginal administration of estradiol: effects of dose, preparation and timing on plasma estradiol levels. *Climacteric*. 2015 Apr; 18(2): 121–34. doi: 10.3109/13697137.2014.947254. Epub 2014 Oct 18.
5. http://patient.info/doctor/hrt-topical
6. https://www.rcog.org.uk/globalassets/documents/guidelines/gtg_58.pdf
7. Jones M.E., Schoemaker M.J., Wright L., et al. Menopausal hormonal therapy and breast cancer: what is the true size of the increased risk? *British Journal of Cancer*. 2016; **115**: 607–15.

Doctor's Notes

Patient   Jacqui Mason   25 years   F
PMH   No information
Medications   No current medications
Allergies   No information
Consultations   No recent consultations
Investigations No recent investigations
Household   No household members registered

Example Consultation — Menorrhagia

Open ☐	Oh dear, tell me more about them. What pain do you experience?
Flags ☐	Do you ever bleed between periods or after sex? Any pain during sex? Do you have pain at other times? Have your periods changed?
History ☐	Tell me about your periods from when you first started them. I'm interested to know more about you … how is your general health? Any medical problems? Any other symptoms? Do you take any medicines? Do they help? Who are the important people in your life? Do you work? Any FH I should be aware of? Or of bleeding conditions?
Impact ☐	How do your periods impact on your life?
ICE ☐	Have you had thoughts as to what could be causing these heavy periods? Is there anything else that you have been wondering? Any other worries? Is there anything particular you were hoping for today?
Sense ☐	I see you feel strongly about seeing a gynaecologist.
Curious ☐	When did you start to think about endometriosis? Why did you think this may be endometriosis? Does anyone you know suffer with this?
O/E ☐	Would you like me to examine you? Your tummy and internally. This may be helpful as your periods changed last year. I may be able to feel a fibroid, a harmless lump in the womb which can cause heavy periods.
Empathy ☐	Your periods are impacting on your life. Especially at work.
Summary ☐	You are concerned about endometriosis and the possible complication with infertility. This is an understandable concern and you want tests to find the diagnosis. Is that correct?
Impression ☐	You are suffering with heavy menstrual bleeding which we call menorrhagia. Reassuringly, you do not have additional symptoms like pain during sex which may suggest endometriosis.
Experience ☐	Do you know any treatment options for menorrhagia?
Explanation ☐	Everyone's periods are different. When women feel their periods are too heavy or they impact on their life, we call this menorrhagia. The clots you mention are blood which has grouped together. There is always the possibility of endometriosis but the operation often needed to diagnose endometriosis carries its own risk. Therefore, without the additional symptoms, I would recommend trying treatment for menorrhagia first.
Options ☐	We could do a blood test to check for anaemia. Meanwhile treat the menorrhagia with either a hormone treatment, the pill, which may reduce your periods, or a tablet called tranexamic acid which reduces the amount of bleeding. Other options include the Mirena coil which can be helpful to reduce heavy painful periods. We could request an ultrasound to check for a fibroid. If we aren't winning, and we'll know soon, then we could think about endometriosis. I appreciate this does not relieve your concern about blockages of the tubes. However, it is reassuring that you have regular periods and if you struggled to fall pregnant we could have a low threshold for referring you to gynaecology. This way we have tried the least invasive route. What are your thoughts?
Empower ☐	Okay, I can see this is important to you. Okay.
Future ☐	Would you like to try a medication in the meantime? Can we arrange a blood test to check for anaemia? I will refer you and, if you do not receive an appointment within a month, inform the secretary please.
Safety net ☐	If your symptoms change – a change to your pain or bleeding pattern– let a GP know.

Gynaecology – 1

Patient's Story — Menorrhagia

Doctor's notes	Jacqui Mason, 25 years. PMH: None. Medications: None.
How to act	A little pushy. Intelligent.
PC	*'It's my periods. They are becoming very heavy.'*
History	Your periods started aged 14 years. They became heavy and painful a year ago.
	The pulling pain starts on the morning of your period in your lower stomach.
	The pain lasts 2 days. Your period cycle is 8/30 with 5 heavy days.
	You are changing a tampon every 2 hours. *'There are clots!'*
	During a period, you have to leave meetings, which is embarrassing.
	Paracetamol doesn't help.
	No IMB or PCB. You have no abnormal discharge.
	Jacob is your boyfriend of two years. No dyspareunia.
	You both had an STI check at the start of your relationship.
	You have never had an STI. You have never been pregnant.
	Your first smear was normal. For contraception you use condoms.
	You are otherwise well. No PMH, medicines or FH.
	No one you know suffers with it. Decline an examination. *'It will be normal.'*
Social	You are a graphic designer. You enjoy your job.
	You rent your home with your boyfriend and have a good relationship.
	You drink alcohol occasionally and do not smoke.
ICE	Two weeks ago you read an article in a magazine about endometriosis.
	It mentioned it causes heavy painful periods and can lead to blockages in the tubes.
	You believe you have endometriosis.
	You are concerned that this could make you infertile.
	You are hoping to get married next year and start a family.
	You do not want hormones as you want your body to be natural.
	You thought the GP may suggest the pill. You want a referral to a gynaecologist.
	Become angry if the doctor does not offer a gynaecology referral.
	You do not want to take medicines without knowing what is wrong.
	You demand to see a gynaecologist. You do not take no for an answer.

Learning Points — Menorrhagia

DUB	Abnormal uterine bleeding in the absence of pregnancy, infection or tumour.
Menorrhagia	'Excessive menstrual blood loss which interferes with the woman's physical, emotional, social and material quality of life'[1] … so ask about impact!
Cause	Dysfunctional uterine bleeding (DUB) if no cause for menorrhagia is found.
	Iatrogenic (e.g. IUD) or psychosomatic disturbance.
	Fibroids, endometrial hyperplasia or cancer, endometriosis or PID.
	Hypothyroidism or blood clotting disorders.
Red flags	IMB, PCB, pelvic pain or pressure – possible structural or histological abnormality.
Examination	'If the history suggests heavy menstrual bleeding without structural or histological abnormality, pharmaceutical treatment can be started without carrying out a physical examination or other investigations at initial consultation.'[1]
Investigations	FBC if symptoms or signs suggest anaemia, structural or histological abnormality.
	TFT if symptoms or signs are present.
	Anticoagulation screen if required.
	If PCB or IMB: View the cervix and refer for colposcopy if abnormal.
	Infection (chlamydia) swab.
	If red flags are present, an USS is indicated.
Imaging and biopsy	'Ultrasound is the first-line diagnostic tool for identifying structural abnormalities.'[1]
	A hysteroscopy ± endometrial biopsy may be required following an USS.
	Indications: Medication not effective or persistent bleeding.
	Women aged 45 years and over.
	IMB, PCB, a change in periods or pain/pressure symptoms.
	Palpable uterus on examination of the abdomen or mass on PV examination. (If 'not obviously uterine fibroids'[2] then 2WW).
Immediate referral	NICE advise 'immediate referral' to a gynaecology specialist if:
	Fibroids are palpable from the abdomen.
	Intracavity fibroids or uterus >12 cm on USS[1]
2WW referral	Consider if a 2WW referral is indicated – ensure you are up to date with all the 2WW criteria for gynaecological cancers in the NICE Guidance for Suspected Cancer[2]
Routine referral	3/12 without a response to treatment, unclear diagnosis (not meeting the above criteria for urgent referrals) or severe anaemia (use clinical judgement).
Management options	Tranexamic acid (side effects include GI disturbance and headaches)
	Ibuprofen/mefenamic acid.
	Hormonal: IUS, COCP or norethisterone.
	Surgical, e.g. endometrial ablation or hysterectomy.
Norethisterone VTE risk	Consider medroxyprogesterone acetate as an alternative to norethisterone to delay menses or in the treatment of menorrhagia in women with additional risk factors for VTE: >35 years and smokers or overweight or personal or FH of VTE. [3]

Gynaecology – 1

Doctor's Notes

Patient   Juliet Perkins   27 years   F
PMH   Acne
Medications   Epiduo
Allergies   No known allergies
Consultations Telephone call 6 months ago to repeat Epiduo treatment for acne.
Investigations No recent investigations
Household   No household members registered

Example Consultation — PCOS

Open ☐	Tell me more about your periods from when they first started.
Sense ☐	I can see that you are worried.
History ☐	When did your periods change? Have you noticed anything else that you don't think is right? I see you have acne in your medical history – how is that now? Have you noticed any hairs on the face or neck? Your general history – do you have any pain – generally or during intercourse? Have you ever been pregnant? Or had an STI? Have you had normal smear tests? Are you in a relationship? Do you live with anyone else? What work do you do? Do you smoke or drink much alcohol?
Flags ☐	Because you haven't had a period I need to double check – is there any chance you may be pregnant?
Risk ☐	Has anyone in your family had trouble with their periods or other women's health problems?
ICE ☐	What has crossed your mind about what may be causing this? Is there anything else you have been wondering? Anything that you are worried about? What did you think I may suggest? Is there anything else you were hoping for?
Curious ☐	What conversations with others have you had about polycystic ovaries?
Summary ☐	To summarise, for several years your periods have been less than monthly which has made you question cysts in the ovaries. You came across this when your friend's sister needed IVF and her diagnosis of PCOS has made you worry about your own fertility.
O/E ☐	May I examine you – have a closer look at your skin and check your weight and height?
Empathy ☐	I appreciate it may be disconcerting not having regular periods and a worry when you have heard that this may be linked to problems with fertility.
Impression ☐	I think you may be right. Polycystic ovaries are when we see cysts on your ovaries. You have mentioned having a scan and I agree this would be helpful. If we see cysts on your ovaries, it is likely that you have PCOS because you have the associated problems, e.g. acne and infrequent periods. There are also some blood tests which can help with the diagnosis.
Impact ☐	I appreciate this may be concerning; what is going through your mind?
Experience ☐	Do you know what doctors suggest if we see cysts on your ovaries?
Explanation ☐	The lining of the womb doesn't tend to get thicker and thicker but the alteration to your hormones can put you at increased risk of womb cancer in the long term.
Options ☐	To protect the womb, we should aim for four to five periods a year or protect your womb with the hormone progesterone. You have questioned whether metformin may be helpful. We should be guided by test results. Metformin is a tablet usually used for diabetes. The manufacturer did not intend it to be used for PCOS which means if prescribed it is off licence, but it has been shown to help with weight, the hair on the face and sugar levels which can creep up in PCOS. It can also help with fertility. However, I suggest waiting until we have your test results back and make the diagnosis.
Empower ☐	Because PCOS can put you at increased risk of raised sugars and cholesterol, which in turn can increase the risks to the health of your heart and blood vessels, keeping active, like you already do with your sport, can protect you in the long term, as can eating a healthy diet. You may find significant lifestyle changes alone prevent the need for metformin. I will provide you with information leaflets on the hormone options we can use to ensure you have five periods a year and we can discuss this when we meet again.
Future ☐	Although it sounds like PCOS, I would like to arrange blood tests to check your testosterone and other hormone levels and make sure there is no other hormonal cause for this by checking your thyroid function and prolactin. I would like to check your general health bloods including your sugar and cholesterol. Shall we catch up again, after your blood test, on the phone? We can then talk about the hormone options and also inducing a withdrawal bleed just before the ultrasound scan which can be a helpful part of the ultrasound test.
Safety net ☐	I don't expect you to experience any new symptoms; however, occasionally cysts can cause pain so if you ever have stomach pain please see a doctor.

Gynaecology – 2

Patient's Story

PCOS

Doctor's notes	Juliet Perkins, 27 years. PMH: Acne. Medication: Epiduo.
How to act	Concerned.
PC	*'I haven't had a period for 4 months.'*
History	Your periods started aged 13 years and have always been every 4–8 weeks until about 3 years ago when they started to range from 1–5 months.
	Your periods are not heavy. You have no IMB, PCB or dyspareunia.
	You have no abdominal pain.
	You have never had an STI.
	You have never been pregnant.
	Normal smear 2 years ago.
	You have no other medical history apart from acne. You have no family history.
Social	You are a teacher for children with learning disabilities.
	You have a female partner of 2 years.
	You drink occasionally <14 units a week and have never smoked.
	You enjoy running and tennis.
ICE	You have heard that you may have polycystic ovaries.
	You are concerned that 4-monthly periods are not normal. You worry that the lining of your womb is getting thicker and thicker; is this dangerous?
	Your friend's sister, aged 33 years, has just started IVF treatment.
	She mentioned that she has PCOS.
	You would like a scan.
	You have been reading and want to know if you can start metformin.
Examination	Mild acne. Some long hairs below the chin. BMI 27.

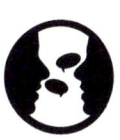

Gynaecology – 2

Learning Points — PCOS

Diagnosis[1]	2 out of 3 of …	
	Hyperandrogenism	*either* symptoms (e.g. hirsutism, acne, alopecia) *or* biochemical (abnormal blood tests).
	Cysts	>12 in 1 ovary or ovarian volume >10 ml.
	Decreased ovulation	Oligomennorhoea or amenorrhoea.
Other symptoms	Weight gain or acanthosis nigricans.[1]	
Investigations	Testosterone, SHBG, LH, FSH, TSH, prolactin, T4, HbA1c and lipids.[1]	
Diagnostic	Hyperandrogenism – Testosterone (increased) and SHBG (low/normal).[1]	
	Elevated LH:FSH ratio also supports the diagnosis.	
Other causes	Premature ovarian failure – increased LH and FSH.[1]	
	Hypogonadotropic hypogonadism – decreased LH and FSH.[1]	
	Hypothyroidism – raised TSH and low T4.	
	Hyperprolactinaemia – however, prolactin may also be mildly elevated in PCOS.[1]	
Complications	Raised glucose and lipids.	
USS	For diagnosis (ovaries).	
	Or if oligo/amenorrhoea	induce a withdrawal bleed (see below) then refer for USS.
		If endometrial thickness >10 mm → endometrial sampling.[1]
Lifestyle	Decrease CV risk – exercise, weight loss and low GI diet.	
Oligomenorrhoea	Prevent endometrial hyperplasia by inducing a withdrawal bleed every 3 months, with either cyclical progesterone or the COCP (unless protected by the IUS).[1]	
For acne	Usual acne Rx or co-cyprindiol for acne and hirsutism.	
For hirsutism	Bleach and electrolysis.	
	Eflornithine cream	May cause skin irritation.
		Review and stop if no effect, e.g. at 4 months.
For weight	General advice and consider metformin and orlistat.	
Complications	Weight gain, CVD, infertility due to anovulation, diabetes, high cholesterol.	
	Endometrial hyperplasia and carcinoma.[1]	
Pregnancy plans	GP – advice about lifestyle and weight loss.	
	Specialists – metformin, clomiphene, gonadotrophins or fertility Rx.[1]	
If pregnant	OGTT <20 weeks.[1] Increased risk of HTN, pre-eclampsia and premature birth.[1]	
Metformin	Unlicensed for PCOS, initiated by a specialist[1], can improve insulin sensitivity, help to normalise menstrual cycle and it may help with weight loss or hirsutism.	
Investigating secondary amenorrhoea		Consider a progesterone withdrawal test.[2]

Gynaecology – 2

Doctor's Notes

Patient	Hilda Rowland	53 years	F
PMH	Mirena coil inserted aged 48 years		
	Menorrhagia		
Medications	No current medications		
Allergies	No information		
Consultations	No recent consultations		
Investigations	No recent investigations		
Household	Brian Rowland	55 years	M

Example Consultation — Post-Menopausal Bleeding

Open ☐ — What's led to this decision? Tell me more about the bleeding? Any pattern? And your periods prior to this?

History ☐ — Is your general health good? Any other medical problems? Do you take any medicines? Tell me more about you? Are you active? Have you had any menopausal symptoms? Have you had children?

Flags ☐ — It is helpful to know if you are sexually active and if there is bleeding afterwards. I always check there is no risk of infection – any discharge? Other sexual partners? Any weight loss?

Risk ☐ — Any family history you are aware of? When was your last smear? Have you had any abnormal smears?

Sense ☐ — You seem relaxed about this bleeding.

ICE ☐ — You mentioned the bleeding is likely due to the coil. Why do you think that? Has anything else crossed your mind? Are you worried about anything? What did you think we may decide today?

Impact ☐ — How has this bleeding impacted on your life?

Summary ☐ — To summarise, you were warned the coil may cause abnormal bleeding and is usually in for 5 years, therefore this bleeding has not come as a shock but has been irritating. You don't want the heavy periods to return but are hoping for a trial without the coil.

O/E ☐ — I do not think we should remove the coil today as I do not yet know the cause of the problem. But I would like to examine you – feel your tummy, have a look with a speculum to see if the bleeding could be coming from the vagina or the neck of the womb called the cervix, and then feel the womb if I may? Would you like a chaperone? Please go behind the curtain, undress from the waist down, get underneath the top sheet and let me know when you are ready … You have no sign of infection but may I check some swabs to be sure? May I check your weight and height?

Impression ☐ — My concern is that you may have gone through the menopause. I say 'may have' because we don't know whether the absence of bleeding is due to your coil. Bleeding after the menopause can be common but needs investigation.

Explanation ☐ — There are many possible reasons for the bleeding: a fibroid which is a harmless lump in the womb; a polyp which is originally harmless but may have the potential to become a cancer; it may be due to the coil, but the coil's hormone usually lasts for 7 years; the bleeding may also be coming from the cervix or vaginal walls which become more fragile as we age but they look fine today. I will send the swabs to also rule out infection. The priority is ruling out a cancer which can cause abnormal bleeding.

Options ☐ — We refer all women who bleed after the menopause urgently for an USS which is a jelly scan to check the womb shows no sign of a cancer. What are your thoughts?

Empathy ☐ — I appreciate me mentioning the possibility of cancer may come as a shock. Especially when the bleeding at the 5-year mark has made sense from what previous doctors have mentioned. As I say, in most cases nothing serious is found; however, I am sorry if this is upsetting and causes worry whilst we consider the possibility.

Future ☐ — Let's now go through what you can expect in the next few weeks. At the ultrasound scan they will insert the probe into the vagina to look at the womb. They may suggest proceeding with a camera into the womb to have a closer look and take biopsies, little samples of the womb. If they do not remove the coil at the hospital, we can do this afterwards. Please make a follow-up appointment with me to go through what they have found, a few days after the ultrasound.

Safety net ☐ — You should be seen within 2 weeks from today. If you have not received your appointment within 10 days let me know. If your bleeding becomes heavier or you have pain let a GP know, please. If you have any questions just leave a message at the front desk and I'll give you a ring. Try not to worry – remember we are being thorough.

Gynaecology – 3

Patient's Story

Post-Menopausal Bleeding

Doctor's notes	Hilda Rowland, 53 years.
	PMH: Menorrhagia. Mirena coil inserted aged 48 years. Medications: None.
How to act	Relaxed.
PC	*'I wondered if we could remove my coil now.'*
History	You had the coil inserted 5 years ago for menorrhagia.
	You stopped being sexually active with your husband a few years ago.
	Over the last 3 months you have started bleeding.
	You have never been on HRT and take no other medication.
	Your last period was 3 years ago. Your smears are up to date.
	You have had no spotting until 3 months ago, with no pattern.
	You have no abdominal pain.
	You have not lost weight.
	You had hot flushes for a couple of years but these stopped a year ago.
	You have no urinary or bowel problems.
	You have been irritated by having to remember to take towels with you.
Social	A headmistress for the local primary school.
	You enjoy walking and you are a well-known member of the community.
	You lead a busy lifestyle with the school and church group charity events.
	You have never smoked and enjoy a sherry on weekends.
ICE	You believe your coil has started to run out which is why you would like it out.
	You are not worried, as you were told you may bleed at random times and it usually lasts for 5 years, so this makes sense to you.
	You expect the doctor will want to remove it today and then it will be sorted.
	Another possibility is that you could have another one. You just worry about the menorrhagia coming back but wonder if you could try without it first.
	If the doctor mentions that this could be cancer react to this …
	'You think I have cancer? You've got me worried now!'
Examination	The vulva, vagina and cervix look healthy. The coil string is visible.
	No palpable pelvic masses.
	Abdomen soft, non-tender and no masses.
	BMI 25.

Gynaecology – 3

Learning Points — Suspected Gynaecological Cancer

Always refer to the full text. Suspected Cancer: Recognition and referral. NICE 2015.

Cervical

When to examine the vagina and cervix with a speculum and palpate the uterus/ovaries:

Every woman with abnormal or post-coital bleeding or pelvic pain.

Do not rely on recent smear tests.

Do not wait for the result of a smear test if there is any abnormality on the cervix. Refer 2WW.

Ovarian

When to request CA125 testing for possible ovarian cancer:

Age	Any woman (>18 years). Especially if over 50 years.
Symptoms	Persistent abdominal distention (bloating), early satiety, loss of appetite, pelvic or abdominal pain, increased urinary frequency or urgency.[1]
Symptom frequency	'Persistent or frequent … particularly more than 12 times per month.'[1]
Consider also if	'unexplained weight loss, fatigue or changes in bowel habit'.[1]
Be aware	> 50 years 'IBS rarely presents for the first time in women.'[1]

CA125 is ≥ 35 IU/ml

Urgently (within 2 weeks) 'arrange an ultrasound scan of the abdomen and pelvis'.[1] If this suggested a cancer the patient would then require a 2WW gynaecology referral.

CA125 is <35 IU/ml OR ≥ 35 IU/ml and the USS is normal

Re-assess for other conditions then safety net for more frequent/persistent or new symptoms.[1]

Endometrial

2WW Gynaecology	≥ 55 years with PMB
	Consider if <55 years with PMB[1]

However, in some areas, e.g. Oxford, GPs have direct access (2WW) to ultrasound (85% sensitivity) as a first-line investigation for PMB. If women also have a normal speculum examination, up to date smear, endometrial thickness of <4 mm and no risk factors (BMI >35, DM, Tamoxifen or previous hyperplasia) then, if the bleeding settles, no hysteroscopy is required.[2] If, however, bleeding persists then the GP should consider referral for a hysteroscopy which may detect a mass not seen on the ultrasound, for example an endocervical tumour.

'**Consider a direct access ultrasound scan** to assess for endometrial cancer in women' ≥55 years with:

Unexplained symptoms of vaginal discharge who:

are presenting with these symptoms for the first time **or** have thrombocytosis **or** report haematuria **or** visible haematuria **and**:

low haemoglobin levels **or** thrombocytosis **or** high blood glucose levels [new 2015].'[1]

Reasons to send a 2-week wait gynaecology referral:

- 'Ascites and/or pelvic or abdominal mass (which is not obviously uterine fibroids) (2011).'[1]
- If an ultrasound suggests cancer.
- Women with PMB – see above and your local guidelines.
- Consider if abnormal appearance of the cervix, vagina or vulva (e.g. lump: ulceration or bleeding).[1]

Doctor's Notes

Patient   Margaret Smith   47 years   F
PMH   2 normal vaginal deliveries.
Medications   No current medications
Allergies   No information
Consultations No recent consultations
Investigations No recent investigations
Household   No household members registered

Example Consultation — Menopause and HRT

Open ☐ — What has been troubling you recently? Anything else you have noticed?

Curious ☐ — What have you read about HRT?

History ☐ — Do you have any other medical problems? When was your last period? What were they like? Any problems with your bowels or waterworks? Any vaginal dryness? How is your mood? Have you tried taking any medicines or herbal medicines to help? What do you do for a living? Do you have a sexual partner? What contraception do you use? How is your libido? We can talk about your options. Do you live together? Have you ever smoked?

Risk ☐ — Have you ever had a blood clot? Any family history of cancers, blood clots, heart conditions or strokes?

Flags ☐ — Any unusual bleeding at all – after sex?

Impact ☐ — How have these symptoms impacted on your life or the relationship? Or your sleep?

Sense ☐ — Do you feel embarrassed at times?

ICE ☐ — What do you put your symptoms down to? How do you feel about HRT? Is there anything else you were wondering about? Any other worries on your mind? What did you hope I may suggest today? Any other thoughts?

Summary ☐ — To summarise, your hot flushes are troublesome and the dryness and a loss of libido are having an impact on your relationship. You have read articles encouraging women to try HRT and are hoping this may be a solution.

O/E ☐ — May I check your blood pressure, height and weight?

Empathy ☐ — I appreciate this has come at an unfortunate time, having recently started a new relationship.

Impression ☐ — It sounds as if you are currently going through the menopause.

Experience ☐ — What do you know about the menopause?

Explanation ☐ — The menopause is where the hormone balance in your body changes. Symptoms may continue for a few years. We say you have reached menopause once you have gone a year without a period. The time when you have menopausal symptoms, but before you have reached a year, is called the perimenopause. In ladies under 50, we still advise contraception for 2 years after the last period.

Options ☐ — HRT is a good option for all your symptoms. With HRT there is a slight increased risk of ovarian and womb cancer, blood clots or a stroke. There is no evidence of an increased risk of breast cancer until the age of 50. As with any medicines, we need to weigh up risk vs benefit. As the symptoms are impacting on your life, you may wish to try HRT. I would certainly support this decision. The safest way to give HRT is with oestrogen patches and the Mirena coil. The coil protects the lining of the womb against cancerous change and provides you with contraception. The patches have the lowest risk of blood clots, but you could have tablets if you prefer. We use the coil as HRT for 4 years. But, if you don't want a coil, we could give you all you need through tablets or patches. However, there are non-hormonal ways of managing flushes and your vaginal symptoms could be treated with oestrogen cream or even lubricants. What are your thoughts? Blood tests are unlikely to be helpful in the run up to the menopause, as they are often normal.

Empower ☐ — Would you like time to think? I could give you some more information. Here is information on HRT, alternatives and the Mirena coil. On the PIL herbal options are mentioned, for example black cohosh. These may help with the hot flushes but, as different preparations are available, their safety is uncertain. Any questions? In the meantime, for dryness you could try Replens or Sylk from the pharmacy. Other advice is to keep cool with cotton clothing, avoid spicy foods and alcohol and, for your bone health, ensure you eat foods containing calcium and do weight-bearing exercises.

Future ☐ — Shall I arrange to call you next week to answer any further questions and discuss the coil if you would like to go ahead?

Patient's Story

Menopause and HRT

Doctor's notes Margaret Smith, 47 years. PMH: 2 normal vaginal deliveries. Medications: None.

How to act Pleasant.

PC *'Years ago they said women shouldn't take HRT, then recently in the news it said they should. I wondered if I should try it. I wanted your advice please.'*

History Your last period was 9 months ago. Prior to this they were every few months.

You have a new partner. You divorced 4 years ago.

Your last smear was a year ago and all smears have been normal.

You have never had an STI. No problems with your bowels or passing urine.

You have had sex a few times and, if the doctor asks, it has been sore.

Because vaginal dryness has been a problem, sex is a little awkward.

No PCB. You don't use contraception. *'Surely there's no need at my age.'*

You have hot flushes. You hide these by opening the fridge for some relief.

You have some night sweats but generally sleep well.

You were speaking to your daughter about it – she suggested you see your GP.

You have no PMH. You have not tried any OTC medicines. No FH of note.

Social You live on your own. You attend yoga with friends.

You work in television behind the scenes.

You drink, on average, a bottle of wine over a week. You have never smoked.

ICE You believe that you have gone through the menopause.

You are concerned about the risks of breast cancer.

You also have no libido. You really hope the HRT will help with this.

You hope that the GP will tell you that HRT is now safe.

You are interested in whatever the GP suggests but would like time to think.

Understanding You are aware HRT may increase the risk of breast cancer.

Recently, however, you have read that it is safe.

Ask the doctor *'Do I need a blood test?'*

Examination BP 118/62. BMI 23

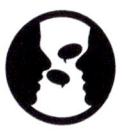

Gynaecology – 4

Learning Points   Menopause and HRT

Symptoms   Flushes, vaginal dryness, mood changes, low libido and urinary symptoms.

FSH testing

'Measurement of FSH is largely unreliable whilst taking HRT.'[1]

'Do not use a serum follicle-stimulating hormone (FSH) test to diagnose menopause in women using combined oestrogen and progestogen contraception or high-dose progestogen.'[2]

'Consider using FSH test to diagnose menopause only: in women aged 40–45 years with menopausal symptoms, including a change in their menstrual cycle or in women aged under 40 years in whom the menopause is suspected.'[2]

FSH testing may be helpful in women with IUS to help guide removal (2 readings >30 IU/L 6 weeks apart suggestive of menopause). If ≥ 50 years the IUS can be removed 1 year after the 2nd raised FSH reading.[1]

General advice Exercise, cotton clothing. Avoid: caffeine, spicy foods, smoking and alcohol.

CBT may be helpful.[2]

Premature menopause

'Diagnose premature ovarian insufficiency in women aged under 40 years based on: menopausal symptoms … and elevated FSH levels on 2 blood samples taken 4–6 weeks apart.'[2]

'Offer … a choice of HRT or a combined hormonal contraceptive.'[2]

In practice, many GPs advise women <45 years to start additional bone protection, e.g. with HRT.

Ensure sufficient dietary calcium intake (blood tests and dietary calcium calculators) and encourage weight-bearing exercises to prevent the risk of osteoporosis and fragility fractures.

Contraception   Do not rely on HRT for contraception.[1]

Options: Mirena (4-year licence if used for endometrial protection) + oestrogen only HRT.

This is the safest combination, especially if HRT (oestrogen) patches are used.

POP + **combined** HRT[1]

'A woman who is under 50 years and free of all risk factors for venous and arterial disease can use a low-oestrogen combined oral contraceptive pill to provide both relief of menopausal symptoms and contraception; it is recommended that the oral contraceptive be stopped at 50 years of age since there are more suitable alternatives.'[3]

SSRIs/SNRIs   Are not recommended as first-line treatment for vasomotor symptoms alone.[2,3]

If not diagnosed with depression, there is 'no clear evidence' this Rx eases low mood.

However in women who are keen to avoid HRT or in whom HRT is contraindicated, citalopram, fluoxetine or venlafaxine can be given for vasomotor symptoms.[4]

'SSRIs paroxetine and fluoxetine should not be offered to women with breast cancer who are taking tamoxifen.'[2]

See Extra Notes for further information on HRT.

Doctor's Notes

Patient   Mildred Lamb   76 years   F
PMH   2 normal vaginal deliveries
                 Carpal tunnel syndrome
Medications No current medications
Allergies   No information
Consultations No recent consultations
Investigations No recent investigations
Household   No household members registered

Example Consultation — Overactive Bladder

Open ☐ — Tell me more about what has been troubling you. Is there a pattern to the problem?

History ☐ — How much do you leak? Does it occur when you sneeze or cough? At night? Have you had any problems passing too much urine or needing to pass urine more frequently? Any pain passing urine or in the tummy? What do you like to do during the day? Do you have a partner? I'm sorry to hear that. Are family or friends close by? Do you smoke or drink alcohol? How much tea and coffee do you drink? Do you open your bowels regularly? Any constipation/straining?

Flags ☐ — Have you noticed any blood in the urine? Is your weight stable? Any accidents with your bowels? Any back pain?

Risk ☐ — Have you had children? How were your labours?

ICE ☐ — Have you had any thoughts about what is causing this? Is there anything that has been worrying you which we haven't discussed? What were you hoping we may decide today? What did you think I may say?

Impact ☐ — How has this problem impacted on day to day life? Are you still walking?

Sense ☐ — I see you feel embarrassed by this. Please don't be. It sounds like it is causing you a lot of bother.

Curious ☐ — When you say 'sagging', have you noticed any part of the vagina pulling down?

O/E ☐ — It would be helpful to examine the vaginal walls and check the strength of what we call your pelvic floor muscle. Would that be okay? Would you like a chaperone? May I also ask for a sample of urine? Thankfully everything seems normal on examination.

Summary ☐ — To summarise, leaking urine has become a real nuisance. You tried squeezing the bladder as you thought the problem may be due to a lack of strength. You are worried I will suggest surgery. Have I got it?

Empathy ☐ — I can imagine it is frustrating and tiring, having to plan for leaks before you go out.

Impression ☐ — We call the leaks you're having urge incontinence, likely due to an overactive bladder.

Experience ☐ — Have you come across or known anybody with this problem?

Explanation ☐ — You are not alone – it is very common but women often hide it. Normally we go to the toilet when a message is sent to the brain from the full bladder. In overactive bladder or urge incontinence, the signals are sent too early and the bladder starts to contract when it is not time. The result is you are caught short.

Options ☐ — You mentioned that you have tried squeezing the muscle around the bladder to make it stronger. This was a good idea. But unlike stress incontinence where the muscle is weak, your muscle isn't weak but contracts too early. Therefore, we suggest different exercises for this: bladder drills. Next time you need the toilet, wait 30 seconds, the next time wait a minute and gradually increase the time you wait.

Empower ☐ — I've got a leaflet which gives you tips on how to do this. It will suggest keeping a diary. Another tip is stop drinking all caffeine, which is a real troublemaker when it comes to incontinence. You may find this makes a big difference. Alcohol is also a culprit. What are your thoughts so far?

Future ☐ — If these are not working, there is the option of medication. There are side effects: dry mouth, constipation and risk of memory problems in the future. On the other hand, it can be very effective. How would you feel about this option? Shall we see how you get on with the bladder drills and avoiding the caffeine and alcohol for a month? I would like you to complete a frequency volume chart for me where you record how often you pass urine and how much over a few days. It will take at least a month, even a few months, until you notice an improvement with the bladder-training drills, but they are often very effective in the end. If we are not making progress, we can ask a continence nurse for help. After this there are surgical options or Botox to the bladder.

Safety net ☐ — If you ever notice any blood or pain – something else is going on – let me know please.

Gynaecology – 5

Patient's Story

Overactive Bladder

Doctor's notes	Mildred Lamb, 76 years. PMH: 2 vaginal deliveries. Carpal tunnel syndrome. Medications: None.
How to act	Embarrassed.
PC	*'It's a problem with leaking, Doctor.'*
History	The problem started about 6 months ago. You have no stress incontinence but have found you can't get to the toilet quickly enough and sometimes leak.
	You had to start wearing liners but now need the thicker pads.
	You have no symptoms of infection. You have no symptoms of a prolapse.
	You wear a pad when you go to bed but it is not often a problem at night.
	No haematuria or weight loss. No back pain.
	You enjoy tea, coffee and 1 glass of wine with dinner.
	You have had 2 difficult labours which required stitches. Your carpal tunnel is now fine.
	You enjoy hill walking with your friends and help out at the League of Friends at the hospital.
	You now always think about where the toilets are, or make sure you have enough pads to hand. It is very disruptive to your day. You have been put off hill walking with your friends due to toilets not being easy to locate.
	If the doctor asks, you don't walk as far now because of this problem.
Social	You live alone after you lost your husband to Alzheimer's 2 years ago.
	Never smoked.
ICE	You believe that everything is *'just sagging and not as strong due to my age'*.
	You are worried the GP may say your only option is surgery.
	You expect the GP will suggest to practise squeezing the bladder, but you have tried this for a few weeks several times a day.
	'No one else has this problem.'
	You don't know anything about the diagnosis the doctor gives you.
	If the doctor recommends medication, ask about the risks.
	You would not want any medication which could put you at risk of dementia.
	You would prefer surgery if this was the case.
Examination	All normal. Normal urine dipstick.

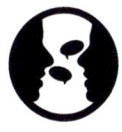

Gynaecology – 5

Learning Points   Overactive Bladder

History	3 days of a bladder diary is helpful (frequency volume chart).
Examination	'Undertake a routine digital assessment to confirm pelvic floor muscle contraction before the use of supervised pelvic floor muscle training for the treatment of UI.'[1]
	Also assess for prolapse. Urine dipstick for infection.
Investigations	USS for post-void residual volume if recurrent UTI or voiding problems.
	Urodynamic studies following conservative treatment.
Refer	'Symptomatic prolapse that is visible at or below the vaginal introitus.'[1]
	Post-void palpable bladder.
	Non-response to conservative or medical treatment.
	Other symptoms (pain, faecal, neurological, previous cancer/surgery – see full list).[1]
	See also NICE Guidance – Suspected Cancer Guidance: recognition and referral. 2015.

Stress urinary incontinence (SUI)

Supervised pelvic floor training	'8 contractions … 3 times a day … for 3 months'[1]
Medical Rx in SUI	'Do not use duloxetine as a first-line treatment for women with predominant stress UI … it may be offered as second-line therapy *if* women prefer pharmacological to surgical treatment … counsel women about its adverse effects.'[1]

Urge urinary incontinence/overactive bladder (OAB)

Conservative	Avoid caffeine/alcohol. Review fluid intake and medication (diuretics).
	Weight loss if BMI >30.[1]
	'Bladder training lasting for a minimum of 6 weeks as first-line treatment to women with urgency or mixed UI.'[1]
Medication	Discuss/review cumulative anticholinergic burden and the increased risk of dementia.[3]
	Rx effect may take up to 4 weeks.[1]
	'Oxybutynin (immediate release), or tolterodine (immediate release), (Oxford use this as first line)[4] or darifenacin (once daily preparation).'[1]
	However 'do not offer oxybutynin (immediate release) to frail older women.'[1,2]
Mirabegron	An adrenergic agonist. Consider 'in whom antimuscarinic drugs are contraindicated or clinically ineffective, or have unacceptable side effects'.[5]
Desmopressin	'may … reduce nocturia in women with UI or OAB'[1,6] – see guidance and cautions.

Mixed incontinence

'If stress incontinence is the predominant symptom in mixed UI, discuss with the woman the benefit of conservative management including OAB drugs before offering surgery.'[1]

See the **Link Hub at CompleteCSA.co.uk** for helpful links to
PIL – OAB – bladder retraining
PIL – OAB – treatment management

Gynaecology – 5

Extra Notes

Endometriosis

Symptoms Cyclical or chronic pelvic or ovulation pain. Pelvic or elsewhere. Chronic fatigue.

Dysmenorrhoea, menorrhagia and deep dyspareunia.

Premenstrual or postmenstrual spotting.

Cyclical or perimenstrual bladder or bowel symptoms.

O/E Likely to be normal. There may be a fixed retroverted uterus or tenderness.

Investigations An USS is likely to be normal. Endometriosis may be identified on MRI but patients are usually offered a laparoscopy for the diagnosis.

GP Treatment NSAID – Mefenamic acid

OCP – may back-to-back (off licence)

Progestogen – Mirena or implant.

Discuss with a specialist other options – GnRH analogues, danazol or gestrinone.

Complications Infertility.

See the **Link Hub at CompleteCSA.co.uk** for helpful links to Organisations for women with endometriosis

'**Consider referring** all women with suspected endometriosis to a gynaecologist to confirm the diagnosis by laparoscopy, and for consideration of medical or surgical treatment. In particular, offer referral for women with unconfirmed endometriosis if:

The woman wishes for referral.

She has severe or long-standing symptoms.

She has concerns about future fertility, or is having problems trying to conceive.

There are abnormalities found on clinical examination or pelvic ultrasound scan.'[1]

Gynaecology

Extra Notes

Ovarian Cyst Management[1-3]

Post-menopausal women

In all post-menopausal women with an ovarian cyst suggest measurement of serum CA-125 in the report

SIMPLE CYSTS	Recommend rescan with CA-125 measurements every 4 months for 1 year.
Simple cyst ≤5 cm	If no change after 1 year (three scans) consider cessation of scanning, if there is no clinical concern.
Simple cyst >5 cm	Recommend an urgent 2-week wait referral to Gynaecological Oncology. MRI assessment should be considered.
COMPLEX CYSTS Any complex cyst	Recommend an urgent 2-week referral to Gynaecological Oncology. Fax report to GP/referring clinician.

Pre-menopausal women

SIMPLE CYST Simple cyst <5 cm	No follow-up is required unless there is clinical concern. A statement to this effect should be included in the report.
Simple cyst 5–7 cm	Rescan in 6–8 weeks. If resolved or decreased in size no follow-up required. If persisting or increased in size suggest gynaecology referral.
Simple cyst >7 cm	Suggest gynaecology referral. MRI assessment should be considered by gynaecologist.
COMPLEX CYSTS	
Any typical **dermoid** cysts	Suggest gynaecology referral.
Haemorrhagic cyst	Rescan in 6–8 weeks to ensure resolution. If not resolved likely to be endometrioma (follow recommendations for endometriotic cysts).
Endometriotic cysts Symptomatic, any size Asymptomatic • Less than 5 cm • Larger than 5 cm	Suggest gynaecology referral. Rescan in 6 weeks. If it persists, suggest gynaecology referral. Suggest gynaecology referral.
Complex cysts with features **suspicious** for ovarian malignancy	Recommend an urgent 2-week wait referral to gynaecological oncology. Fax report to GP/referring clinician. Recommend measurement of CA-125. (Also LDH, α-FP and Beta-hCG if patient <40 years of age.) Any woman/girl before the 19th birthday should be managed jointly by Paediatric and Gynaecology Oncology MDT.

With thanks to Miss Natalia Price for permission to include this Oxford University Hospitals NHS Foundation Trust guidance. N. Price, Z. Traill, M. Goldstein, et al. Management of ovarian cysts. Joint PCT/ Radiology/ Gynaecology/Gynae Oncology guidelines. As guidance updates, the link can be found at the **Link Hub at CompleteCSA.co.uk**

Gynaecology

Extra Notes — HRT Risks

VTE risk — 'Consider transdermal rather than oral HRT for menopausal women who are at increased risk of VTE, including those with a BMI >30 kg/m². Consider referring menopausal women at high risk of VTE to a haematologist.'[1]

CVD risk — 'The presence of cardiovascular risk factors is not a contraindication to HRT as long as they are optimally managed. … HRT with oestrogen alone is associated with no, or reduced, risk of coronary heart disease. … HRT with oestrogen and progestogen is associated with little or no increase in the risk of coronary heart disease.'[1]

HRT 'does not increase CVD risk when started in women younger than 60 years.'[1]

Stroke risk — 'Oral (but not transdermal) oestrogen is associated with a small increase in the risk of stroke.'[1]

T2DM risk — 'HRT is not generally associated with an adverse effect on blood glucose control.'[1]

Breast risk — 'HRT with oestrogen alone … little or no change in the risk of breast cancer.'[1]

'There is no evidence of an increased risk of breast cancer in women on HRT under the age of 51 years compared with menstruating women of the same age.'[2]

Note a recent study suggested the risk of breast cancer from combined HRT has been underestimated.[7]

Dementia risk — 'The likelihood of HRT affecting their risk of dementia is unknown.'[1]

How given — HRT is available as tablets, skin patches, gels, nasal spray or a vaginal ring.

Preparations — If the woman has had a hysterectomy – oestrogen only.

If still having periods – a cyclical combined HRT to avoid random spotting.

If periods have stopped – a continuous combined HRT product.

Safety net — If leg swelling/pain, or any sign of stroke, seek immediate help.

Inform of the importance of BP monitoring and provide breast awareness advice.

F/up — 3 months, then 6-monthly.

Side effects — Nausea, breast pain, leg cramps. Skin irritation from patches. See the BNF.

Stopping HRT — Can be either immediate or gradual. Tip – patches can be cut down in size gradually.

'Gradually reducing HRT may limit recurrence of symptoms in the short term.'[1]

Vaginal dryness — Oestrogen pessary for vaginal atrophy combined with Replens for dryness.

'Consider vaginal oestrogen for … whom systemic HRT is contraindicated, after seeking advice.'[1]

Contraindications to use of topical oestrogens are active breast cancer and undiagnosed vaginal or uterine bleeding.[3,5] 'They are otherwise safe. The amount systemically absorbed is very low.'[4,5] A year's supply of topical oestrogen is equivalent to having one tablet of standard HRT.[5]

See the **Link Hub at CompleteCSA.co.uk** for Useful PILs in gynaecology
Especially the link to self-managing vulval skin care[6]!

Gynaecology

CHAPTER 9 OVERVIEW
Men's Health

	Cases in this chapter	Within the RCGP curriculum: Men's Health RCGP Curriculum Online March 2016[1]	Learning points in the chapter include:
1	Erectile Dysfunction	'Know that men may be both more reticent and less articulate about their health than women, and describe strategies to compensate for this during the consultation' 'Know that men may present with more than one health problem at a time and that men may mask mental/emotional health problems with physical symptoms' 'Know that erectile dysfunction is an early warning for many conditions including coronary vascular disease'	ED investigations and management The well man check
2	Gynaecomastia	'Utilise the consultation to help change behaviour so that male patients are confident in behaving differently on subsequent occasions ...' 'Know about overweight and obesity issues in men and where to refer them for weight management'	Causes, investigations and management of gynaecomastia
3	PSA Test Result	'Know that men from different cultural backgrounds may have widely differing attitudes towards health and expectations of the doctor'	Bladder outflow obstruction PSA levels
4	Prostatitis	'Know that men may need more encouragement both to attend surgery and to articulate the full extent of their health problems during consultation'	Acute and chronic prostatitis
5	Overactive Bladder	'Demonstrate a non-judgemental, caring and professional consulting style to minimise embarrassing male patients'	Overactive bladder management
	Extra Notes	'Intervene urgently with suspected malignancy'	BPH Prostate cancer PSA screening UTI in men Haematuria

1. http://www.rcgp.org.uk/training-exams/gp-curriculum-overview/online-curriculum/caring-for-the-whole-person/3-07-mens-health.aspx

CHAPTER 9 REFERENCES

Erectile Dysfunction
1. http://www.njurology.com/_forms/shim.pdf
2. http://patient.info/doctor/erectile-dysfunction
3. https://www.relate.org.uk/
4. NICE Guidelines. NG12 Suspected cancer: recognition and referral. Jun 2015.

Gynaecomastia
1. Porter K. GP management of gynaecomastia. Feb 2012. http://www.gponline.com/gp-management-gynaecomastia/cancer/womens/article/1118276

PSA Test Result
1. NICE Guidelines. NG12 Suspected cancer: recognition and referral. Jun 2015.
2. http://www.uptodate.com/contents/screening-for-prostate-cancer
3. Oxford University Hospitals NHS Trust. 2WW referral form for prostate cancer.
4. Carter H.B., Pearson J.D., Metter E.J., et al. Longitudinal evaluation of prostate-specific antigen levels in men with and without prostate disease. *JAMA*. 1992; 267: 2215.
5. http://patient.info/doctor/prostate-specific-antigen-psa
6. NICE. http://cks.nice.org.uk/urinary-tract-infection-lower-men#!scenario. Revised Oct 2013.

Prostatitis
1. NICE. http://cks.nice.org.uk/prostatitis-acute. Revised Aug 2014.
2. NICE. http://cks.nice.org.uk/prostatitis-chronic. Revised Feb 2015.

Overactive Bladder
1. NICE. http://cks.nice.org.uk/luts-in-men. Revised Feb 2015.

Benign Prostatic Hypertrophy
1. http://patient.info/doctor/benign-prostatic-hyperplasia
2. http://www.nhs.uk/Conditions/resectionoftheprostate/Pages/Risks.aspx
3. Cyproterone-acetate. http://www.cancerresearchuk.org/about-cancer/cancers-in-general/treatment/cancer-drugs/cyproterone-acetate. Jun 2016.

UTI in Men and Haematuria
1. NICE. http://cks.nice.org.uk/urinary-tract-infection-lower-men#!scenario. Revised Feb 2015.
2. NICE Guidelines. NG12 Suspected cancer: recognition and referral. Jun 2015.
3. NICE Guidelines. CG 182. Chronic kidney disease in adults: assessment and management. Jul 2014.

Doctor's Notes

Patient   Kevin Barton   57 years   M
PMH   Hypertension
Medications   Indapamide 2.5 mg OD
Allergies   No information
Consultations No recent consultations
Investigations No recent investigations
Household   No household members registered

Example Consultation — Erectile Dysfunction

Open ☐	Good. Thank you for coming. Do you have thoughts about what we should include in your check?
Sense ☐	Any other changes in the body or worries?
History ☐	I see you have high blood pressure. Are you otherwise well? Do you live alone? Do you work? Any stress in your life at the moment? How is your mood? Do you worry about your health?
Risk ☐	Do you smoke? How much alcohol do you drink? Any family history?
Flags ☐	Any pain in your chest, legs or breathing problems? Any problems going to the toilet? Do you check your testes for lumps? Any problems with erections? Do you have any erections? Is this a problem maintaining erections or do you struggle to have an erection in the first place? Are you worried about anything else; for example, when you ejaculate? Do you have any erections on your own or in the morning?
Impact ☐	How has the impotence affected you or your relationship?
Curious ☐	How is your relationship? What does your husband think? Have you had any other sexual partners? When was this? Tell me more about this person? Male or female?
ICE ☐	Has this been worrying you? What has been going through your mind? What is your biggest fear? Is there anything specific you were hoping I would do today?
Impact ☐	Has anything else in your life changed since? Your mood? How are you and David?
Curious ☐	You mentioned David encouraged you to attend – is he worried about you?
Flags ☐	Do you have any symptoms that may suggest an infection?
Summary ☐	To summarise, you are troubled with impotence and you fear you may have an infection. You are feeling low in mood and fear this may affect your marriage.
Empathy ☐	Impotence can often be frustrating and can increase the stress in your life.
O/E ☐	It would be helpful to examine you with a chaperone present to ensure the skin of the penis is healthy, then check your blood pressure and weight. Is this okay?
Experience ☐	Have you read or heard about anything that may cause impotence?
Explanation ☐	Stress or low mood or conditions that affect the vessels can cause impotence. For an erection, blood needs to flow into the vessels in the penis.
Impression ☐	Your BP or even the indapamide may be contributing to impotence. It's reassuring that you are sometimes able to have erections, which makes me believe it is most likely due to your recent worries.
Options ☐	If you wish, we could check for infections and also swab the penis and take a urine sample. The other option is that you visit the GUM clinic and they are able to provide a thorough assessment for infections quickly. There is a walk-in clinic this afternoon. Shall I give you the details of where to go? We could try stopping indapamide to see if this helps. You may be interested in talking to a relationship counsellor or trying sildenafil (also called Viagra), which increases the blood flow to the penis. Out of these options, what is right for you? I can give you information on Relate, our relationship counsellors.
Empower ☐	Have a think if there are any changes you could make to your lifestyle that may help your vessels. You have stopped playing squash but exercise is very important. We can check your cholesterol and blood sugar which can affect vessels. We could also check a prostate cancer blood test. I will give you an information leaflet to read about the test and its limitations. We can discuss this when we meet again.
Future ☐	I suggest meeting in a month to discuss your blood results and see how things have been. I recommend waiting to have sex until your sexual health screen is clear and, if you do need treatment, both you and David will require a completion of treatment before you have sex. Here is a prescription for 50 mg sildenafil. Take one an hour before you plan to have sex. There is no rush as it works for hours. It will only cause an erection when you become aroused. It may cause a headache.
Safety net ☐	If your mood deteriorates or anything else worries you, see me sooner.

Men's Health – 1

Patient's Story

Erectile Dysfunction

Doctor's notes Kevin Barton, 57 years. PMH: HTN. Medications: Indapamide 2.5 mg OD

How to act Embarrassed. You do not give much away unless pushed.

You do not mention you have a problem with ED until the doctor asks directly.

Then call it impotence.

PC *'I would like a well man check please.'*

History Your friends have had a well man check.

You are unsure what this is exactly.

You have no symptoms of bladder outflow obstruction.

You have had problems with impotence.

You have morning erections and find masturbation easier.

You are well and healthy. You exercise. You do not smoke.

You drink 1 pint of lager a night.

You have no other medical history and no family history.

Social You married your male partner, David, 3 years ago.

David has encouraged you to go to the GP.

You had an affair a year ago with a male friend from the squash club and for which you feel guilty. You do not disclose this until the doctor explores your sexual history.

This has put stress on your marriage.

You no longer see this friend or play squash.

ICE You fear you have an STI and that one day your husband will discover this.

You fear your relationship with your husband ending if he ever found out.

You fear you have let him down and are struggling to forget what you did.

You would like blood tests for a general check-up but don't insist on a prostate test.

You would like to try Viagra.

Examination NAD genitalia. BP 134/78, BMI 24.3.

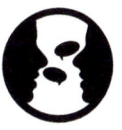

Men's Health – 1

Learning Points — Erectile Dysfunction

Causes of ED

Vascular disease	Risk factors include: HTN, smoking, hypercholesterolaemia and DM.
Structural	Surgery within the pelvis. Peyronie's disease.
Skin disorders	Foreskin problems (lichen sclerosis, balanitis, xerotica obliterans).
Neurological	Tumour, spinal cord disease, MS, Parkinson's, stroke, peripheral neuropathy (DM).
Hormonal	Hypogonadism, Cushing's, thyroid, hyperprolactinaemia.
Drug induced	Diuretics, SSRIs, GnRH analogues and antagonists, antipsychotics.
Alcohol and recreational drugs	
Psychological causes	Stress, depression, anxiety, relationship difficulties, performance anxiety.
SHIM	Sexual health inventory for men[1] score may be useful.

Tailor investigations to the likely cause depending on symptoms, age and risk factors.

The patient may have their own terminology in a sexual health history. Use words they have chosen.

Make no assumptions Ask about other sexual partners and confirm their partner's gender.

Management options

Sildenafil	CI include: already on a nitrate, unstable angina, recent MI or stroke, optic neuropathy
	Side effects: headaches, flushing, N&V, dizziness and visual disturbances.
	Interactions: no alpha blocker within 4 hours.
Other options:	2nd line tadalafil (Cialis) with a longer duration of effect.
	Vacuum pumps. MUSE (alfraprostadil per urethra) and cavaject.[2]

Relationship counselling[3] or a referral to psychosexual medicine may be helpful.

Show you have recognised the opportunity for health screening and promotion.

The well man check	CVD RFs, prostate and testicular screening, weight and bowel changes, stress/mood.
PSA screening	Offer all men with ED PSA screening.[4]

Men's Health – 1

Doctor's Notes

Patient	Craig Mason	46 years	M
PMH	No medical history		
Medications	No medications		
Allergies	No information		
Consultations	No recent consultations		
Investigations	No recent investigations		
Household	Carolyn Mason	45 years	F
	Julianne Mason	15 years	F
	Thomas Mason	13 years	M

Example Consultation — Gynaecomastia

Sense ☐	I can see you are worried.
Open ☐	Anything else that you have noticed? Or are concerned about?
Flags ☐	Have you felt any lumps in the breast? Or elsewhere, for example the testicles? Any other symptoms elsewhere? For example, are your bowels normal? Any symptoms in the chest or tummy?
Risk ☐	Is it painful? Do you have a cough or any breathing problems? Any pain in the chest? Or weight loss? Do you smoke?
History ☐	You are otherwise well? Have you taken any medications or any supplements? What is in this supplement? How much alcohol do you drink? I'm interested to know more about you. Do you work? Do you live with anyone?
ICE ☐	What has gone through your mind regarding what may have caused this? Is there anything you fear this could be? Is there anything in particular you thought I might suggest?
Impact ☐	Has this affected you or your relationship?
Curious ☐	What led you to start taking supplements?
Summary ☐	So to summarise, you have noticed your breasts have enlarged and this started after the addition of a body-building supplement. You are otherwise well with no symptoms. In the back of your mind you fear this could be a cancer, or that I may suggest you need to go to a breast team. Have I understood correctly?
O/E ☐	I would like to examine your chest, on the couch with your shirt off, if that is okay? There are a few possible causes for this – may I feel your liver and neck please? Would you like me to check that the testes are normal? Okay, that's fine; we could do this another time if you wish. May I check your height and weight?
Empathy ☐	I can see this has been a fright.
Impression ☐	Breast tissue growth in men is called gynaecomastia.
Experience ☐	Have you come across this?
Explanation ☐	It has many different causes. In your case I believe it has been caused by the supplement. There is no sign of a cancer.
Empower ☐	I would expect the breasts to go back to normal a month or two after stopping the supplement. I appreciate you wanted to increase your tone but taking a supplement has risks, especially if from the Internet and we do not know what is in the product.
Options ☐	Do you think you will talk to your wife about our consultation today? Can you think of other ways to improve your fitness? Eating a varied diet that contains natural proteins and gradually improving your fitness is healthy. If the problem hasn't resolved in a couple of months, we could check a few blood tests.
Future ☐	You seem interested in your general health; would this be something you would like to talk more about? Is there anything specific that worries you about your general health? What tests did you have in mind? We can ask the nurse to see you for a cholesterol and blood pressure check. Let's catch up in a month to see if there has been improvement. However, sometimes it takes up to 12 months to settle completely. You can cancel this if the problem has gone, but you may prefer to return to discuss your general health again. Do you think reducing the amount of fat in your diet and increasing exercise is something you could do? Is there anything else that you were hoping for today?
Safety net ☐	If you notice anything new, symptoms or lumps then tell me straight away please.

Men's Health – 2

Patient's Story

Gynaecomastia

Doctor's notes	Craig Mason, 46 years. PMH. None. Medications: None.
How to act	Concerned.
PC	*'I'm worried that my chest has grown. It's like I have breasts.'*
History	Your breasts have started to appear in the last few months.
	They are not painful. You have no PMH.
Social	You live with your wife and two children. Estate agent. Minimal alcohol. No stress.
	You started using a body-building treatment 6 months ago.
	Your wife encouraged you to go to the gym and tone up.
	You do not know what is in the supplement, you get it from the Internet.
ICE	You think it may be fat as you have put on weight.
	At the back of your mind you hope it's not breast cancer.
	Your fear would be being sent to a clinic full of women.
	You have no idea what the doctor may suggest.
	Late in the consultation, say you were worried about a decline in your health.
	You hope the GP offers a check-up including blood pressure and cholesterol.
	You decline a genital examination.
Examination	Bilateral gynaecomastia, no lymphadenopathy.
	No hepatomegaly and no palpable thyroid.
	BMI 26.

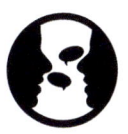

Men's Health – 2

Learning Points — Gynaecomastia

Causes of gynaecomastia[1]

Idiopathic	
Physiological	In teens and elderly
Infection	Mumps
Tumours	Lung (there may be an increased β-hCG) and testicular
Systemic disease	Liver, thyrotoxicosis
Iatrogenic	Drugs, steroids, PPIs, TCAs
Hormonal:	Hyperprolactinaemia, hypogonadism
Alcohol	

Examination[1]

- Breast examination and lymphadenopathy
- Signs of hyperthyroidism or goitre
- Chronic liver disease
- BMI
- Testicular examination

Investigation

Not required in:	Teens, if typical senile changes, or if obvious iatrogenic cause.[1]
Consider	TFT, LFT, GGT, U&E, testosterone, prolactin, LH, β-hCG, oestradiol, DHEA, SHBG.[1]
If lung cancer suspected	CXR
Testicular pain or mass	USS testes
Mammography	Only if cancer is suspected.
Genetic cause suspected	Chromosomal karyotyping.
Management	Treat the cause, stop the drug and f/up in 1/12.
Prognosis	Usually 1–12/12 to resolve after treating the cause.

'In patients with physiological gynaecomastia, especially adolescent boys, reassurance can be given that most cases are transitory, with more than 90% resolving within three years.'[1]

See the **Link Hub at CompleteCSA.co.uk** for a useful article on Gynaecomastia

Doctor's Notes

Patient	Remigio Sánchez	47 years	M
PMH	No medical history		
Medications	No medications		
Allergies	No information		
Consultations	2 years ago for a soft tissue injury of the ankle		
Investigations	PSA 4.5 ng/mL		
Household	Perla Sánchez	48 years	F
	Sosimo Sánchez	16 years	M
	Manuela Sánchez	14 years	F
	Pilar Sánchez	10 years	M

Example Consultation

PSA Test Result

Open ☐	What has led to this test being taken? I see we haven't seen you for a long time.
Experience ☐	Tell me more about your father and brother's experience. What is your understanding of the PSA test? Has a doctor explained?
Sense ☐	I can see you are keen to know the result.
Impression ☐	The result is slightly raised; however, activities such as running, cycling, ejaculating or intercourse can all increase this result. In the week prior to the test, did you do any of these activities? That is helpful to know. This result cannot be interpreted and I would expect your result to be raised if you have done those activities. I would like to repeat the test.
History ☐	Are you well? Any medical problems? Tell me more about you – your work and home. Do you notice any problems when passing urine? What is the flow like? Is it painful? Do you have to race to the toilet? Do you go frequently? Any fever? Any pain in the sides? How many times do you pass urine at night? Is the flow okay? Do you have to wait because it dribbles at the end? Afterwards do you feel your bladder isn't quite empty? Are you always thirsty? Any problems with erections?
Flags ☐	Have you seen any blood in the urine? Have you noticed any new back pain? Have you lost weight? I'm pleased you have no symptoms.
Impact ☐	Coming for a result can be worrying. How did you feel prior to coming today?
Curious ☐	You mentioned 'I haven't got time to be ill.' Is this something that has been on your mind? If this result were raised, have you had thoughts about how it may affect you?
ICE ☐	Is there anything else on your mind? What are you most fearful of? What did you think I might suggest today?
Empathy ☐	I appreciate that, with your family history and fear of the impact a diagnosis may have on your life, this result is very important to you.
Summary ☐	So to summarise, your brother and father have prostate cancer and you have arranged this test in the hope that if there was a cancer you are catching it early. You fear how a diagnosis of prostate cancer would impact on your health and ability to provide for your family. This has been very stressful for you.
O/E ☐	I would like to examine your prostate if I may. It would involve lying on the couch behind the curtain, then I would insert one finger into the back passage as this is where we can feel the prostate. It is usually uncomfortable but not usually painful. I would also like to feel your abdomen. Is that okay? I will ask for a nurse chaperone if that is okay? I'm pleased to say that the examination is normal.
Explanation ☐	The PSA level can be raised in prostate cancer. But it can also be raised in harmless growth of the prostate. If the PSA level was raised, we would need a biopsy to diagnose or exclude a cancer. The biopsy is taken through the back passage; therefore, it can be an uncomfortable procedure with the risk of infection.
Future ☐	Please see the doctor again after your next blood test. Because you have had the prostate examination today, please wait 7 days until your next blood test. Avoid sex, ejaculation and exercise for 48 hours before the test. If it is raised, we normally do a further test whilst checking your urine and kidney function before referring you to the urologist.
Safety net ☐	If in future you have any problems passing urine, or any new pain, let a GP know.

Men's Health – 3

Patient's Story

PSA Test Result

Doctor's notes Remigio Sánchez, 47 years. PMH: PSA 4.5 ng/mL, nil else. Medications: None.

How to act Eager to know what will happen to you.

PC *'I've come for my PSA result.'*

PMH You asked for the test as your brother has been diagnosed with prostate cancer.

You made an appointment with the phlebotomist and told her you needed the test.

You have never had any problems with your health.

Your father also had a total prostatectomy for prostate cancer.

You haven't noticed any symptoms.

You attended the gym prior to the test being taken.

You understand the PSA test will tell you if you have prostate cancer.

Social *'I haven't got time to be ill.'*

You moved from Argentina 6 years ago for work on oil rigs.

You spend a lot of time away from home.

Your work would not be sympathetic if you needed time off.

They often make people redundant. You feel the pressure of finances at the moment with three children who want to go to university.

ICE You assume you have prostate cancer too and want to catch it early.

You are worried that you will need chemotherapy.

You couldn't sleep last night because of fear of the result.

You expect the doctor to send you for a biopsy. You have had no UTI symptoms.

Examination Prostate and abdomen are normal.

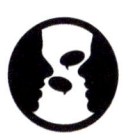

Men's Health – 3

Learning Points

PSA Test Result

Consider a PSA test to check for prostate cancer in

   Associated LUTS[1]

   Visible haematuria[1]

   Erectile dysfunction[1]

   The patient interested in the test after counselling (even if asymptomatic*)

*Prostate cells adjacent to urethra (transitional zone of the prostate) commonly change to become hyperplastic (BPH) whereas prostate cancer arises in the peripheral zone of the prostate – the part you can feel on DRE. Hence men with early prostate cancer are usually asymptomatic. Men who present with LUTS due to prostate cancer often have locally advanced disease. However, BPH and prostate cancer can coexist. Occasionally tumours arise from the anterior portion of the gland, and are impalpable.

Symptoms from bladder outflow obstruction (from BPH or cancer of the prostate) may include:

   Urgency, frequency, incontinence or nocturia

   Hesitancy, poor flow or post-micturition dribbling

Symptoms of metastases may include back or bone pain, haematuria or weight loss.

Erectile dysfunction is not usually caused by prostate cancer but completes a well man history.

Men with low back pain: always consider a PSA test (as well as a myeloma screen and kidney/ureteric disease).

2WW referral

1. Abnormal PSA levels (various thresholds are available[2-4] and we have chosen the lowest threshold)
   - 40–49 years   PSA >2.5 ng/mL[2]
   - 50–59 years   PSA >3 ng/mL[3]
   - 60–69 years   PSA >4 ng/mL[3]
   - >70   PSA >5 ng/mL[3]
2. Suspicious prostate on DRE[1]
3. Bone pain with malignant characteristics – direct assess 2WW MRI lumbar/sacral spine
4. Recurrent UTI[3,6]
5. Retention (consider catheterisation and acute admission)[3]

Significant rise in PSA   >0.75 ng/mL/year[2,5]

Halve the abnormal PSA thresholds per age group (above) if the patient is taking an alpha reductase inhibitor (finasteride).[3]

Refer after two raised values 2 weeks apart, but if concerned refer with one value.[3]

Prior to referring check creatinine and MSU.[4]

If a UTI is present repeat the PSA after 4–6 weeks.[3]

PSA rises in   Cancer, BPH, UTI, exercise (e.g. cycling), ejaculation, urinary retention or surgical intervention, e.g. flexible cystoscopy.

Doctor's Notes

Patient	Arthur Smalling	49 years	M
PMH	Hypertension		
	Irritable bowel syndrome		
	Depression		
Medications	Amlodipine 5 mg OD		
	Mebeverine 135 mg TDS		
	Citalopram 20 mg OD		
Allergies	No information		
Consultations	No recent consultations		
Investigations	No recent investigations		
Household	Patricia Smalling	42 years	F

Example Consultation — Prostatitis

Open ☐ — Please don't be embarrassed. Could you tell me a little more about your symptoms?

History ☐ — Some specific questions about your symptoms … Some of the questions are a little personal. How long have you had this pain? What sort of pain is it? Does anything bring it on or make it worse? How are your bowels? Have you passed any blood? Any mucus? How are your waterworks? Any pain passing urine? Going more often or in the night? Do you have to rush to the toilet? Does the urine flow start straight away or is there a pause? How is the stream? Does the flow stop and start? Do you get dribbling at the end when you think you have finished? Have you had a water infection before? Have you had any problems sexually?

Flags ☐ — Have you ever seen blood in your urine? Or blood in your semen? Have you had a fever? Or any weight loss? Any new sexual partners?

Impact ☐ — How have these symptoms been affecting you?

Curious ☐ — You mentioned being saddle sore. Have you been cycling a lot recently?

ICE ☐ — Have you had any thoughts about what could be causing your symptoms? Are you worried about anything in particular? Were you hoping I would do anything specific today?

Summary ☐ — So you have been experiencing pain in your back passage, pain between your privates and bottom and discomfort passing urine. You have also noted that your stream isn't as fast as it used to be and have had some sexual issues and pain on ejaculation. You wondered if your symptoms were caused by cycling a lot but the symptoms didn't improve with a month off cycling. You haven't had a fever or passed blood and your bowels are working normally.

O/E ☐ — It would be really helpful if I could examine your tummy, testes and back passage. This will help me with the diagnosis. Would that be okay? Would you mind if a chaperone was present? Could I check your temperature, BP and HR? It would also be really helpful if you could provide a urine sample for testing; could you manage to do a sample?

Impression ☐ — It think you may have chronic prostatitis.

Experience ☐ — Do you know much about the prostate?

Explanation ☐ — The prostate is a gland found in every man and is located in the pelvis. Prostatitis is a condition where the prostate becomes inflamed. Sometimes it's due to a bacterial infection but sometimes there is no obvious reason why the prostate becomes inflamed. It is not a form of cancer and isn't usually caused by sexually transmitted infections. Classic symptoms are pain in the region between your scrotum and anus – called the perineum – pain in the back passage and problems passing urine or with intercourse. Because the symptoms have been there for more than 3 months, we call the condition chronic. Unfortunately, it can be tricky to treat, but most men notice an improvement within 6 months.

Future ☐ — First of all I would like to send a urine sample off to check for bacteria. It would be helpful if you could complete a couple of questionnaires to identify how the symptoms have been affecting you. One is called the International Prostate Symptom Score and the other is the National Institutes of Health – Chronic Prostatitis Symptom Index. We would normally treat this condition with a month of antibiotics. Do you have any allergies? I would like to start you on ciprofloxacin 500 mg BD (check local guidance), is that okay? Could we meet next week to review your questionnaires and urine test? Then we'll decide if you need any blood tests to check the kidney and prostate levels. If we are not making progress, we will ask a specialist to see you.

Safety net ☐ — Should your symptoms worsen or you develop a fever or pass blood, please let me know straight away.

Men's Health – 4

Patient's Story

Prostatitis

Doctor's notes	Arthur Smalling, 49 years. PMH: HTN, IBS, Depression. Medications: amlodipine, citalopram, mebeverine.
How to act	Embarrassed.
PC	*'Hello Doctor, I'm rather embarrassed, I've been getting a lot of pain in my bottom.'*
History	For the last 4 months you have been experiencing pain in your rectum. The pain can be sharp or a burning pain. You have been opening your bowels normally, passing a soft stool each day. No PR bleed or mucus. You have also had discomfort when passing urine for a number of weeks. You feel tender in the region between your *'privates'* and anus. Your stream isn't as good as it used to be but isn't too bad. You get up 1–2 times a night to pass urine. Until 4 months ago you hadn't noticed any frequency or urgency in the daytime. You have not seen blood in your urine. You don't suffer with hesitancy or terminal dribbling. You have had a couple of episodes of erectile dysfunction which you thought were due to your age (and possibly cycling) but you have also had pain during ejaculation which you thought was odd. No weight loss. No fever. No history of UTIs. You have been married for 25 years and have not had any other partners.
ICE	You are a keen cyclist so initially thought cycling may be causing your symptoms. You have been training for a 100-mile bike ride for charity. You stopped cycling 4 weeks ago but unfortunately you haven't got any better so you thought you should get checked out.
	'I thought I'd got a little saddle sore!'
O/E	Temperature 36.3°C. HR 68 bpm. BP 136/88
	Abdomen soft and non-tender
	Testicular examination normal
	Tender perineum
	Tender slightly enlarged smooth prostate on rectal examination
	Urine dipstick – leuco ++, protein +, blood trace, nitrite negative

Men's Health – 4

Learning Points — Prostatitis

Acute prostatitis[1]

Symptoms	Febrile illness, urinary symptoms + perineal/suprapubic pain.
Examination	Exquisitely tender prostate, leucocytes on urine dipstick.
Investigations	MSU and STI screening.
Acutely unwell	If severely ill or acute urinary retention admit to hospital.
Urgent referral	Immunocompromised, diabetes, pre-existing urological condition or catheterised.

Chronic prostatitis (2 types)[2]

1. Chronic bacterial prostatitis (10%)
2. Chronic prostatitis/chronic pelvic pain syndrome (CPPS = 90%)

   Although prostatitis suggests infection and inflammation, the pathology is poorly understood. The histology does not always reflect the symptoms or treatment response. Chronic bacterial prostatitis is thought to be caused by recurrent UTIs, undertreated acute bacterial prostatitis, ascending urethral infection or lymphatic spread from the rectum. The cause of CPPS is unclear.

Symptoms:

Pain	Perineum, inguinal, suprapubic, penis, scrotum, testes, rectum, lower back or abdomen.
LUTS	Hesitancy, urgency, poor stream, terminal dribbling, frequency, nocturia or dysuria.
Sexual	ED, painful ejaculation, premature ejaculation or decreased libido.

History needs to identify/exclude: a UTI, acute prostatitis, haematospermia (may be prostatitis but also prostate cancer or STI), IBS (present in up to 30% of men with chronic prostatitis).

Duration of symptoms – minimum of 3 months.

Assess symptom severity using the National Institutes of Health – Chronic Prostatitis Symptom Index or IPSS.

Assess for depression/anxiety if cues to suggest this.

Examination: observations (rule out acute infection/sepsis), abdominal examination (tenderness, bladder distension or retention), external genitalia (urethral discharge, phimosis, meatal stenosis, penile cancer), digital rectal examination (prostate size, lumps? and tenderness).

Differential: acute prostatitis, prostatic abscess, UTI, urethritis, pyelonephritis, epididymitis, benign prostatic hyperplasia, cancer of prostate/bladder/colon, urethral stricture, obstructive calculus in urinary tract or foreign body and pudendal neuralgia.

Investigations	Urine dip and MSU (try sending MSU after DRE to increase microbiology yield).
	Consider full STI screen (esp. if <35 years or new partner).
	Bloods: Consider PSA testing and routine bloods, e.g. FBC, U&E and CRP.

NB: MSU may be negative in chronic bacterial prostatitis so look for old MSUs.

Management	4–6 weeks antibiotic (check local guidance).
	NICE – ciprofloxacin, ofloxacin or trimethoprim if quinolones not tolerated/allergy.
	Trial alpha-blocker if LUTS present.
	Paracetamol +/– NSAID, laxatives if constipation also present.
Refer	If diagnosis in doubt.
	Severe symptoms or if chronic bacterial prostatitis is suspected.

Men's Health – 4

Doctor's Notes

Patient	Angus McLaughlin 72 years M
PMH	Chronic obstructive pulmonary disease
	Ischaemic heart disease
	Hypertension
Medications	Salbutamol PRN
	Tiotropium 18 mcg OD
	Aspirin 75 mg OD
	Isosorbide mononitrate 20 mg BD
	Atorvastatin 80 mg nocte
	Bisoprolol 5 mg OD
	Ramipril 2.5 mg OD
Allergies	No information
Consultations	No recent consultations
Investigations	No recent investigations
Household	No household members registered

Example Consultation — Overactive Bladder

Open — Could you possibly tell me a little more about your symptoms?

History — How long have you had these symptoms? How often are you passing urine during the day/night? Do you have to rush? Do you have any episodes where you don't make it to the toilet in time, causing a leak of urine? What is the flow of urine like? Does the flow of urine ever take time to get going? Do you ever dribble urine after you think you have finished? How are your bowels? Do you drink much tea or coffee? How much alcohol do you drink? Have you avoided drinking fluids?

Flags — Is it painful to urinate? Any blood? Weight loss? Tummy or back pain? Recent angina?

Sense — I sense these symptoms have become a real nuisance to you.

Impact — Have you had to stop doing anything that you enjoy? I'm sorry to hear that this is stopping you getting out. How is your mood? Have the symptoms been disrupting your sleep?

ICE — You mentioned having to rush to the toilet; is there a particular concern you have? You also mentioned your prostate at the beginning; is that something you have been worrying about? Were you hoping that I'd do anything particular today?

Summary — So for several months you have been passing urine every hour during the day and every couple of hours at night. You get a sudden urge to go and sometimes don't make it to the toilet quick enough and leak some urine. You find it difficult to rush to the toilet due to breathlessness and you fear bringing on an angina attack. Unfortunately, you have had to stop going to the pub as you worry about having an accident. You also worry about smelling of urine if you have an accident. You thought your symptoms may be due to your prostate as you're aware that prostate problems cause waterworks symptoms and particularly fear prostate cancer.

O/E — It would really help me assess your symptoms if I could examine you. I would like to examine your abdomen, if possible your genitals and your prostate – this involves placing a finger into your rectum. Are you happy for me to do this examination? I will ask a chaperone to be present for the intimate examinations if that's okay with you?

Impression — Thankfully I don't think there is a problem with your prostate. I think you have something called 'overactive bladder'.

Experience — Have you heard of overactive bladder?

Explanation — Overactive bladder is a condition where the bladder is sensitive and empties suddenly, often when it's not even very full. It's not a harmful condition although it can cause troublesome symptoms. The main treatment is 'bladder training' but sometimes medications can help.

Empower — There are some simple things you can do to help. Reducing caffeine and alcohol often improves symptoms as these both irritate the bladder and have a diuretic affect which means they make you pass more urine. Although reducing fluid intake may sound like a sensible thing to do, actually this can make the problem worse as concentrated urine can irritate the bladder. We can check the prostate blood test. If the level is raised, we would repeat the test. You may need a biopsy. I will give you information to read and we can discuss this next time.

Future — I would like to send a urine sample off to ensure that there is no water infection causing your symptoms. It would be really helpful if you could complete a 'frequency volume chart' for me. This simply means recording on a chart, which I will give you, each time you go to the toilet to pass urine and if possible measuring the volume of urine passed. Some people will buy a cheap plastic measuring jug to do this. Would it be possible for you to do this? Then we can have a look at the chart together and discuss the bladder training techniques. Would you like me to ask our district nurses to supply you with some pads you could use in the meantime – just in case?

Safety net — Could we catch up in a couple of weeks? If your symptoms worsen, you develop pain or blood in your urine, please let me know straight away.

Men's Health – 5

Patient's Story

Overactive Bladder

Doctor's notes Angus McLaughlin, 72 years. PMH: COPD, IHD, HTN. Medications: Salbutamol PRN, Tiotropium 18 mcg, Aspirin 75 mg, ISMN 20 mg bd, Atorvastatin 80 mg, Bisoprolol 5 mg, Ramipril 2.5 mg.

How to act Concerned.

PC *'Doctor, I'm having trouble getting to the toilet. Do you think it's my prostate?'*

History For several months you have been having difficulty passing urine. You feel that you have to go every hour during the day and every couple of hours during the night. You suddenly get the urge to pass urine and if you don't find a toilet quickly you will often have an accident. You are often short of breath due to your COPD so find it difficult: *'I have to rush to the loo.'* As a result you have started to avoid going out so that you can stay close to the toilet. You were fond of meeting friends in your local pub for a beer but now feel you can't do this. You worry that you'll have an accident and will smell of urine *'like an old man'*. You know some of your friends had difficulty with their waterworks and one needed an operation on his prostate. You drink 2 cups of tea in the morning and have another before bed.

No dysuria. No hesitancy or terminal dribbling. Good stream. No intermittency. No erectile dysfunction. Normal bowel habit. No haematuria. No weight loss.

Social You are a retired miner. Your wife passed away 3 years ago so you live alone now. You feel a bit lonely and isolated now you feel you can't go out.

Ex-smoker. Drink 2 pints of ale a day.

ICE You are worried you may have prostate cancer.

You worry about getting angina attacks if you have to hurry but this has not happened.

You have heard about prostate cancer and fear having an operation. You expect the doctor to examine your prostate. You hope the doctor will arrange some tests.

Examination Abdominal examination normal.

Prostate smooth and normal size.

Men's Health – 5

Learning Points

Overactive Bladder

NICE advice – Overactive bladder[1]:

Take a full history of the symptoms as with other lower urinary tract symptoms. Look for drugs and lifestyle factors which may be exacerbating the symptoms. Ask about the impact on life.

Examination should include abdominal, genital and digital rectal examination.

Suggest patient completes a 'frequency volume chart'. The patient is asked to record the number of times they pass urine, the volume of urine passed each time and any other significant information such as episodes of incontinence, what they drink, how much and when. This helps to quantify the patient's symptoms and highlights problems such as nocturia.

Management

Conservative measures:

- Bladder training.
- Avoid caffeine and alcohol. Carbonated soft drinks and fruit juice may aggravate symptoms.
- Avoidance of dehydration (concentrated urine can exacerbate the problem).
- Weight loss may help.
- Pelvic floor exercises may help men, especially if history of stress incontinence as well.
- Offer containment devices, e.g. pads or external sheaths to help whilst problem is being investigated.

Drug treatment

Offer anticholinergic – usually oxybutynin 1st line either immediate release or modified release (cheapest!), tolterodine (Detrusitol) or solifenacin (VESIcare) are also frequently prescribed. Fesoterodine (Toviaz) is also used.

Common side effects of anticholinergics: dizziness, drowsiness, dry mouth, blurred vision, constipation, headache, indigestions and abdominal pain.

Second line (if anticholinergic contraindicated or ineffective): mirabegron. Also consider this if the patient already has a high anticholinergic burden with the other medications they take, due to increased risk of Alzheimer's. (Even warfarin has anticholinergic effects.)

An anticholinergic can be used alongside an alpha blocker in patients with both voiding and storage symptoms.

Refer if above measures are unsuccessful.

For assessment of LUTS in general use:

The International Prostate Symptom Score (IPSS) questionnaire to assess severity and impact on quality of life.

See below for more details about lower urinary tract symptoms and BPH.

Extra Notes — Benign Prostatic Hypertrophy

BPH management

Conservative — Reduce caffeine and alcohol. Bladder exercises.

Alpha-blocker[1] E.g. tamsulosin

Explanation to patient: *'Acts by relaxing the prostate.'*

Side effects include drowsiness, light-headedness from low BP and retrograde ejaculation which some men find very troublesome. Review after 4–6 weeks.

5-alpha-reductase inhibitor[1]

E.g. finasteride

Explanation to patient: *'Acts by blocking the conversion of testosterone to a stronger hormone which increases the size of the prostate.'*

Side effects: loss of libido, ED, ejaculation problems and gynaecomastia.

Review in 3–6 months but can take up to 6 months to work.

Reduces PSA so avoid use if watchful waiting.

Transurethral resection of the prostate

90% risk of retrograde ejaculation. Other risks: incontinence, infection, retention, need for re-TURP, ED, strictures, bleeding, TURP syndrome and death.[2]

Tadalafil — Helps with ED and outflow symptoms.

Prostate cancer specialist management

Conservative — Watchful waiting (usually frail elderly) or active surveillance (regular MRIs ± biopsies) – usually in men with low-risk cancers.

Hormonal — Bicalutamide or Cyproterone acetate prior to giving goserelin analogue.[3]

Goserelin – Check LFTs 6 monthly

Chemotherapy (increasing role of chemotherapy in metastatic prostate cancer) and radiotherapy.

Total/Radical Prostatectomy.

Counselling for PSA testing … an example

'The prostate is a gland that helps make semen. It is located near the bladder and rectum. As men get older it can become cancerous. Prostate cancer is the most common cancer in men, in fact 80% of men in their 80s have evidence of prostate cancer. Most prostate cancers are slow growing, especially in more elderly gentlemen and the cancer may be so slow growing that these men may never be affected by the cancer in their lifetime. Therefore, some men prefer not to know. However, in other men prostate cancer may be fast growing and spread to other areas like the bones in the back. There is a blood test called a PSA test which can be helpful in identifying prostate cancer in some patients. It checks for a chemical released from the prostate, called PSA. If this is high, it may be a sign of prostate cancer but may just be a sign of a large prostate, which is harmless. Because PSA can be raised when there isn't cancer, this can mean men having unnecessary tests done. Also around 20% of prostate cancers have a normal PSA. To help find these cancers we also feel the prostate through the rectum to see if it feels abnormal. Any questions so far? If either PSA or examination are abnormal we refer men to the urologists who would usually perform a biopsy. This biopsy, which means taking small pieces of the prostate, is taken through the back passage and is therefore an uncomfortable procedure and has a risk of causing an infection or bleeding in the prostate. You have/do not have symptoms of prostate problems but symptoms do not necessarily correlate with the cancer. You are welcome to take reading material home to think about it, or have you already made a decision? … If you would like the test I suggest I examine your prostate, then we'll do the blood test in 1 week. I suggest waiting a week as examining the prostate can falsely increase the PSA level. So can exercise, cycling, sex and ejaculation. I will give you information on when to stop these activities prior to the test.'

Men's Health

Extra Notes — UTI in Men and Haematuria

Differential diagnosis[1] Urethritis   Pyelonephritis   Kidney cancer
                Calculi   Epididymitis   Bladder cancer   Prostate cancer

Investigations   Urine dipstick AND urine culture

If microscopic haematuria is detected in a man ≥ 60 years without dysuria and the MSU returns as negative → FBC

Complications   Pyelonephritis, prostatitis and some bacteria increase the risk of stones.[1]

Treatment   1 week of treatment, e.g. trimethoprim / nitrofurantoin – see local guidance.[1]

When to refer to Urology for further investigations:

UTI fails to respond to antibiotics[1]

Recurrent UTI – 2 or more in a 3-month period[1]

Even if >60 years – NICE advise this is a non-urgent referral[2]

However, if recurrent UTI with haematuria present – see below.

Genitourinary history suggests a cause or risk factor:

e.g. stones, operations, bladder outflow obstruction.[1]

Persistent microscopic haematuria and normal renal function.[1]

If renal function impaired or proteinuria – refer to renal.[1]

Refer 2WW through the suspected cancer (for urological/renal cancer) pathway if:

>45 years   Unexplained visible haematuria (asymptomatic or negative MSU).[2]

Visible haematuria which persists or recurs despite Rx for UTI.[2]

>60 years   Unexplained non-visible haematuria (negative MSU) AND EITHER dysuria OR ↑ serum WCC.[2]

Mass   Is identified (clinically or on imaging).[1]

Remember to use dipstick (not microscopy) to assess for haematuria and if one dipstick is positive → TWO more dipsticks are required. If EITHER of these shows a haematuria → refer (speed of referral depends on age as above).[3] 1+ on dipstick or more is significant. Routine referral if persistent non-visible haematuria which doesn't meet the above criteria for suspected cancer pathway referral.

Haematuria follow-up 'Persistent invisible haematuria in the absence of proteinuria should be followed up annually with repeat testing for haematuria, proteinuria or albuminuria, GFR and blood pressure monitoring as long as the haematuria persists.'[3]

CHAPTER 10 OVERVIEW

Sexual Health

	Cases in this chapter	Within the RCGP curriculum: Sexual Health RCGP Curriculum Online March 2016[1]	Learning points in the chapter include:
1	Fertility Work-up	'Take a sexual history … private and confidential, non-judgemental' 'Make timely, appropriate referrals to specialist services … reproductive health'	NICE Guidance. CG156. Fertility problems: assessment and treatment. 2013
2	Contraception – Combined	'Be aware of the legal aspects of providing contraception and sexual health advice in under-16s' 'Refer to the UK Medical Eligibility Criteria for Contraceptive Use'	Fraser Guidelines Missed pill rules UKMEC Evrapatch Nuvaring
3	Contraception – POP	'Demonstrate a working knowledge of: contraception'	POP
4	Pelvic Inflammatory Disease	'Apply the information gathered from the patient's sexual history and examination to generate a differential diagnosis and formulate a management plan'	PID IMB
5	Long Acting Reversible Contraception	'Demonstrate a working knowledge of: contraception'	Implant Injection IUS/IUD
Extra Notes	Emergency Contraception	'Know when urgent intervention is needed in sexual health'	Emergency contraception Quickstarting
	Stopping Contraception		FSRH guidance Sterilisation

1. http://www.rcgp.org.uk/training-exams/gp-curriculum-overview/online-curriculum/applying-clinical-knowledge-section-1/3-08-sexual-health.aspx

CHAPTER 10 REFERENCES

Fertility Work-up
1. NICE Guidelines. CG156. Fertility problems: assessment and treatment. 2013.
2. Chief Medical Officers for the United Kingdom. Vitamin D – advice on supplements for at risk groups. Cardiff, Belfast, Edinburgh, London: Welsh Government, Department of Health, Social Services and Public Safety, The Scottish Government, Department of Health; 2012. [http://www.scotland.gov.uk/Resource/0038/00386921.pdf].
3. NICE Guidelines. CG62. Antenatal care. 2008.
4. Oxfordshire CCG, et al. Assisted reproductive services for infertile couples. November 2013. http://www.oxfordshire ccg.nhs.uk/wp-content/uploads/2013/03/TV-Assisted-Reproduction-Services-policy-November-2013-FINAL.pdf

Contraception – Combined
1. British Medical Association (BMA). Consent Toolkit (4th ed.). London, UK: BMA, 2008.
2. http://www.fsrh.org/pdfs/ceuGuidanceYoungPeople2010.pdf
3. http://www.fsrh.org/pdfs/CEUStatementMissedPills.pdf
4. http://www.fsrh.org/pdfs/ukmecsummarysheets2009.pdf
5. http://www.fsrh.org/pdfs/UKMEC2009.pdf
6. http://www.fsrh.org/pdfs/CEUGuidanceCombinedHormonalContraception.pdf
7. Killick S.R., Eyong E., Elstein M. Ovarian follicular development in oral contraceptive cycle. *Fertil Steril*. 1987; 48: 409–13.
8. Schwarz J.L., Creinin M.D., Pymar H.C., Reid L. Predicting risk of ovulation in new start oral contraceptive users. *Am Coll Obstet Gynecol*. 2002; 99: 177–82.
9. Darnforth D.R., Hodgen G.D. 'Sunday start' multiphasic oral contraception: ovulation prevention and delayed follicular atresia in primates. *Contraception*. 1989; 39: 321–30.
10. http://www.fsrh.org/pdfs/CEUGuidanceQuickStartingContraception.pdf
11. http://patient.info/health/contraceptive-patch
12. http://patient.info/health/contraceptive-vaginal-ring

Contraception – POP
1. http://www.fsrh.org/pdfs/CEUGuidanceProgestogenOnlyPill09.pdf
2. http://www.fsrh.org/pdfs/UKMEC2009.pdf

Pelvic Inflammatory Disease/Intermenstrual Bleeding
1. http://patient.info/doctor/intermenstrual-and-postcoital-bleeding

LARC and Sterilisation
1. http://www.fsrh.org/pdfs/CEUGuidanceProgestogenOnlyImplants.pdf
2. http://www.fsrh.org/pdfs/CEUGuidanceProgestogenOnlyInjectables.pdf
3. http://www.fsrh.org/pdfs/CEUGuidanceintrauterineContraceptionNov07.pdf
4. http://www.fsrh.org/pdfs/ukmecsummarysheets2009.pdf

Emergency Contraception
1. http://www.fsrh.org/pdfs/CEUguidanceEmergencyContraception11.pdf
2. Piaggio G., Kapp N., von Hertzen H. Effect on pregnancy rates of the delay in administration of levonorgestrel for emergency contraception: a combined analysis of four WHO trials. *Contraception*. 2011; 84: 35–9.
3. NICE. http://cks.nice.org.uk/contraception-emergency#!scenariorecommendation:5. Revised Feb 2015.
4. Faculty of Family Planning and Reproductive Health Care Clinical Effectiveness Unit. UK Selected Practice Recommendations for Contraceptive Use. 2002. http://www.fsrh.org/admin/uploads/Final%20UK%20 recommendations1.pdf [Accessed 14 June 2011].
5. HRA Pharma UK Ltd. ellaOne: Summary of Product Characteristics (SPC). 2010. http://www.medicines.org.uk/emc [Accessed 14 June 2011].
6. Wilcox A.J., Dunson D., Baird D.D. The timing of the 'fertile window' in the menstrual cycle: day specific estimates from a prospective study. *Br Med J*. 2000; 321(7271): 1259–62.

Stopping Contraception
1. http://www.fsrh.org/pdfs/ContraceptionOver40July10.pdf
2. Sivin I., Stern J., Coutinho E., Mattos C.E.R., el Mahgoub S., Diaz S., et al. Prolonged intrauterine contraception: a seven-year randomized study of the levonorgestrel 20 mcg/day (LNg 20) and the copper T380 Ag IUDs. *Contraception*. 1991; 44: 473–80.
3. Díaz J., Faúndes A., Díaz M., Marchi N. Evaluation of the clinical performance of a levonorgestrel-releasing IUD, up to seven years of use, in Campinas, Brazil. *Contraception*. 1993; 47: 169–75.
4. http://www.fsrh.org/pdfs/MaleFemaleSterilisation.pdf

Sexual Health

Doctor's Notes

Patient   Miranda Butler   33 years   F
PMH   No information
Medications   No current medications
Allergies   No information
Consultations No recent consultations
Investigations No recent investigations
Household   No household members registered

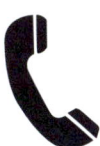

Example Consultation   Fertility Work-Up

Open That is disappointing. Now is a good time to discuss this.

History Tell me more about you. Are you well? Any medical problems? Or medication? Do you work? How about your partner? Do you exercise? Have you ever been pregnant? Are your smears up to date? What are your periods like? Any pain or abnormal bleeding between your periods? Has your husband had children?

Risk Does either of you smoke or drink? Do you know your weight? And height? Do you feel your weight is normal or high? Have you had an STI? Tell me more about that. How quickly was it treated? Are you under pressure or stress at the moment? Thinking about your hormones, do you suffer with acne or facial hair?

ICE I'm wondering what you think may have led to struggling to conceive? Have you been worrying about the chlamydia? Has anything else been worrying you? Your husband does not have to be told. What would you like us to decide today?

Empathy Falling pregnant can be difficult. All the stars need to align – for many couples this doesn't always happen quickly.

Curious You mentioned your friend. What does she think? Does your husband know you have called today?

Impact Has trying for a baby changed your relationship or your mood?

Summary To summarise, you have been trying for a baby for 18 months, this has changed your relationship as you now have sex routinely in the middle of your monthly cycle. You are worried the chlamydia may be a reason. You do not want your husband to know. You would like to proceed with fertility treatment.

Sense I am sorry to hear you have struggled and I sense the chlamydia has been weighing on your mind.

Impression It sounds like the infection was treated quickly, which reduces the chances of scarring. There are many other reasons why you may not have fallen pregnant.

Experience What do you know about how to increase your chance of falling pregnant?

Explanation Your friend advised sex is most important on day 14. Sperm lasts for 7 days. Once released, an egg needs to be fertilised within 24 hours. This is why it is so hard to fall pregnant. Having sex every two days, especially the week prior to ovulation, increases your chances of a sperm being ready to meet that egg.

Options If you make these changes you may fall pregnant now. But let's proceed anyway. The fertility team requires a series of tests. First, bloods to test your hormones, thyroid and immunity to rubella and chickenpox. Please arrange the first blood test 1 or 2 days after your next period begins. Then we need another blood test on day 21 to check you have ovulated. I will also arrange an USS which takes up to 6 weeks. Meanwhile do you think you can ask your husband to do a semen analysis sample through his GP? Ask his GP to send the result to me. We also need an up to date chlamydia test with the nurse please. Would that be okay?

Future When all of this is done, contact me and I'll send the referral and results to the fertility team. Do be aware that sometimes the chlamydia result may be a false positive. Have you come across this term in the labs?

Empower In the meantime being active, eating well and maintaining a healthy weight and avoiding alcohol are important when trying to fall pregnant, for both you and your partner. Are there any steps you could take regarding your lifestyle here? I would also recommend taking folic acid and vitamin D supplements that you can buy from the pharmacy. These supplements are important for the health and spine development in a baby. Any questions? How do you feel about the plan? If you have any further questions do call me.

Sexual Health – 1

Patient's Story

Fertility Work-Up

Doctor's notes Miranda Butler, 33 years. PMH: None. Medications: None.

How to act Slightly nervous on the phone.

PC *'Doctor, we've been trying for a baby for 18 months now. I wondered if I could have some tests please.'*

History You have never been pregnant. Your husband has never had children.

You have been married for 3 years and your relationship is very good.

Your coil was removed 18 months ago.

You have light periods and 5/28 regular cycles.

You have no IMB or PCB. No dyspareunia, no discharge or abdominal pain.

Smear last year was normal and no abnormal smears.

You know you are slightly overweight. You are 70 kg and 5 foot 3 inches.

If asked how you may lose weight, suggest you would like to start jogging.

You have no PMH and take no medicines. You have no FH.

Social You are a lab technician and your husband is a plumber.

Neither of you feels stressed.

You have a sedentary lifestyle and are happy.

You rarely drink and have never smoked.

ICE You believe your tubes are blocked from the chlamydia you had when you were 19 years old. Do not give this information away in your medical history unless asked directly or about your concerns.

The chlamydia was treated within a month of having UPSI.

Your husband does not know that you had chlamydia and you would prefer not to have to tell him but fear he will find out. If he knew, you think he would be disappointed in you and may think of you differently.

He has never been keen to talk about previous relationships.

You are hoping that the doctor will refer you for fertility treatment.

'I know falling pregnant takes time. It did for my friend.'

You understand that you need to have sex on day 14 of your 28-day cycle so you always do and have sex three times a week mid-cycle. Your friend told you that her fertility test kit lit up when she had ovulated on day 14, which meant she needed to go and have sex. (False health belief.)

There has been an impact on your relationship. Sex has become a mid-month routine, rather than spontaneous and fun.

Your husband is aware you are calling the doctor today.

Learning Points   Fertility Work-Up

Relationship — Frequency of intercourse

History
- Previous pregnancies and children
- Period cycle
- Smear history
- PCOS symptoms

Stress — Lifestyle, work and other stressors

Risk factors
- Alcohol and smoking history
- STIs
- BMI
- PCOS
- Other gynaecological history/surgery

Vaccinations — Rubella + varicella status

Investigations
- Days 2–4   LH, FSH, TFT, testosterone, DHEA, SHBG, prolactin
- Day 21/28 Progesterone – 7 days before the next period is due (if short or long cycle)
- Chlamydia screen
- TVUSS
- Semen analysis
- Smear if not up to date

Advise
- Ideal BMI 20–25 and avoid alcohol
- Start folic acid 0.4 mg /day[1] and vitamin D 10 micrograms/day[2,3]

Who is entitled?
- Look at your local guidance
- E.g. In Oxford the criteria is <35 years, BMI 19–29.9 and non-smoker and 'Infertility of at least two years' duration, including one year of expectant management in primary care'.[4]
- NICE recommend <40 years.[1]

Chlamydia test — Chlamydia test. Be aware that false positives are possible. Always counsel women as the result can have an impact on a relationship.

Sexual Health – 1

Doctor's Notes

Patient	Gemma Briggs	15 years	F
PMH	No information		
Medications	No current medications		
Allergies	No information		
Consultations	No recent consultations		
Investigations	No recent investigations		
Household	Simon Briggs	47 years	M
	Davina Briggs	48 years	F

Example Consultation — Contraception – Combined

Open ☐ — What's led to this decision? How did you meet your partner?

Flags ☐ — I can help today but I need to ask a few personal questions to make sure we make the right choice for you and, as you are under 16, I have to make sure you are not at risk. Is anyone forcing you to have sex? How old is your boyfriend? As you tell me you are in no danger then what you say to me is confidential. Have you had sex already? Is there any possibility you might be pregnant now? Would you have sex if you were not on the contraceptive pill? What is your relationship like with your parents? Could you tell them? What might they say? Is there anyone else you could talk to, an older sister or auntie perhaps? When was your last period? Do you have a regular cycle? Before we proceed I would just like to check you have no other medical problems that would prevent you from taking the pill.

Risk ☐ — Have you or anyone in your family ever had a blood clot? Do you suffer with migraines? Have you ever had a headache which caused a problem with your vision or arms or legs? Has anyone in the family had breast cancer?

History ☐ — Do you have any health problems? Take any medicines? Do you smoke?

ICE ☐ — Do you have any worries about starting the pill? Was there anything else you were hoping for?

O/E ☐ — I'd like to check your BP, weight and height if I may.

Experience ☐ — What do you know about the pill?

Explanation ☐ — The OCP is taken for 21 days then you have a 7-day break when you will have your period. Side effects can include breast tenderness or mood changes. There are risks to consider when taking the pill. Rarely, women can have a stroke or a blood clot due to the pill. The COCP also slightly increases your risk of breast and cervical cancer; however, it is protective against ovarian and womb cancer. No contraception is 100% protective against pregnancy and the pill does not protect you against STIs. Can I please check I have been clear; what are the risks of the pill? That's correct.

Options ☐ — More reliable options include a hormone matchstick under the skin, an injection or a coil in the womb. Are you interested in any of these? You can start the pill on the first day of your next period. Do you feel you can wait until then? If you miss one pill then that is okay, just take it when you remember, even if that means taking two in a day. However, if you miss a second pill within the month then you will need to use condoms for 7 days. If this happens in the first week of the pill packet and you've had sex since the LMP, you will need emergency contraception. If this occurs in the third week of the pill packet, don't have a pill break but start the next packet straightaway and remember to use condoms for 7 days. So if you forgot 2 pills after 5 days into your pill packet what would you do? What about if you forgot the last 2 pills in your packet?

Empathy ☐ — I know this is a lot to take in. If you're ever unsure what to do, please phone us for advice. There is a leaflet in the pill packet which can also help and you should read it now and keep it safe.

Experience ☐ — Can I check I have been clear? Can you explain to me how to take the pill?

Empower ☐ — I will send you a PIL so you have further information regarding what to do if you are unwell. For example, if you have vomiting or diarrhoea. Remember, only condoms protect you from STIs. You should always encourage your partner to have an STI check. Do protect yourself as STIs can cause long-term pain or infertility.

Future ☐ — Here is your prescription; the pill is called Microgynon. There is nothing to pay: even when you become 16, the pill is free if you tick the 'free of charge contraceptive' box on the back of the prescription. Wait until your next period starts and start taking the pill on the first day. Please see the GP again in 3 months and call if you have any questions in the meantime.

Safety net ☐ — If you ever have a painful swollen leg or a severe headache see a doctor immediately.

Sexual Health – 2

Patient's Story

Contraception – Combined

Doctor's notes	Gemma Briggs, 15 years. PMH: None. Medications: None.
How to act	Mature and intelligent.
PC	*'I would like to go on the pill.'*
History	You have a new boyfriend. You met at school in your class.
	No one is forcing you. You have not had sex yet.
	You would also use condoms.
	You would still have sex even if you were not prescribed contraception.
	You get on well with your parents but will not tell them. It would just be too awkward. However, you will tell your older sister, who is 22 years.
	No PMH or other medication.
	You have read a little about the pill on the Internet but would like the doctor to explain again. A friend of yours has a contraceptive implant but you don't like how it feels under the skin. You aren't keen on regular injections and wouldn't like anything inserted into your womb.
	You started your periods when you were 12, they are usually regular 7/30.
	Your LMP was 3 weeks ago, you expect to start again in about 5 days' time.
	You do not plan to have sex prior to your period and are happy to wait.
ICE	You have no concerns.
Social	In year 10 at school. Living with parents and your older sister lives with her partner. Never smoked.
Examination	BMI is 22. BP 90/50.

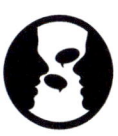

Sexual Health – 2

Learning Points Contraception – Combined

To meet Fraser Guidelines the patient …
- Will not tell her parent/carer despite encouragement from the doctor
- Understands the advice
- Is likely to have sex if the contraception is not prescribed
- Her mental or physical health may be at risk if not prescribed
- It is in her *best interests*[1,2]

In practice you should document all this clearly in the notes.

'Is this confidential?' A suggested answer begins with 'yes' – *'Yes … so long as you are not in danger.'*

Understanding the OCP missed pill (>24 hours) rules

'No indication for EC if the pills in the preceding 7 days have been taken consistently and correctly (assuming the pills thereafter are taken correctly and additional contraceptive precautions are used).'[3] Therefore the week prior to and following the pill-free-week is the most risky time as 7 days could be extended. Although the standard advice suggests 1 pill can be missed anywhere in the pack, if the woman was to take her next pill late (but not missed), the risk of ovulation and therefore pregnancy is increased. The woman may choose to have a 4 day pill-break to minimise this risk.

The advice for backup contraception for 7 days following two missed pills 'may be overcautious in the second and third weeks, but the advice is a backup in the event that further pills are missed.'[3]

UKMEC guidelines[4]	Contraception cautions and contraindications
	'Each UK category should be considered separately (it is NOT appropriate to consider Category 1 and 2 safe and 3 and 4 unsafe.'[5]
Alternative regimes	The woman does not have to have a period every month!
	She may prefer to tricycle 3 packets (without pill-free days) or back to back packets until breakthrough bleeding occurs then have 4–7 pill-free days.[6]
Commencing the OCP	'COCs containing ethinyl estradiol can be started up to and including Day 5 of the cycle without the need for additional contraceptive protection.'[6-9]
Risk of OCP to a foetus	Studies are limited but with no consistent data to support serious abnormalities. Read more at 'Effects of foetal exposure to steroid hormones'[10] within the reference.
Benefits	Decreased risk ovarian/endometrial/colorectal cancer.[9]
	May reduce menopausal symptoms.[9]
Thrombosis risks	>3 hr flight – 'should be advised about reducing periods of immobility'.[9]
	>7 days at >4500 m altitude – 'consider switching to an alternative method'.[9]
Increased risks	Breast and cervical cancer, thrombosis and stroke[9] – read more within the reference.
Evra Patch	Weekly for 3 weeks then a patch-free week. If falls off >48 hours – apply a new patch, condoms for 7 days and ECP if sex within the previous 5 days.[11]
Nuvaring	Insert for 3 weeks then remove for 1 week.
	If it falls out, no need for condoms or ECP if replaced within 3 hours.[12]

Doctor's Notes

Patient	Emma Brown	28 years	F
PMH	No information		
Medications	Rigevidon		
Allergies	No information		
Consultations	No recent consultations		
Investigations	3 months ago	BP 108/62	
		BMI 23.3	
	6 months ago	normal smear	
Household	No household members registered		

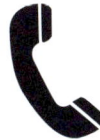

Example Consultation — Contraception – POP

Open ☐ — Any problems on the pill? What are your periods like?

Risk ☐ — Can I check there are no reasons why you shouldn't be on the pill; any FH of blood clots or breast cancer?

Flags ☐ — Do you ever forget a pill? Any bleeding in between periods or after sex? Do you smoke? Any headaches? Tell me more about the headaches. Do they affect your vision? Or affect your arms or legs?

ICE ☐ — What do you think caused the headache? Are you worried about anything? Apart from your pill today was there anything else you were hoping for?

History ☐ — Any medical problems? Tell me more about you. You mentioned you had been feeling stressed? What do you do for a living? Are you in a long-term relationship?

Summary ☐ — To summarise, you have been pleased with the pill but have had headaches which affect your eyesight and give you tingling. You felt this was likely to be due to the stress of work at the time. Is that correct?

Impression ☐ — Your headaches are called focal migraines – bad headache which affects the body.

Experience ☐ — Can you remember the risks of the pill?

Explanation ☐ — One risk of the pill is having a stroke. Migraines that affect your eyesight or cause tingling are often warning signs that you may be at a high risk of having a stroke if you continued with the pill. We should change your contraception and take away the oestrogen that causes this risk.

Sense ☐ — I appreciate this is not what you were expecting.

Options ☐ — There are many options still available to you which only contain progesterone hormone, which is safe. Options include the tablet, injections, the implant or coil. Are you interested in these other methods?

Curious ☐ — What is your friend's experience? She had a hard time with it.

Empathy ☐ — I appreciate why you feel frustrated, then. But the risk of having a stroke is real and I do not want to put you in danger. We should change your pill. I'm sorry you are disappointed. What is going through your mind? It does sound like your skin is important to you. If it became a problem, there are lots of treatments that we can try. Women take the pill for different reasons. What is the most important benefit of the pill for you? Okay – protection and secondly skin? How is your skin now? We will aim to keep it that way so at the first sign of things getting worse let me know. Okay?

Explanation ☐ — All progesterone-only methods may cause erratic bleeding in 40% of woman. Forty per cent have regular periods and 20% no bleeding at all,[1] which is safe. We cannot predict which group you will be in. Often bleeding settles to an extent after 3–6 months. The progesterone hormone may cause skin or mood changes but remember this hormone, progesterone, is present in the pill you have been taking. No contraception is 100% and if you did fall pregnant on the POP there is an increased risk of an ectopic pregnancy which is a pregnancy in the wrong place, but overall the risk is small. There are non-hormonal options, the copper coil or the diaphragm.

Empower ☐ — So out of the all the options, which one is best for you?

Future ☐ — With the tablet there are two options, a stronger progesterone with a 12-hour window to remember or the mini-pill with a 3-hour window. Overall the 12-hour window pill may be safer but if this affected your skin we could rethink. Which do you prefer? When was your last period? Have you missed any pills this month? You can start taking the new POP today and you are protected from pregnancy because you have taken your other pills this month. Remember to take it every day at the same time, without the 7-day break – put it with your toothbrush. The new pill is called Desogestrel. Why don't we catch up in 3 months? But do get in touch if it isn't suiting you. Any questions? If the headaches return, see a GP.

Safety net ☐ — You have 12 hours to remember the pill and, if you forget, use condoms for 48 hours. If you've had sex, contact us as you may need the ECP.

Sexual Health – 3

Patient's Story

Contraception – POP

Doctor's notes Emma Brown, 28 years. PMH: None. Medications: Rigevidon.
BP 3 months ago 108/62. BMI 23.3. Last smear 6 months ago (normal).

How to act You are in a hurry and have come out of a meeting to take the call.

PC *'I'd just like my repeat pill please.'*

History You have been taking the pill for 6 months. You are keen to continue.

Your bleeding is normal 7/28 with no IMB or PCB.

You sometimes forget your pill but have not forgotten this month.

You have a hectic lifestyle so don't always take it at the same time.

You have no vaginal discharge and are in a stable relationship of 2 years.

You had a negative chlamydia test after starting the relationship.

You have never been pregnant.

Only if asked directly about headaches do you disclose you have experienced headaches which gave you tingling down the right side.

Your vision also changed to flashing lights during the headache.

These headaches have not been present for 4 months. Usual onset was late afternoon.

You found that lying down and taking ibuprofen relieved the headache.

You have heard about the POP, and if the POP is mentioned, freely give the information *'My friend took the POP so yes I've heard about it.'*

If asked about the friend's experience, she bled every day and told you not to get it. You are at first happy to take the risk with the OCP as your headaches have not been present for months.

You don't want anything which will make your skin worse – it is currently good.

You agree to the POP once you are informed that the GP can no longer prescribe the OCP; however, you remain unhappy with the GP. You do not want any other form of contraception.

Social You work as a solicitor and live alone. You do not smoke.

ICE You thought the headaches were due to stress. You had work deadlines at the time.

You are worried that changing pills will put you at risk of pregnancy.

You had sex yesterday. You have not missed a pill for the past 18 days.

The main thing you want from your pill is reliability.

You also want to have nice skin.

Sexual Health – 3

Learning Points   Contraception – POP

Norethisterone	350 micrograms (e.g. Micronor and Noriday)	Alters cervical mucus
Levonorgestrel	30 micrograms (e.g. Norgeston)	Alters cervical mucus
Desogestrel	75 micrograms (e.g. Cerazette or Cerelle)	Also inhibits ovulation
Side effects:	Erratic bleeding, low libido, vaginal dryness, acne, bloating and mood changes.	
Risks:	Ectopic pregnancy.	
Prescriptions:	May prescribe for 12 months from the first prescription.[1]	
Window	12 hours for desogestrel and 3 hours for norethisterone and levonorgestrel.[1]	
Missed pill	Extra precautions for 48 hours after missed pill is taken and ECP if sex during this time.[1]	
Cautions	Refer to UKMEC guidance.[2]	
Erratic bleeding	If they return with erratic bleeding *the most likely cause is the POP*.	
but always:	**Rule out a pregnancy**	or ectopic pregnancy with a urine β-hCG
	Rule out infection	symptoms of STI/PID and arrange a chlamydia test
	Consider cancer	ask about PCB, consider looking at the cervix and consider a TVUSS for older women.

Sexual Health – 3

Doctor's Notes

Patient	Stephanie Smith	24 years	F
PMH	No information		
Medications	Cilest		
Allergies	No information		
Consultations	No recent consultations		
Investigations	No recent investigations		
Household	No household members registered		

Example Consultation — Pelvic Inflammatory Disease

Open ☐	Tell me more about this spotting? Anything else that is new? How are your periods?
History ☐	Do you have any medical problems? Allergies? Remember your pill? Tell me more about you. Are you in a relationship? Is that a long-term relationship?
ICE ☐	What has gone through your mind as to what may be causing this bleeding? Is there anything specific that you worry is causing it? Any other thoughts? What did you think I may suggest today?
Impact ☐	How has the bleeding impacted on day-to-day life or the relationship?
Sense ☐	I can see that you are keen to get to the bottom of this and I hear how bothersome this is for you.
Risk ☐	I'm wondering about clues in your sexual history – have you ever had an STI? Could you be at risk? When did you first have sex? Have you had a check-up since restarting your relationship? Has any family member had any women's health problems? When was your LMP? Was the period due? Was it a normal period?
Flags ☐	Have you had any: fevers? Bleeding after sex? Pain during sex? Discharge? Smell? Burning passing urine? Or going more frequently? How are your bowels? How do you feel in yourself? Any stomach pain?
Curious ☐	Have you spoken to your partner about relationships you have had during your time apart?
Summary ☐	To summarise, spotting for 2 months is starting to impact on everyday life. You have had lower stomach pain including during intercourse. You are not sure what has caused this or what to expect today.
O/E ☐	May I examine you? I'd like to take your temperature and pulse, feel your tummy and feel the womb through the vagina, as pain may suggest an infection. May I look at the neck of the womb with a speculum, a plastic tube, which fits into the vagina? It can be uncomfortable but will allow me to check the cervix and take swabs for infection including general bacteria, thrush, chlamydia and gonorrhoea. Does this sound okay? Would you like a chaperone? May I have a urine sample for a pregnancy and infection test?
Impression ☐	I believe you may have an infection, possibly chlamydia, causing pelvic inflammatory disease.
Experience ☐	Have you come across either of these?
Explanation ☐	Before the chlamydia result returns I would prefer to treat for what I suspect is inflammation from an infection. If not treated, you could become unwell or have problems with fertility in the future. Two antibiotics, metronidazole and ofloxacin, are taken twice a day for 14 days. Use paracetamol/ibuprofen for pain relief.
Options ☐	You cannot drink alcohol during this treatment as you will be unwell on this antibiotic. If the bleeding persists then we will review your pill.
Empathy ☐	Do you think you will be able to tell your boyfriend? What might he say?
Empower ☐	Does this plan sound okay so far? You should both complete the sexual health screen at the GUM clinic. Do not have sex again until you have both completed treatment with antibiotics. Your smear test, which screens for cancer of the cervix, is due next year. Any questions? The risk of chlamydia is infertility so it is important to protect yourself.
Future ☐	Please arrange to speak to the doctor again about your test results.
Safety net ☐	If your period is late, please repeat the pregnancy test. If you start to feel unwell, the stomach pain feels worse, you have a fever or if the symptoms and bleeding have not started to improve within 48 hours, please see the doctor straight away as infections can be serious if you don't respond to the antibiotics. May I clarify you are happy with when you need to speak to the doctor again?

Patient's Story

Pelvic Inflammatory Disease

Doctor's notes	Stephanie Smith, 24 years. PMH: None. Medication: Cilest.
How to act	Very pleasant.
PC	*'It's my periods. I don't bleed just during my period but other times too.'*
History	2 months of bleeding – spotting randomly throughout the month.
	Occasional PCB.
	You are very well in yourself and have no prescribed medications.
	LMP almost 4 weeks ago.
	Your LMP was a 5-day period surrounded by the spotting.
	Periods have always been regular. You are a good pill taker. No FH.
	No medicines apart from the OCP which you commenced 18/12 ago.
	You have had deep pain on intercourse but you didn't make the connection.
	You have had some lower abdominal pain and thought this may be your bowels.
	You occasionally need a Fybogel for mild constipation.
	You have no urinary symptoms.
	No PV discharge. You have never had an STI check.
	You have never had an STI or a smear test. You have never been pregnant.
	You split up from your boyfriend 8 months ago.
	The relationship restarted 3 months ago.
	During the break you both had one other sexual contact using condoms.
	Since the age of 18 years you have had 2 other sexual relationships in total.
	The bleeding has been too light to comfortably use tampons and you don't like the smell of wearing liners. You have also had to avoid intercourse.
	You will tell your partner what the GP says today.
	You realise you should have both been to GUM.
Social	You did a Master of Business Administration.
	Now you are an investment banker.
	You are enjoying your job and thrive on the pressure of the work.
	You are happy in your relationship. All is going well.
ICE	You have no idea why you are bleeding. It is just very irritating.
	You are not concerned about anything particular. Only that it may continue.
	You have no idea what the GP will suggest.
O/E	Abdomen. LIF pain. No palpable mass. No guarding or rebound tenderness.
	PV – left adnexal tenderness and cervical excitation. No masses.
	Speculum – normal-looking cervix.
	HR 70 bpm and apyrexial. BP 120/60. Urine dipstick negative.
	Pregnancy test negative.

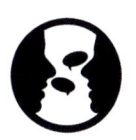

Sexual Health – 4

Learning Points — Intermenstrual Bleeding

Causes
- Physiological — 2% spot around ovulation.[1]
- Pregnancy — Miscarriage or ectopic.
- Smear/trauma
- Infection or vaginitis
- Structural/histological — Cancer, polyps or ectropion.
- Any contraception — Especially low oestrogen content.
- ↓ Contraception efficacy — Secondary to interactions, e.g. tamoxifen, steroids, SSRIs, warfarin, St John's wort.[1]

History
- Menstrual history — Onset, LMP, IMB, PCB and cycle pattern.
- Gynaecological history — Smears, contraception, operations and FH.
- Obstetric history — Gravida and parity.
- Sexual history — Age became sexually active, partners and infections.
- General health — Feeling unwell or fevers, urinary/bowel symptoms.

Risk factors
- Endometrial cancer — Obesity, PCOS, nulliparity and late first child.
- Cervical cancer/STI — Early sexual activity and multiple partners.

Examination
- Abdomen — Tenderness and masses.
- Pelvic examination — Masses, adnexal tenderness and cervical excitation.
- Inspection and speculum — Vulva, vagina and cervix (ectropion/polyps/ulceration).
- Swabs — Chlamydia if at risk and triple swabs if signs of PID.
- Observations — If possibility of infection/sepsis.

Investigations
Pregnancy test (instruct the patient to do this at home).
If negative it needs to be repeated 3 weeks after last UPSI.
Urine dipstick. Swabs. FBC/TFT.
Consider TVUSS to assess the endometrium and if abnormal/ongoing concern (especially if >40 years) a hysteroscopy for biopsies.[1]
Be sure the woman does not meet the criteria for a 2WW gynaecology cancer referral.

Gynaecology rule

The same rule applies to both abnormal PV bleeding or pelvic pain.

   Consider/rule out pregnancy, infection and structural/histological causes.

Structural/histological causes include polyps, fibroids, cancer or ovarian cysts.

Remember no contraception is 100% so do not be reassured if they are taking a contraception.

If the cause of abnormal bleeding (especially in a young woman) is most likely secondary to her hormone Rx, you may decide to change Rx as a trial first before investigating (but do exclude pregnancy and chlamydia).

The IMB may be due to the strength of the OCP, especially if menses occurs early but remains regular. Consider changing the progesterone or increasing the dose of the ethinylestradiol to 30–35 mcg and the next step may be a triphasic OCP. Remember the ↑ risk of the OCP with increasing strengths of ethinylestradiol.

PID
Symptoms may include: Dyspareunia, discharge, abnormal bleeding, pain and fevers.
Signs: Adnexal tenderness ± cervical excitation ± fever or tachycardia or low BP.
Treat immediately as per local guidance before waiting for swab results.
Admit if systemically unwell or no improvement in 48 hours or pregnant.

Sexual Health – 4

Doctor's Notes

Patient   Fedora Baros   38 years   F
PMH   No information
Medications   Ovranette
Allergies   No information
Consultations No recent consultations
Investigations No recent investigations
Household   Domenic Baros   42 years   M

Fedora attends with her husband Domenic who is also registered at the practice and has no known medical history.

Example Consultation — LARC and Sterilisation

Open ☐	Please tell me about what has led to this decision. What are your thoughts so far?
History ☐	I'm interested to know more about you both. Fedora, do you have any medical history? Have you ever been pregnant? Do you have regular periods? Do you take any tablets?
Flags ☐	Would you mind, Domenic, if I spoke to Fedora alone for a couple of minutes? Fedora, because you are my patient today, I just wanted to make sure that you have not been encouraged by anyone to make a decision you are not comfortable with.
Risk ☐	Before thinking about the coil, have you had any abnormal bleeding in between periods or after sex, or heavier bleeding or discharge? Any pain on intercourse or infections in the past 3 months? Are your periods manageable or painful?
ICE ☐	What is the right thing for you? Did you have any concerns at all? Or worries about either procedure? How would you feel if you did fall pregnant? It sounds as if this would be stressful for you. What did you expect us to decide today? Is there anything else you were wondering? Or would like to discuss today?
Impact ☐	How is your relationship? We should consider your risk of regret if your husband had a permanent procedure. You should be at peace with a vasectomy being irreversible.
Sense ☐	You were not expecting me to say that? Does this change things? Is your mood okay?
Curious ☐	How would Domenic feel if you fell pregnant? Is there anything you want to ask whilst we are alone? Would you like to finish this consultation with the two of us or invite your husband back in? Are you happy for me to share your concerns with Domenic?
Summary ☐	Hello Domenic. To summarise, you have both made the decision to not have children together. Fedora, you feel that this would put you under financial pressure. You are currently looking for work. You are fed up with taking the pill. You are both happy, therefore, with the plan for a vasectomy. However, Fedora you were not aware that this should be seen as irreversible. We started to discuss the risk of regret; for example, if you did find work, life became less stressful and you decided you wanted children. The other option you have considered is the coil but you do not want erratic bleeding and you feel comforted by regular periods.
Impression ☐	You would like a reliable form of contraception which you can forget about and is free from hormones, but is reversible should things change. You wondered about the coil.
Options ☐	Other options include using condoms or a diaphragm if you wish to avoid all hormones, continuing with the pill or hormones in the form of an injection or skin implant.
Experience ☐	What do you understand about how the coil works? And the risks?
Explanation ☐	There are two types of coil – the copper coil which has no hormones and usually gives regular periods but you may have heavier and longer periods. Or the hormone coil which is the one which can give erratic bleeding or no bleeding at all. As you have manageable periods you may find you tolerate heavier periods with a copper coil. No contraception is 100% but the coil is a very good form of contraception. If you did fall pregnant, however, there is an increased risk of ectopic pregnancy, a pregnancy not in the womb which is dangerous. There is the risk of pushing an infection through to the womb and if this occurred you may become very unwell, but we minimise this risk by recommending swabs to check for infection a week before we fit the coil, and it is a sterile procedure, which means we use equipment which is very clean. There is a 1 in 20 chance the coil may fall out, especially in the first few months. When we put it in, your blood pressure may drop or you may be in pain. Usually the pain is like a period cramp which settles. There is a 1–2/1000 chance of the coil going through the womb.
Empower ☐	Have you made a decision or may I provide you with information to explain further?
Empathy ☐	It is a lot of information and a big decision. Domenic, what are your thoughts?
Future ☐	Would you like to call me when you have made a decision or if you have further questions? I will also print out some information on vasectomies.

Sexual Health – 5

Patient's Story

LARC and Sterilisation

Doctor's notes		Fedora Baros, 38 years. PMH: None. Medications: Ovranette.
		Husband Domenic Baros, 42 years, is also present.
How to act		Very pleasant.
PC		*'We would like to discuss whether the coil or vasectomy is the best option.'*
History		You have decided not to have children.
		This is a decision you have made together.
		You have been married for 2 years.
		Domenic has three children from a previous marriage.
		Fedora has not been married before and has no children.
		You are both very well and have no medical history. You take no medicines.
Social	**Fedora**	You are currently unemployed. Money is tight and you are looking for work.
		You used to work as a cleaner. You have decided you are not able to afford having a child. You believe you are happy with this decision.
	Domenic	You are a security guard. You see your three children twice a month. You would be very happy to have children if this is what Fedora wanted. However, she has decided that with life's stressors you should not have more children.
		Neither of you smokes or drinks.
ICE	**Fedora**	You would prefer Domenic to have a vasectomy.
		You are fed up with taking the OCP. You don't want any hormones in your body and feel comforted by a monthly period. You have concerns about the coil as you have heard that it is painful.
		You expect the doctor will arrange a vasectomy for Domenic today.
		You believe that if you did change your mind the vasectomy can be reversed by putting the tubes back together.
		If asked about your risk of regret, you become unsure.
		Your main concern about the coil is erratic bleeding. You like monthly and regular periods.
		If the doctor explains how the coil is inserted and discusses the risks, you decide you feel comfortable to have this procedure.
	Domenic	You are happy to have a vasectomy if this is what Fedora wants.
		You decided to attend together, however, to discuss all options.
		You expect the doctor will arrange a vasectomy for you today.

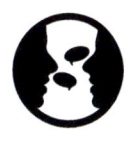

Sexual Health – 5

Learning Points — Long Acting Reversible Contraception

Contraceptive implant[1]

Implant indication	LARC or dysmenorrhoea.
How to take	Insert day 1–5 of cycle. Repeat within 3 years.
Side effects	Acne, bleeding changes, mood or libido changes and headaches reported although 'no evidence of a causal association'.[1] No osteoporosis risk.
Bleeding risk	<1/4 regular periods, 1/3 infrequent bleeding, 1/5 no bleeding, and 1/4 frequent/prolonged bleeding.[1]
Lost implant	If impalpable implant, use additional contraception and arrange an USS.
Problematic bleeding	Exclude pregnancy, chlamydia and malignancy (view cervix).
	Consider an additional hormone off licence (COCP or POP) for 3 months.[1]
	Use judgement: risk unknown with longer use and see guidance.

Injection[2]

Side effects	The same as other progesterone contraceptives and 'associated with weight gain'.[2]
Fertility	Can be delayed for up to 1 year after discontinuation.[2]
BMD	Small loss of BMD usually recovers after discontinuation. Review 2-yearly.[2]
Caution/CI	Maximum recommended age of 50 years. Caution in CVD.[2]

IUS (Mirena)/IUD (Copper)[3]

Indication	IUS = LARC, progesterone cover for HRT and menorrhagia.
	IUD = LARC and EC
Mode of action	IUS prevents implantation. IUD prevents fertilisation and implantation.
Risks	Infection, perforation, failure rate, ectopic, expulsion and cervical shock.
Contraindications	Must be 'reasonably certain'[3] she is not pregnant. See page 7 of reference.[3]
	See also UKMEC guidance.[4]
Side effects:	IUS: erratic bleeding. Small risk of systemic progesterone side effects.
	IUD may give longer/heavier periods.
	Tampons can be used
Licensing of duration	Mirena = 5 years
	= 4 years if the indication is endometrial protection for HRT
	Jaydess = 3 years
	Copper = depends on the device – 5 or 10 years so check the device.

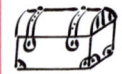

> See the **Link Hub at CompleteCSA.co.uk** for a link to **UKMEC guidance** which should be followed when commencing contraception.

Extra Notes

Emergency Contraception

Levonorgestrel (LNG) 1.5 mg
Prevents/delays ovulation. Licence = up to 72 hours.

Efficacy demonstrated up to 96 hours[1,2] and if other EC is not an option consider prescribing up to 120 hours (off-licence use).[3]

If vomiting occurs within 2 hours of ingestion then repeat the LNG dose.[4]

Double the dose (off licence) if liver enzyme inducing drugs have been taken within 28/7.[1]

Ulipristal acetate (UPA) = EllaOne 30 mg
CI: Pregnancy, hypersensitivity to UPA and severe asthma.[1]

Caution in 'hepatic dysfunction, hereditary problems of galactose intolerance, the Lapp lactase deficiency or glucose-galactose malabsorption',[1,5] if liver enzyme inducing drugs have been taken with 28/7,[1,6] or if taking antacids and H2/PPIs.[1]

Prevents/delays ovulation. Licence = 120 hours.

If vomits <3 hours repeat UPA.[5]

IUD
CI if there is a risk that implantation has already taken place.

Licence: Can be inserted up to 5 days after SI or up to 5 days after ovulation (only if regular cycles) – whichever event is the latest.

Prevents fertilisation and implantation.[1]

'All eligible women presenting between 0 and 120 hours of UPSI or within 5 days of expected ovulation should be offered a Cu-IUD because of the low documented failure rate.'[1]

Quickstarting contraception is off licence after an emergency contraceptive pill
Advise to check a pregnancy test 3 weeks later or if there is a delayed period.

After LNG use condoms for 7 days with OCP, or 2 days with POP, or 9 days for Qlaira[1].

After UPA, use condoms for 14 days with OCP, or for 9 days with POP, or 16 days with Qlaira[1].

'UPA is a progesterone receptor modulator that blocks the action of progesterone and therefore in theory could reduce the efficacy of contraceptives containing progesterone.'[1,5]

Case: 'I've already taken LNG this cycle'
UPA and IUD not an option as there is already a risk of implantation.

Therefore, may use second LNG off licence.[1]

LNG 'is not thought to be harmful to the fetus if accidental exposure occurs'.[3]

Case: 'I've had UPSI earlier this month but didn't take any EC'
If requested before 5 days after expected ovulation, the IUD would be recommended.[1]

Sexual Health

Extra Notes   Stopping Contraception

Non-hormonal method   ≥50 years

    After 1 year of amenorrhoea.[1]

    <50 years

    After 2 years of amenorrhoea.[1]

Progesterone only   ≥50 years and amenorrhoea for a year

    *If 2 × FSH level tests ≥30 IU/L (6 weeks apart).

    … Stop 1 yr after the second raised FSH level.[1]

IUS   Inserted ≥45 years:

    Women may leave the Mirena in situ >5 years but this is off licence.

    Research has shown there is contraceptive cover for 7 years.[2,3]

    If amenorrhoeic for 1 year consider removing the coil aged 55 years.[1]

IUDs (copper)   Inserted ≥40 years and if Cu-IUD containing ≥300 mm^2 copper.

    Can retain the device 'until the menopause'.[1]

    If amenorrhoeic for 1 year consider removing the coil aged 55 years.[1]

Progesterone injection   ≥50 years an alternative contraception is advised.[1]

COCP   ≥50 years an alternative contraception is advised.[1]

The POP cannot replace the progesterone in HRT but can be used with combined HRT.

'FSH is not a reliable indicator of ovarian failure in women using combined hormones, even if measured during the hormone-free interval.'[1]

*The FSRH advise FSH monitoring may be used for women on progesterone only methods; however, as discussed in the Gynaecology chapter, Menopause and HRT learning points, NICE advise GPs not to rely on FSH to confirm the menopause in women taking high-dose progesterones.

Sterilisation

What has led to this decision?

How has this decision been made?

What is the risk of regret?

Is the family complete?

Do both partners agree?

Female   If tubal occlusion is performed at the same time as a caesarean section, counselling and agreement should be given at least 2 weeks in advance of the procedure.[4]

Male   Semen sample at 12 weeks.

    A routine second sample is not required if azoospermia in the first sample.[4]

Sexual Health

CHAPTER 11 OVERVIEW
End-of-Life Care

	Cases in this chapter	Within the RCGP curriculum: End-of-Life Care RCGP Curriculum Online March 2016[1]	Learning points in the chapter include:
1	DNACPR Discussion	'Co-develop with the patient, carers and family an effective plan to manage the full range of their physical, psychological, socioeconomic, cultural and spiritual needs'	DNACPR discussion – an example
2	Discussion with a Relative	'Communicate effectively with the patient, their family and carer(s) regarding difficult information about disease progression and prognosis' 'Describe how to provide and manage 24-hour continuity of care through various clinical systems'	Confidentiality Example consultation structure when discussing end-of-life care with a relative
3	Treatment Refusal	'A holistic and personalised assessment of needs'	Capacity PE and Wells' Score
4	End-of-Life Discussion	'Apply best practice principles for end-of-life care in community settings, such as those described in the Gold Standards Framework' 'Prescribe effective drugs and suitable combinations of drugs, pre-empting likely side-effects'	Difficult questions from a patient
5	Palliative Care Symptoms	'Counsel and explain for patients, families and their carers: symptom control advance care planning'	Pain management Palliative care Team input Carers Financial help Anticipated complications Ceiling of care Safety Netting

1. http://www.rcgp.org.uk/training-exams/gp-curriculum-overview/online-curriculum/caring-for-the-whole-person/3-09-end-of-life-care.aspx

CHAPTER 11 REFERENCES

Discussion with a Relative
1. Howell-Jones R., de Silva N., Akpan M., et al. Prevalence of human papillomavirus (HPV) infections in sexually active adolescents and young women in England, prior to widespread HPV immunisation. *Vaccine*. 2012 Jun 6; 30(26): 3867-75. doi: 10.1016/j.vaccine.2012.04.006. Epub 2012 Apr 16.

Treatment Refusal
1. http://www.mdcalc.com/wells-criteria-for-pulmonary-embolism-pe/

Doctor's Notes

Patient	Ernest Platt	72 years	M
PMH	Parkinson's disease		
	Depression		
	Discharged 2 days ago from hospital following admission with aspiration pneumonia		
Medications	Madopar		
	Selegiline		
	Baclofen		
	Citalopram		
	Discharge medication co-amoxiclav to complete 5 days		
Allergies	No known drug allergies		
Consultations	Home visit 2 weeks ago – admitted with pneumonia		
Investigations	Discharge 2/7 ago	Admission	
	CRP 32 mg/L	CRP 128 mg/L	
	Hb 142 g/L	Hb 148 g/L	
	WCC 12.3×10^9/L	WCC 17.3×10^9/L	
	Neutrophils 9.2×10^9/L	Neutrophils 15.1×10^9/L	
Household	No household members registered		

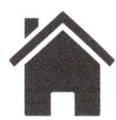

Example Consultation — DNACPR Discussion

Open ☐ — Good idea ... and how do you feel you are doing? Is there anything else we should discuss today?

Sense ☐ — It is a big question and, if that has been on your mind, we should certainly talk about it to help you reach a decision which you feel is right for you.

History ☐ — This is the first time we've met. I'm interested to know more about you and your medical history. I also see you have suffered with depression; how is your mood at present? The medicines I have listed for you are ... when do you take them? Tell me more about when you 'seize up'. What were the symptoms that caused you to go into hospital? Has this happened in the past? How is your breathing now? Are you still worried about your chest? Tell me about you at home. Does anyone give you support? What do your specialists say?

Empathy ☐ — It sounds as if you have been through quite a difficult time with your health.

Impact ☐ — How does your Parkinson's impact on your life? Are there any everyday tasks in the home that you struggle with, such as cooking, washing or getting to bed? What do you miss?

Flags ☐ — Do you ever struggle to call for help should you need it?

ICE ☐ — What goes through your mind regarding your health? What has been through your mind since the discussion with the doctor when you were admitted? What is your greatest fear? Do you worry about anything else? What is important to you regarding your future health? What were you hoping I would suggest today? Is there anything else that you need? I'm wondering about carers during the day; what are your thoughts?

Curious ☐ — Have you talked to anyone else about your thoughts? What do they think?

O/E ☐ — I would like to examine your chest, feel your pulse and take your temperature, breathing rate and oxygen level if I may.

Summary ☐ — To summarise, you frequently have frightening moments where you seize up. Your fears are further infections and not being able to call for help. You have also been wondering whether you would want to be resuscitated should your heart stop. Have I understood you correctly?

Experience ☐ — What is your understanding of the 'do not resuscitate' document?

Explanation ☐ — This is usually a decision made when someone feels their health has deteriorated to a stage where, if their heart were to stop, resuscitation is unlikely to be successful or if it were successful, their health is expected to deteriorate afterwards. It does not mean that we would stop treating things like infections; all other care would continue as normal. How do you feel about this? Would you like me to complete this document? Okay.

Options ☐ — You mentioned that your greatest fear would be lying on the floor not able to reach for your phone. So I could send a request for you to have a pendant alarm if you wish? I also wonder about you having a carer, at least at night to make sure you are okay getting to bed. Does this sound like something you could arrange?

Empower ☐ — Would you like some doxycycline at home to treat signs of a chest infection early? Would this be reassuring?

Future ☐ — When is your next hospital appointment?

Safety net ☐ — If you ever feel unwell, develop a cough, fever or any new symptoms please let us know. Here is a prescription for the doxycycline if you experience your usual chest infection symptoms, but do also let a GP know if you feel unwell. I'm glad you are on the mend from your recent infection but do not hesitate to get in touch with the doctor early if you are concerned.

End-of-Life Care – 1

Patient's Story

DNACPR Discussion

Doctor's notes	Ernest Platt, 72 years. PMH: Parkinson's disease and depression.
	Discharged from hospital following aspiration pneumonia 2 days ago.
	Medications: Madopar, Selegiline, Baclofen, Citalopram and Co-amoxiclav 5 days.
How to act	Polite.
PC	*'The hospital doctor said I should see you to check my lungs were improving.'*
	Mention very early on: *'I wondered if I should have a DNACPR?'*
History	You were diagnosed with Parkinson's disease 8 years ago. You have had multiple episodes where you have seized up, recently, and you also have muscle spasms for which you find baclofen helpful. You find these seizing-up episodes frightening. You have not felt depressed for 2 years since starting the citalopram. At that time your disease had started to progress but you have found peace with your condition and way of life now. You sleep well and you eat. You saw your hospital specialist last month and the Parkinson's Specialist Nurse is your first point of call if you have a question about your medications. They know you and look after you well. You discussed that the current combination of medications is the best for you at present. You are aware the disease will progress.
Social	You live alone. Most days you can walk to the shops 200 yards away between 11 am and noon as this is your window when your medications are most effective. You always carry your mobile phone with you and your ex-wife also checks in on you every day. You have remained good friends. Your daughter also visits several times a week. An OT has made adjustments to your home. You used to be a builder and a keen gardener. You have, on occasions, lain on the floor at night as you struggled to get to bed.
ICE	You want to make sure the infection is improving. You think it is improving as your temperature settled a few days ago and your chest and breathing feel easier. You no longer have pain.
	You want to talk about what the hospital doctor mentioned when you were admitted. She asked if you had a DNACPR. At the time you were horrified but it has been on your mind since. You want to ask the GP what he thinks. After discussion, this is what you want.
	You fear that the aspiration pneumonia will happen again. You fear lying there after you have seized up but so far you have managed to reach for the mobile in your pocket. You call your ex-wife, if it's not too late at night. You have had several courses of antibiotics in the past year for a chest infection. Co-amoxiclav or doxycycline works well if taken quickly. You would have carers if this was suggested.
	You have talked to your family about the DNACPR and they say it is your decision.
Examination	Few crackles lower left base but vesicular breaths with good air entry,
	RR 15, Saturations 97%, HR 72 regular and apyrexial.

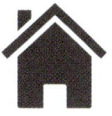

End-of-Life Care – 1

Learning Points   An Example Care Plan Discussion – COPD

'You have just had a serious chest infection. I wonder if you would like to talk about how we can prevent another serious infection but also what you may want to do if this happened again. Before I make some suggestions, do you have any thoughts? Now you are home again, is there anything else you would like at home to make life easier? I'm wondering about meals on wheels, carers, hand rails and a pendant alarm should you struggle to reach a telephone. What support do you have? How do you feel physically? How do you feel mentally and emotionally?

I think you should have a supply of antibiotics and steroids at home to try to get on top of a new infection straight away. We can also supply you with the nebulisers you found helpful in hospital. You should also contact the doctor early if you feel unwell. I can arrange for oxygen to be delivered to your house. So there is lots we can do for you in your home. How does this sound?

It is important that others involved in your care – for example, doctors who may be called to you on a weekend – are aware of not only your medical conditions but also what you need and what is important to you. One way of communicating this is through a care plan which you keep in your home and we can also send this to the out of hours' doctors. Within the care plan, it will ask me about your wishes for the future. The questions I need to ask are very sensitive but important questions. Do you feel ready to discuss your options? Does your faith help us with these decisions? Is there anyone else you would like to include in this discussion?

Do you have any questions about a care plan? May I document your wishes in a care plan and send it to my colleagues just in case they are called to you when I am not available? We can always change it. Before I ask questions, is there anything specific you would like me to write down in the care plan?

If you became unwell again you have options. My priority as your doctor is to ensure that you have what you need, to respect your wishes and to give you the information to help you make informed choices. I can advise you if you wish based on what I believe is in your best interests.

The first question is about antibiotics if the ones I have given you today don't work. It is common that, at the end of life, a pneumonia may happen because the body is so weak. If you had a serious infection which was not responding to the antibiotics you have, I'm wondering would you want more antibiotics to try to fight the infection or would you not want this? Okay, I will make your wishes clear in the plan.

The second question is this: if you were still unwell and antibiotics had not worked at home, would you want to go to hospital, which would be through the emergency department, or go to the community hospital only, or would you prefer us to keep you at home and do all we can for you at home to keep you comfortable? There may be other reasons why you become unwell. Would you always want your care to be at … or does it depend on the situation?

The medicines that prevent problems in the future, like your cholesterol treatment, shall we stop these now or would you like to keep taking them? Have you thought about where you would like to be in your final hours? Why would you like to be there? Have you thought about other options, which are …?

There is one last question which is another difficult question. When your heart does stop, would you like an ambulance to be called and receive chest compressions to try to restart the heart, or at that moment would you want to be left in peace? I can see you are struggling to answer this and you can think about this. Would you like my thoughts? My feeling is that you are already very poorly. Therefore, this is unlikely to be successful and if it was successful you are likely to be more frail. I think, therefore, that to maintain your dignity not resuscitating may be in your best interests. But I will be guided by you. I have a leaflet that may help you when thinking about this. Shall we meet again next week?'

End-of-Life Care – 1

Doctor's Notes

Patient	Mrs Louise Barker	33 years	F
PMH	Metastatic cervical cancer diagnosed 5 months ago		
	Last hospital letter – TAH followed by chemotherapy. Now palliative care		
	Normal vaginal delivery 2 years ago		
	Ex-smoker		
Medications	Cyclizine		
	Ibuprofen		
	Paracetamol		
	Codeine phosphate		
	Metoclopramide		
Allergies	No known drug allergies		
Consultations	1 week ago with GP – abdominal pain. Codeine commenced		
Investigations	No recent tests completed at the practice		
Household	James Barker	35 years	M
	Megan Barker	2 years	F

Husband has arranged an appointment to discuss his wife.

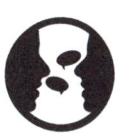

Example Consultation — Discussion with a Relative

Open ☐ — Hello Mr Barker, my name is Dr Blount. What would you like to talk to me about today? What has been going through your mind?

History ☐ — May I clarify what you understand about Louise's health? How is Louise physically? How is she coping emotionally? How are you coping? How is your mood at present? Who else is at home? Do you have any other support? Are you at work? Who is involved in Louise's care at present?

Sense ☐ — I can see that you are devastated and I hear that you have lots on your mind.

ICE ☐ — When you are on your own what thoughts do you have? Anything else that you have been wondering? All kinds of emotions occur at a time like this: sadness, fear, guilt, hopelessness. I'm interested to know what you have been feeling. Is there anything else that makes you feel anxious or worried? What would be helpful to you and your family? Is there anything else that you need or you are hoping for?

Impact ☐ — Do you feel responsible for Louise's care day to day?

Curious ☐ — When you say she will no longer be breathing … what else is going through your mind? What are your thoughts when you think of life without her? 'Back in time', what do you mean? What do you think is on Louise's mind? Have you shared how you feel with each other? Have you discussed going to a hospice?

Empathy ☐ — You have many thoughts and emotions, whilst it sounds as if you are trying to be brave for your family.

Summary ☐ — You have had fears of finding Louise no longer breathing and hope that when Louise is very poorly she will be in a hospice. You have had feelings of guilt and you can't imagine, at present, life with Megan without Louise, especially when you work and your family live 5 hours away. Have I understood you correctly?

Explanation ☐ — You are correct that the virus that causes this infection can be sexually transmitted but this virus is so common, over a third of people your age will have this virus,[1] which is far higher than other STIs. Louise has been extremely unlucky. Most women with the virus will remain healthy.

Options ☐ — You mentioned that you would like someone to talk to, about how to talk to Megan. Would it be okay if I spoke to the palliative care nurses? They could talk to you and Louise about options for the future but also about talking to Megan.

Empower ☐ — Could you talk to any friends or family about who may be able to help you with Megan?

Future ☐ — I'm just wondering about when we should meet again. What are your thoughts? Can we arrange for Louise and you to come back together?

Safety net ☐ — If, in the meantime, you or Louise ever need help day or night, do you know who to call? If we are open please contact us or Louise's palliative care nurse. During the night you can call 111 for a doctor. Do you have all the telephone numbers to hand?

End-of-Life Care – 2

Patient's Story

Discussion with a Relative

Doctor's notes   Mr Barker has arranged an appointment to discuss his wife.

Mrs Louise Barker, 33 years. PMH: metastatic cervical cancer diagnosed 5 months ago. Last hospital letter; TAH followed by chemotherapy and now palliative care. NVD 2 years ago. Medicines: Cyclizine, Ibuprofen, Paracetamol, Codeine and Metoclopramide.

How to act   Quiet and polite.

PC   *'I just thought I should come and talk to you, Doctor.'*

Be slow to give information.

'There's so much in my mind I can't concentrate sometimes.'

History   You understand your wife was diagnosed with metastatic cervical cancer 5 months ago. She has had a TAH and the last scan showed the chemotherapy was not successful. Originally she had bleeding and pain for months but put this down to her POP and IBS. She missed her smear because of the baby and then she forgot. Currently Louise is able to manage at home on pain relief but you worry about how you will look after her and Megan, who is now 2 years old, as Louise's disease progresses. The palliative care team has not visited as currently Louise's symptoms are controlled. Louise is strong emotionally with family but cries at night.

Social   Louise's family live locally and are around most days. Your family lives 5 hours away. You are signed off work for 3 months. You are a surveyor. You met Louise 3 years ago and within a year you were married. Prior to life with Louise, life was centred around work and friends but once Megan arrived, life dramatically changed. You have no medical or psychiatric history. You do not feel depressed but incredibly sad. You eat and sleep but have many upsetting thoughts which are distracting. You have no thoughts of harming yourself or another.

ICE

'I can't stop thinking that she won't be breathing.' You mean you are frightened about finding Louise dead. Every morning you wait until you can feel her breathe before you turn to look at her.

'How will I cope without her?' By this you mean how you will care for Megan alone. You feel full of sadness when thinking about your future life. No one has brought up the subject of life after Louise as they don't want to upset you but you think it would be a relief to discuss this and will talk to the family.

'You know, if life could go back in time.' You feel guilty with your thoughts. You sometimes wish you had never met Louise, then you wouldn't be going through this. You also believe this is your fault. You read that the virus that leads to the cancer is sexually transmitted and you fear this was passed on from you. Louise told you 'not to be silly'. You cry with Louise if ever you talk about your feelings but you don't tell her things that you fear may upset her. You think Louise feels guilty that she will leave you and Megan alone.

You hope the doctor will visit Louise and talk to her about a hospice so she will be around nurses *'when it happens'*. You feel you need someone to talk to about how to talk to Megan about her mother. You need someone to help you with Megan after she has gone.

End-of-Life Care – 2

Learning Points

Discussion with a Relative

Confidentiality Unless the patient has given consent, no information can be **given** to the NOK. However, you can speak in general terms about a condition or likely outcome, e.g. 'often in similar situations the hospice can offer support'.

You cannot give new information to the relative but can discuss what they already know, again be general to avoid any confidentiality issues; e.g. in this case you can discuss cervical cancer in general (such as links to HPV) but not the specifics of Louise's case.

Do not Do not presume you understand their concerns. Explore their thoughts.

Do Ensure the relative feels understood – summarise their ICE!

Reassure they will receive the help they need specifically related to their concerns.

Example consultation structure when discussing end-of-life care with a relative

Allow the person to do the majority of the talking, be flexible with what they hope to discuss. The following structure may be helpful.

1. Silences, exploring thoughts or stating what you sense can help initiate a sensitive consultation.
2. Check their understanding of the situation.
3. Collect all thoughts, concerns, fears, anxieties and expectations.
4. Be curious. Explore any cues they may have hinted. Silences or repeating words to encourage further discussion may be useful here.
5. Understand the relative; are they well, their mood, their responsibilities as a carer, other stressors in their life, the impact of the situation.
6. Summarise the ICE. A powerful way to help the relative feel understood and also focuses the management plan.
7. Empathise. The immensity of the situation and its potential impact on the person.
8. Enquire about communication between the relatives and patient.
9. Provide options/suggestions to manage each concern in turn.
10. Consider if other professionals or support groups may be helpful.
11. Empower with regard to their concerns.
12. Plan future meetings. Is anything required in the meantime?
13. Safety net: rescue treatment and contact numbers in the event of sudden deterioration.

If appropriate – in the event of death, do they know who to call? Usually the GP or OOH GP to certify death, followed by the undertaker.

Doctor's Notes

Patient   Raymond Styles   86 years   M
PMH   Ankle fracture placed in cast 3 weeks ago
                     Prostate cancer
Medications   No current medications
Allergies   No known drug allergies
Consultations   No recent consultations
Investigations   No recent investigations
Household   No household contacts registered

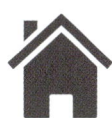

Example Consultation — Treatment Refusal

Open ☐ — I'm pleased your carer called. Tell me more about this pain. Is there anything else you have noticed?

Flags ☐ — Do you feel breathless? Are you coughing up anything? Any blood? Have you had a temperature?

Sense ☐ — You don't seem worried.

History ☐ — How is your leg? How are you in general? Do you have any other family?

ICE ☐ — What do you think has caused your pain? Is there anything you fear it may be? What do you think we should do?

Curious ☐ — Tell me more about your experience of hospital.

Impact ☐ — Things must have been hard since you lost Maggie. How do you spend your days?

O/E ☐ — May I examine you, check your pulse, breathing rate and oxygen level, look at your legs and listen to your chest?

Empathy ☐ — I hear that you do not want to have the same experience as your wife and will not go to hospital.

Empower ☐ — No one will force you. I must explain to you what I think so you can make an informed decision, but you are in charge.

Impression ☐ — I believe you have a blood clot in your lung that has travelled from your leg. There is a good chance we can fix this but without treatment your pain and breathing could get worse or you could die from this. In hospital I would expect them to do a scan and a blood test, give you oxygen and blood-thinning injections. If I were to explain to the medical staff your previous experience in hospital and explain to them you would want to be discharged as soon as possible, would this be okay?

Options ☐ — What about if we asked the community hospital, which is a smaller local hospital, to see you instead? May I give you blood-thinning injections and then tablets called warfarin at home? If your heart were to stop, would you want a paramedic to try to restart the heart? May I give you medicines to make you feel more comfortable?

Experience ☐ — Can I check that we have understood each other correctly? You are aware that I believe you should go to hospital, and not going to hospital or receiving treatment at home may mean ongoing pain or breathing problems and you could die from this. Can you repeat to me what we have just talked about so I can check you understand? Thank you.

Explanation ☐ — I understand and respect your wishes. I would like to ask the hospital at home nurses to have a look at you tonight to assess your oxygen level and pain again, would that be okay? Are you frightened?

Future ☐ — I will arrange for oxygen and pain relief. I suggest taking paracetamol, 2 tablets regularly. We can try a half dose of codeine too. If this isn't strong enough we can increase it or add morphine. Does that sound okay? I will ensure you are also sent some anti-sickness tablets. If you find you are struggling with tablets then don't worry I will ensure medications that can be given under the skin are prescribed and available.

Safety net ☐ — If you change your mind, or your pain or breathing gets worse, or if you want to talk to me again, call the surgery, or 111 if the surgery is closed. If you feel very unwell and would like to go to hospital you can phone 999. I will communicate your wishes to the out of hours' doctors and leave some paperwork in your carer's file so everyone is aware of your wishes. I will arrange for a doctor to be in touch to see how you are tomorrow. Please call if you need anything.

Patient's Story

Treatment Refusal

Doctor's notes Raymond Styles, 86 years.

PMH: Ankle fracture placed in cast 3 weeks ago. Prostate cancer. Medications: None.

How to act Respectful and apologetic. Dismissive of your symptoms.

Under no circumstances are you going to hospital.

You don't want any treatment to thin your blood.

PC *'Doctor, I'm sorry they called you out. I'm fine now.'*

History You have prostate cancer. You were offered but declined hormone treatment for this but are currently not troubled by it.

Your carer called the doctor because you complained of chest pain.

You feel a little cross about this as you don't like to waste the doctor's time.

The pain is sharp and catches you when you take a breath in.

You first noticed it yesterday. You do feel more breathless than usual. You do not have a cough or any sputum. No fever. You have no confusion.

You have never felt this pain before. *'I must have pulled a muscle.'*

Social You live alone with four times daily care at present whilst your leg is in cast.

You have no family.

ICE You do not know what has caused the pain. You suspect it may be serious.

If asked about any negative experiences: your wife, Maggie, died in the hospital and you do not want to have the same to happen to you. Refuse to go to hospital whatever the doctor says. You would not like paramedics to attempt to restart your heart should it stop.

You do not want anything to thin the blood. You will accept palliative care.

Examination Sats 88%, RR 18, HR 108 bpm. Chest exam normal. Apyrexial. Left leg in cast.

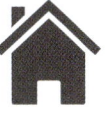

End-of-Life Care – 3

Learning Points

Treatment Refusal

Capacity

This case is testing your ability to clinically assess a patient but also your ability to assess capacity. To do this you need to ensure that the patient:

1. understands the information
2. is able to remember the information long enough to make a decision
3. is able to weigh up the risks and repeat these to the doctor
4. is able to communicate his/her decision.

If a patient has capacity, is aware of risk to life and all the risks of not following advice and you cannot persuade them, you must respect the patient's autonomy. You should ask about involving family members and consider how else you can help the patient including end-of-life and DNACPR discussions. However, you should not simply wash your hands of the patient because they have ignored your advice. Think about ways you can still help the patient, keep them safe and allow them the opportunity to change their mind.

Patients may refuse to go to hospital for many reasons. Their reason should be explored in detail and the doctor should give an explanation of what they expect will happen in the hospital.

Caring for others or even dogs/cats is a common reason to refuse hospital admission. Know your local emergency care team. There are also organisations that can help with pets, e.g. Dogs Trust.

PE

Pulmonary embolism (PE) is a medical emergency and requires admission. Pleuritic chest pain, low oxygen saturations and tachycardia should raise your suspicion of PE, particularly if there are any risk factors (e.g. immobility, lower leg fractures, COCP, long-haul flight, cancer, family or personal history).

Wells' score PE[1]

- Signs and symptoms of DVT
- PE is the most likely diagnosis or equally likely
- HR>100 bpm
- Immobility 3/7 or surgery past 1/12
- Previous PE or DVT
- Haemoptysis
- Malignancy or Rx within 6/12

Double-check oxygen saturations. A useful test may be exercising an able patient. Retest saturations which may then show hypoxia after they have paced around the surgery.

Doctor's Notes

Patient   Elsie Brooks   87 years   F
PMH   Advanced Alzheimer's dementia
                   Multiple urinary tract infections
Medications   No current medications
                   Previous medications   Trimethoprim × 4 in the past 3 months
                                          Nitrofurantoin × 2 in the past 3 months
Allergies   No known drug allergies
Consultations No recent consultations
Investigations 3 × mixed growth urine cultures in past 3 months
Household   No household contacts registered

You have been led to a room where Elsie's daughter is sitting. Elsie is in the next room.

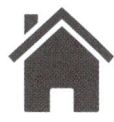

Example Consultation — End-of-Life Discussion

Open ☐ — Please tell me why you and the staff are concerned about your mother today.

Risk ☐ — Has this happened before? I see she has been given many antibiotics. Can you tell me more about what her symptoms were like at the time? Did they help? Has she fallen or hit her head?

History ☐ — This is the first time I have met your mother. Can you tell me more about her? Has she changed? What is she like each day? Does she talk to you? Does she have a faith? Do you have support or siblings? Before she became so unwell, did she ever express any wishes for the future with regards to treatment or hospital admission? Do you know if she ever wrote her wishes down in something called an advanced directive or living will?

Sense ☐ — I can see this is very distressing for you. She is your mum and you want to do all you can for her.

Impact ☐ — Are you currently away from work to be with your mother? How are you emotionally?

ICE ☐ — What are your thoughts as to what may have caused this? Is this the worst your mother's health has been? What is important to you regarding the decisions we make for your mum's care? Before I came today did you have any thoughts about what I may suggest or what you feel we should do?

O/E ☐ — I would like to examine her now, top to toe, to see if I can find a cause for this change.

Summary ☐ — To summarise, your mother has been deteriorating over months but especially in past weeks. She has not improved despite many antibiotics. She is comfortable but distressed by people around her, is that right?

Impression ☐ — I believe your mother is very poorly and, due to progression of her dementia, it is likely that she is approaching the end of her life.

Empathy ☐ — That must be very hard to hear.

Experience ☐ — Have you had a discussion with a doctor about how your mother's dementia may advance?

Options ☐ — There is no sign of infection and previous good antibiotics have not helped. As she is already so frail, at this stage my feeling is that I should concentrate on her comfort and only give medicines if she is in discomfort. We can be guided by what you feel and what we both think is in your mum's best interests. What are your thoughts? My thoughts are that sending her to hospital is not in her best interests as the surroundings can be frightening when disorientated. What are your thoughts about that? If her heart were to stop I would suggest we maintain your mother's dignity and not try to bring her back with chest compressions as she is already very poorly and I would not expect this to be successful. How do you feel about this? In which case I will ensure that these instructions are clear in her notes. So to clarify what we have talked about, because your mother is frail and it appears her dementia has advanced, we will do all we can to ensure that she is comfortable within the care home. Do you have any questions or concerns?

Empower ☐ — What you can do to help your mother is to offer her sips of fluid frequently and let the staff know if you detect she is in any discomfort. I can ensure medicines for pain, sickness, agitations or lung secretions are immediately available for your mother, should she require them.

Future ☐ — I will ask the doctor to call again tomorrow to see if we need to make any changes to the plan.

Safety net ☐ — If at any stage your mother becomes distressed, or you or the care staff are concerned or need any help, you are welcome to call the surgery or the 111 team who will be sent information regarding the discussion we have had today. Is there anything else you need or would like to talk about?

Patient's Story

End-of-Life Discussion

Doctor's notes Elsie Brooks, 87 years. PMH: Advanced Alzheimer's dementia and multiple urinary tract infections.

Medications: None. Previous medication: Trimethoprim × 4 and Nitrofurantoin × 2 in the past 3 months. MSU results: 3 × mixed growth. The GP has been led to a room where you, Elsie's daughter, are sitting. Elsie is in the next room.

How to act Distressed and anxious for your mother to be given treatment initially. However, when the doctor discusses options with you, you soften and with sadness believe keeping your mother comfortable is in her best interests. You also initially ask whether hospital would be appropriate but seem relieved when the GP suggests keeping her where she is.

PC *'Doctor, I think she needs antibiotics again for a water infection.'*

History Elsie was diagnosed with Alzheimer's 3 years ago and was transferred to the care home where she has gradually been deteriorating.

In the past 2 months she has stopped recognising the staff and usually doesn't recognise you. She does not interact with anyone. She shouts out in the night although she doesn't seem to be in pain; she is just generally quiet and has stopped talking. She pushes the staff away and shouts at them when they come near her. She has been in bed for 4 weeks and prior to this she would wander. She is not eating but is drinking sips of fluids with encouragement. She has had no falls for months. Many GPs including the OOH GPs have prescribed antibiotics after the carers said there were 'leucocytes' in her pad urine. The antibiotics never help. Elsie is passing urine normally, her bowels are normal, she has no pressure sores and she is not coughing. Her breathing is currently normal. In the past Elsie did mention not wanting to go to hospital unless it was really necessary, so you suspect she would rather be treated at the care home. She does not have an advance directive.

Social You have no siblings. You are very busy working in your own business but see your mother twice weekly when you can. Your husband doesn't have time to visit Elsie. Neither you nor Elsie have a faith.

ICE You are aware that your mother is unwell. Because many doctors have prescribed antibiotics for a urine infection, you wonder if this is the problem now. You initially request, and expect, that Elsie receives stronger antibiotics. However, with discussion you realise this may be a progression of her dementia and agree with the doctor to manage her comfort only, a DNACPR and for all care to be kept at the care home.

Examination Elsie looks quiet and comfortable but shouts and kicks and punches if anyone is near her. You manage to listen to the back of her lungs and assess her hydration which are normal. She is moving all limbs pain free and has no sign of bruising or head injury. No leg swelling. No abdominal distention. There is no smell of urine.

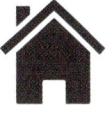

End-of-Life Care – 4

Learning Points

End-of-Life Discussion

Difficult questions from a patient

Be ready for the difficult questions/discussions. Have a think about how you might answer the following:

1. If/how to mention the possibility of cancer if a patient presents with a red flag.
2. 'You think I've got cancer, Doctor?'
3. 'Do you think this will kill me?'
4. 'How long have I got, Doc?' Establish what they already have been told, how they feel their illness is progressing and the reason for them asking this.
5. 'How long does my mother have?'
6. Relative saying: 'I don't want you to tell my mother about the cancer. She won't cope.'
7. Relative saying: 'I don't want you asking my father about resuscitation … he will give up if you do.' Although you may be ready with your answer, which involves explaining their father's autonomy, an angry and insistent relative can be tricky – but there is a way to approach this respecting everyone's feelings by seeking the patient's wishes and 'rules'. See case Palliative Care Symptoms for more detail.
8. Relative saying: 'I don't want you to tell my father that I have talked to you today.'
9. Relative or patient asking for resuscitation when you feel it is not in their best interests.
10. 'He's not drinking. Will you give him fluids, Doctor?' In the setting of a nursing home.
11. The relative of the patient with advanced Alzheimer's dementia: 'I want him to get all the antibiotics to make him better.' Or 'I just don't want anything to happen to him.'
12. 'I am a doctor myself …' The relative who is a doctor may feel the burden of making decisions. Establish his/her agenda, whether he/she would like this responsibility or to be relieved of organising the end-of-life care. The use of signposting can demonstrate you plan to discuss what is required and that you are 'on the ball'.

Some example answers to try

When asked about prognosis – it is very difficult to know as all patients are different and can surprise us by deteriorating quickly or living a long time. As a general rule, if you notice deterioration in a person over months, we are probably talking of months. However, if they are deteriorating over weeks or days, they may pass away in weeks or days.

When asked about artificial nutrition/fluids – as a person becomes sicker, their body begins to shut down. We often first notice this as they do not eat or drink very much, then over time will stop eating and drinking altogether. This usually corresponds with the person being sleepier. If a patient shows any sign of thirst or interest in food or drinks, these should of course be offered frequently. However, as the patient approaches the end of life, the body starts to shut down as part of the natural process of dying. At this time it is less likely that they feel hunger or need food. Sips of water and mouth care will help keep the person comfortable and avoid a dry mouth.

These are difficult and very sensitive areas. Be guided by your judgement, the illness, the clinical situation, the family's wishes and the timing/rate of decline.

Doctor's Notes

Patient	Dennis Richards 88 years M
PMH	Congestive Cardiac Failure, COPD, Chronic Kidney Disease, Osteoarthritis in the lumbar spine, knees and hips.
	Do not attempt resuscitation form completed with Mr Richards' consent.
	Ex-smoker 20/day
Medications	Bisoprolol
	Ramipril
	Furosemide
	Paracetamol
	Codeine
	Salbutamol
	Eklira inhaler
Allergies	No known drug allergies
Consultations	No recent consultations
Investigations	Hb 142 g/L
	eGFR 27 ml/min/1.73 m^2
	Na 129 mmol/L (stable for 5 years)
	K 5.1 mmol/L
Household	Judy Richards 79 years F

Example Consultation — Palliative Care Symptoms

Open ☐ — Thank you for coming in. What would you like to discuss with me today?

Curious ☐ — I'm sorry to hear you don't feel well. What has led you to come now? What do you need?

History ☐ — Tell me about your medical conditions. Do you know your diagnosis? The medicines you have are … When do you take them? What symptoms are you troubled with? How do you spend your days? Is there anything else that you are struggling with? Do you have a carer? Who else is in your life? Is Judy well? How is the relationship? Is Judy managing? Do you have a faith? Do you smoke/drink?

Flags ☐ — Do you have pain in the day or at night? Are you eating/losing weight? How often do you use your inhaler? How many pillows do you sleep with? Do you ever feel as if you are gasping at night? How are your legs?

Impact ☐ — How has your life changed recently? Are you low in spirits? Do you sleep? Feel anxious?

ICE ☐ — What goes through your mind? Any other frightening thoughts? What did you think I may suggest? What is important to you? Is there any treatment/test you do not want? Should we try to keep you at home to manage your symptoms? Would you go to hospital? At the end, where would you like to be?

Curious ☐ — When you say you do not want stronger pain relief, why is this?

O/E ☐ — May I examine you: your heart, lungs, neck vessels, legs, your pulse and breathing rate and oxygen level?

Experience ☐ — Can you tell me, please, what discussions you have already had with other doctors?

Explanation ☐ — It can be a difficult balance, your legs and lungs want less fluid but your kidneys want more.

Sense ☐ — You seem keen to be informed and make decisions about your future. Are you keen to know everything or is there anything you don't feel ready to discuss?

Empathy ☐ — It must be frightening when you feel you are struggling more and feel less independent.

Summary ☐ — To summarise, over the last few months your breathing has become more difficult and your mobility is also a struggle with the arthritis and fluid in your legs. You are mostly concerned about your breathing and suffering at the end. You hope I can talk to you about what is available for you at this time. Have I understood you correctly?

Options ☐ — For your breathing, we can ask the specialist nurses to see you. They are likely to discuss the option of oxygen and help you monitor how much fluid is in your body, to keep the balance just right. For your pain, we should choose medicines that are safer to use with CKD, therefore I would suggest changing codeine to tramadol and some ibuprofen gel may also be helpful. How does this sound?

Empower ☐ — You can help us by measuring your weight at the same time each day. If you notice that you have gained 2 kg over a couple of days, let the doctor know. Do you think you could also keep a record of your fluid intake? I suggest a maximum of 1.2 litres per day at first then recheck your kidney blood test in a week. Does this sound okay?

Future ☐ — You also wanted to also talk about the end of your life. I want to reassure you that if you had any pain, restlessness or breathlessness, doctors would give you medicines to keep you comfortable. You also said you wanted to be in hospital at this time. Can I write your wishes on a care plan so my colleagues are aware in case I am not here?

Safety net ☐ — I can leave you with information about who to call if you need any help or your symptoms deteriorate. Do you want to bring your wife in next week after the blood test to see if she has any questions?

End-of-Life Care – 5

Patient's Story

Palliative Care Symptoms

Doctor's notes — Dennis Richards, 88 years. PMH: Congestive Cardiac Failure, COPD, Chronic Kidney Disease, Osteoarthritis in the lumbar spine, knees and hips. Ex-smoker 20/day. Medications: Bisoprolol, Ramipril, Furosemide, Paracetamol, Codeine, Salbutamol and Eklira inhaler. Results: Hb 142 g/L, eGFR 27 ml/min/1.73 m^2, Na 129 mmol/L and K 5.1 mmol/L.

How to act — Keen to be involved in your care.

PC — *'Doctor, I have come for my review.'* When asked further you can say …

'I would like to talk about my future. I know I'm not well.'

History — Your breathing has gradually been deteriorating over the past 6 months. You no longer go out of the house unless you are in your wheelchair. You use a walking frame around the home due to arthritis and you require pauses for your breathing. Your pain is around the lower spine, hips and knees and worse on movement. You are able to sleep. Your pain is currently controlled but you fear that your breathing, mobility and pain control are deteriorating. The reason you have come today is because you had a fright when you couldn't catch your breath and it took 8 puffs of the inhaler to calm your breathing. You have no features of infection. You use your salbutamol usually twice daily. You are compliant with medicines. You don't smoke or drink alcohol.

You would want to go to hospital if you were unwell (e.g. for intravenous antibiotics) but only if the symptoms could not be controlled at home. You want to die in hospital as this would be easier for your wife Judy.

Social — You live in a bungalow with Judy, your carer, who is well. Judy is not with you today. She copes well. Your son dropped you at the GPs. You have a son and a daughter who live locally and are good support. You read the paper and listen to the radio during the day.

ICE — You have a good understanding of your medical diagnosis. Last time, when you were admitted for medicines in the veins, you told the doctor you do not want resuscitation.

You have been keen to discuss your future health with the doctor and find out if there are any other medicines that may be able to help you. You are concerned that you will be breathless and want reassurance that the doctor will make sure you feel comfortable when your time comes. You hope the doctor will be honest with you today and 'plan the end' as you do not feel that you have got long to live. You have never discussed the future with a previous doctor.

'I don't want any stronger pain relief.' You have been told by a doctor it will accumulate in your body because of your kidneys.

Examination — Oxygen sats 89%, HS ESM radiating to the carotids, crackles to mid zones in the chest bilaterally, RR 19, expiratory wheeze with prolonged expiration. Apyrexial. HR 92 regular. JVP raised 3 cm and pitting oedema to below the knees.

End-of-Life Care – 5

Learning Points — Palliative Care Symptoms

Below is a list of points to consider when looking after patients at the end of their life.

Pain

Types of pain	Neuropathic
	Skeletal muscle spasm
	Bone pain
	Smooth muscle spasm (colic)
Pain assessment	SOCRATES
	The cause, the impact on: sleep, mood, mobility, ADL and independence.
Associated symptoms	Nausea, low mood, loss of appetite and poor sleep.
Pain management	World Health Organization Pain Ladder.
Side effects	Constipation, nausea, drowsiness, delirium, itching and gastritis.

Palliative care

Problem list	Nausea, vomiting, breathlessness, cough, hiccups, secretions, thrush, bowels (constipation or diarrhoea), lymphoedema, itching, anxiety, panic, depression, hydration and pressure sores.
Examination	Hydration, oedema, sign of LRTI, DVT, hypoxia and pressure sores.
Treatments/medicines	For problems
	Underlying cause: radiotherapy, chemotherapy, surgery
	For other long-standing conditions
	For anticipatory problems
Other treatments	Oxygen, physiotherapy, antidepressants, anxiolytics, sedatives, nebulisers.
Equipment	Hospital bed, nebulisers and syringe drivers.
Multi-team input	DNs, specialist nurses, hospital at home and Community Matron.
Carers	Respite and the local carer support team should the carer be taken ill.
Financial help	DS1500, disabled badge and attendance allowance.
Ceiling of care	Infections, hydration, investigations and hospital admissions.
Documentation	DNACPR discussion/form, care plan, anticipatory medication prescription for District Nurse administration and a 'Message in a Bottle' paper trail to guide paramedics.
Anticipated complications	Hypercalcaemia, acute renal failure, anaemia, cauda equina, SVC or airway obstruction, ascites, GI and other haemorrhage.
Safety net	Cauda equina, DVT, sudden new symptom (PE) and symptoms of hypercalcaemia

> See the **Link Hub at CompleteCSA.co.uk** for a helpful link to a **Palliative Care Online Handbook** – Palliative Care Adult Network Guidelines.

It is a good idea to familiarise yourself with a palliative care guide – your own Trust may have guidelines you can access. Alternatively, there are online handbooks. These guides can help with specific symptom management and some of the more complicated aspects of palliative care such as switching between strong opiates and between routes of delivery.

End-of-Life Care – 5

CHAPTER 12 OVERVIEW

Mental Health

	Cases in this chapter	Within the RCGP curriculum: Mental Health RCGP Curriculum Online March 2016[1]	Learning points in the chapter include:
1	Anxiety	'Be aware of the dangers of medicalising distress …' 'Understand the range of psychological therapies available …'	NICE guidelines. (CG113) Generalised anxiety disorder and panic disorder in adults: management. 2011 CBT model
2	Depression	'An exploration of physical, psychological, social, cultural and spiritual issues should be integrated into both the consultation and the management of illness …' 'Understand specific interventions and guidelines for individual conditions using, … NICE guidelines'	NICE guidelines. (CG90) Depression in adults: recognition and management. 2009
3	Personality Disorder	'Enable people who are experiencing mental health problems to engage as much as possible in understanding their difficulties and negotiate appropriate, acceptable management' 'Be able to assess and manage risk/suicidal ideation'	NICE guidelines. (CG78) Borderline personality disorder: recognition and management. 2009
4	Postnatal Psychosis	'Be aware of the need to promote hope and demonstrate compassion and their use as resources to aid healing'	NICE guidelines. (CG192) Antenatal and postnatal mental health: clinical management and service guidance. 2014
5	Eating Disorder	'Use communication skills that enable your patients who are distressed to feel comfortable enough to disclose their concerns' 'Recognise early indicators of difficulty in the psychological well-being of children and young people and respond quickly to concerns raised by parents'	NICE guidelines. (CG90) Eating disorders in over 8s: management. 2004

1. http://www.rcgp.org.uk/training-exams/gp-curriculum-overview/online-curriculum/managing-complex-care/3-10-mental-health-problems.aspx

CHAPTER 12 REFERENCES

Anxiety
1. NICE Guidelines. CG 113. Generalised anxiety disorder and panic disorder in adults: management. Jan 2011.
2. Williams, C.J. (2001) *Overcoming Depression: A Five Areas Approach*. London: Arnold.
3. Williams C., Garland A. A cognitive–behavioural therapy assessment model for use in everyday clinical practice. *Advances in Psychiatric Treatment*. May 2002; 8(3): 172-9. http://apt.rcpsych.org/content/8/3/172

Depression
1. NICE Guidelines. CG 90. Depression in adults: recognition and management. Apr 2016.

Personality Disorders
1. http://patient.info/doctor/emotionally-unstable-personality-disorder
2. NICE Guidelines. CG78. Borderline Personality Disorder – recognition and management. Jan 2009.
3. http://www.nice.org.uk/news/article/new-standard-to-improve-the-care-of-people-with-personality-disorders. June 2015
4. http://www.rcpsych.ac.uk/healthadvice/problemsdisorders/personalitydisorder.aspx

Postnatal Psychosis
1. http://www.rcpsych.ac.uk/healthadvice/problemsdisorders/postnataldepression.aspx
2. NICE guidelines. CG192. Antenatal and postnatal mental health: clinical management and service guidance. Dec 2014.
3. http://patient.info/doctor/postpartum-psychosis-pro

Eating Disorder
1. NICE guidelines. CG9. Eating disorders in over 8s: management. Jan 2004.

Doctor's Notes

Patient	Stephen Harper 42 years M
PMH	Irritable bowel syndrome
Medications	No current medications. Previous medications include mebeverine.
Allergies	No information
Consultations	GP consultation 5 weeks ago. Intermittent bloating. No red flags. Impression IBS.
	A&E attendance with chest pain – discharge letter, tests all normal and reassured.
Investigations	FBC, U&E, LFT, TFTs, GGT, CRP, HbA1c, ESR and coeliac screen all normal 1 month ago.
Household	Judith Harper 43 years F
	Bridget Harper 15 years F
	Aidan Harper 14 years M

Example Consultation — Anxiety

Open ☐ — Can you tell me more about your bowels? Anything else you have noticed? Do you feel well?

History ☐ — Any other problems in the past? Have you taken any medication? Did it work? As it's the first time we've met, please tell me more about you. How are things at home? Work?

Flags ☐ — Any change in your bowels? Any bleeding? Any weight loss? Any pain? What is your sleeping pattern? Your appetite? Are you able to enjoy activities? What comes to mind when you think about the future?

Sense ☐ — You seem quiet today; is there anything else on your mind?

ICE ☐ — What do you think is the main problem? Is there any other diagnosis that has crossed your mind? What were your thoughts regarding what we may decide today? Any other thoughts about this? What is your biggest fear?

Curious ☐ — I'm interested to know what you mean by 'turning 40 … a mid-life crisis'. Where do you think this has come from? Has a terminal illness happened to anyone you know?

Impact ☐ — What triggers these thoughts? Does it make you feel unwell? Then what do you do?

Risk ☐ — Any thoughts of hurting yourself or suicide? How much alcohol do you drink? Any other drugs?

Impression ☐ — There are no worrying bowel symptoms. There is no weight loss, bleeding or change in your bowels and I see your blood tests were reassuring. I am a cautious doctor but I am confident that we do not need a colonoscopy. My feeling is that anxiety is driving your symptoms and fears, causing panic attacks. What are your thoughts about all this?

Experience ☐ — Has anyone else you know suffered with anxiety? Do you know of ways to help?

Explanation ☐ — Everyone has negative thoughts, but when these start to impact on your life we need to help you recognise the triggers and help you find ways to manage them. Panic attacks occur when normal hormones in the body get released inappropriately. These hormone reactions are normal when we are in dangerous situations but, when you have anxiety, they can occur in everyday situations when there isn't any danger. Your symptoms of a racing heart, breathlessness etc. are real but are triggered by a psychological process.

Options ☐ — When it comes to anxiety there are things that you can do, things I can help with and things others can help too. You may find relaxation exercises helpful. You could contact MIND who will advise on local support groups. I can help with providing suggestions, monitoring and prescribing medication if needed, but help which doesn't involve medication can be just as powerful or more so. Other people who can help may include family, friends or professionals. Therapists for anxiety can be helpful. There are other useful resources, websites such as FearFighter.com and, on the Mindfulness website, there is a 'three-minute breathing space' exercise. There are also books: do you enjoy reading? I recommend *Mindfulness: A practical guide to finding peace in a frantic world*. I have a list of all of these suggestions for you to think about, and contact numbers.

Empathy ☐ — Anxiety can have a huge impact on one's life. Here is an explanation of the therapy called CBT. If anyone thinks they have terminal illness, we would expect the *emotional* and *physical* responses. These are natural. The *behaviour* response and initial *thought* is where the CBT can help, over time, gradually giving you tools to step out of the circle.

Empower ☐ — Do any of these suggestions sound like they might work for you? Who else could help?

Future ☐ — I would recommend that you have a look at the information. Recognising that your symptoms are anxiety can help you feel more in control but, if next time we meet we need more help, I would recommend calling Talking Space to arrange CBT. Shall we meet again in a month to see how you are getting on? Earlier if you need to.

Safety net ☐ — If you feel your mood drops or you have new symptoms, for example your bowels change, you lose weight or see blood in the stool, please tell a doctor.

Mental Health – 1

Patient's Story

Anxiety

Doctor's notes	Stephen Harper, 42 years. PMH: Irritable bowel syndrome. Medications: No current medication. Past medication: Mebeverine.
	GP consultation 5 weeks ago. Intermittent bloating. No red flags. Impression IBS.
	A&E attendance with chest pain – discharge letter, tests all normal and reassured.
	FBC, U&E, LFT, TFTs, GGT, CRP, HbA1c, ESR and coeliac screen all normal 1 month ago.
How to act	Hesitant and quiet.
PC	*'It's my bowels again, Doctor.'*
History	You go to the toilet three times every morning.
	Your bowels are loose (not watery) but then they settle down. No other GI symptoms.
	No red flags – no weight loss, no bleeding and no change in bowels.
	You have seen previous doctors and *'they said it is irritable bowel'*.
	You have been struggling with financial pressures.
	Your children want to go to university.
	You have no thoughts of hurting yourself or anyone else.
	You have no features of depression, only worry. You eat and sleep okay.
Social	You work at an electronics store. At work, your concentration is good.
	You exercise to keep healthy. Your parents are elderly, which upsets you.
	Your relationship with your wife is good. She knows you worry.
	Children aged 15 and 14. You do not drink much alcohol. No drugs.
ICE	Deep down you think this must be due to stress.
	You often think when alone and especially on waking.
	Thoughts include financial worry and waiting to be told you have a life-limiting illness.
	Lots of things remind you of this: adverts and articles.
	You think about death a lot and it frightens you. It can make you cry.
	Your chest can become tight, you feel sweaty and can feel breathless. You recently had an episode of chest pain which frightened you, so you went to A&E and were told it was muscular. You had a mild pain in your lower chest which had no features of cardiac, gastric or respiratory disease. You accepted this but you fear you have bowel cancer, perhaps near the top of the tummy because of the recent chest pain.
	If the doctor senses you are quiet say: *'Well, you get to forty.'*
	If asked what you meant you say: *'A mid-life crisis.'* If asked about it further tell the doctor – *'You hear of people going to the doctor and 6 weeks later they are dead.'*
	No one you know has had this happen. You don't know what to do.
	You wondered whether you should have a colonoscopy.
	You expect the doctor will restart your mebeverine. It doesn't help.
	You would follow any guidance from the doctor.
Examination	If the doctor examines you the abdomen is normal. Observations normal.

Mental Health – 1

Learning Points — Anxiety

Open questions help the real problem to surface. Red flags steer diagnosis. Risk assessments guide management. **'Has anything else crossed your mind?'** was useful here to avoid missing his multiple ICE. There were no red flags for lower GI symptoms, but this fear needed to be acknowledged and resolved.

NICE Guidance – the stepped care model for the management of generalised anxiety.[1]

Step 1   'Identification and assessment; education about GAD and treatment options; active monitoring.'[1]

Step 2   'Low-intensity psychological interventions: individual non-facilitated self-help, individual guided self-help and psychoeducational groups.'[1]

Step 3   'High-intensity psychological intervention (CBT/applied relaxation) or a drug treatment.'[1]

SSRIs. Side effects: upset stomach and may increase anxiety initially.

Propranolol may be required in addition. Care of contraindications, e.g. asthma.

Alternative drug treatments: SNRI and pregabalin.

Benzodiazepines may be used for crisis management only.

Step 4   'Highly specialist treatment, such as complex drug and/or psychological treatment regimens; input from multi-agency teams, crisis services, day hospitals or inpatient care.'[1]

A simplified version of the CBT model adapted from Williams et al.[2,3] which can be used in whole or in part within the 10-minute consultation after excluding red flags for the physical causes. This model helps patients to visualise why their physical symptoms are linked to their anxiety and not a sign of something sinister. It is also a great way of summarising and demonstrating you have listened.

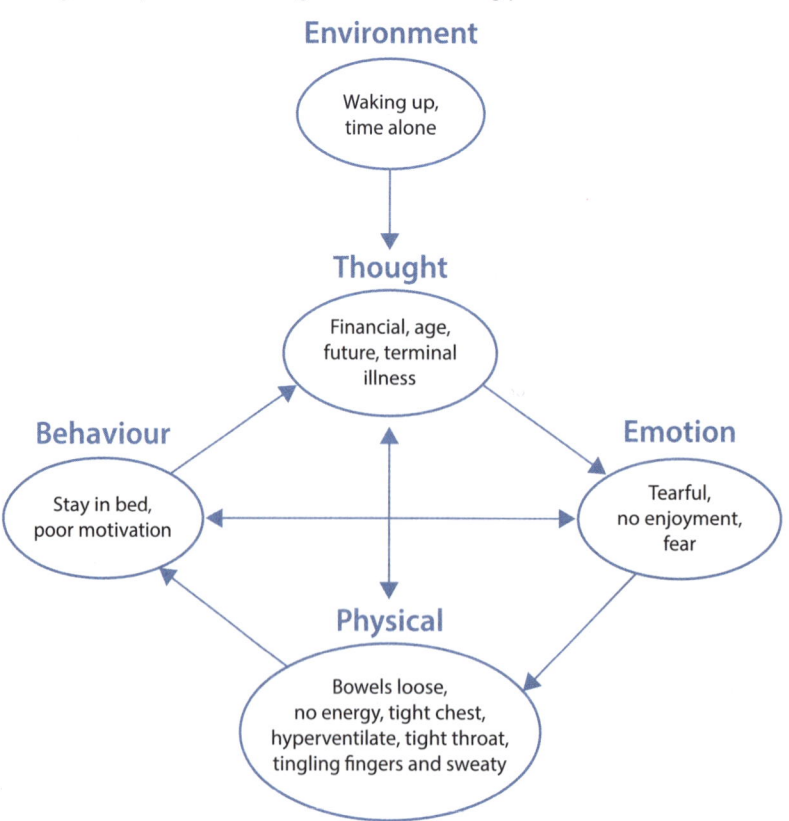

Environment
Waking up, time alone

Thought
Financial, age, future, terminal illness

Behaviour
Stay in bed, poor motivation

Emotion
Tearful, no enjoyment, fear

Physical
Bowels loose, no energy, tight chest, hyperventilate, tight throat, tingling fingers and sweaty

Mental Health – 1

Doctor's Notes

Patient   Jessica Miller   24 years   F
PMH   No medical history
Medications No current medications
Allergies   No information
Consultations No recent consultations
Investigations No recent investigation
Household   No household members registered

Example Consultation — Depression

Open ☐	Can you describe what you've noticed isn't right? Do you feel poorly?
Sense ☐	You seem very quiet.
ICE ☐	What has been going through your mind? Are you worried about anything? Is there anything particular you were hoping I would suggest today?
History ☐	When do you think you started to feel this way? What was happening in your life at the time? How is the job going? Do you have family? Are you close to them? Can you confide in anyone? Do you live with anyone? Have you felt this way before? Tell me what happened then. What helped? Do you have any medical problems or medicines?
Curious ☐	What does your mum think? What have you told her? What haven't you told her? Are people at work aware?
Flags ☐	What is your sleeping pattern like? Do you wake with an alarm? Are you able to enjoy activities? How is your concentration? What comes to mind when you think about the future? Are you eating? Any thoughts of not wanting to be alive? Hurting yourself or suicide? Have you ever hurt yourself or tried to end your life? Have you made any plans to? Do you think you might? Could you tell someone about these thoughts if they became stronger? Any thoughts of hurting another person? How much alcohol do you drink? Do you take any drugs? Have you heard or seen anything that others may not be aware of?
Impact ☐	How do you spend your days? And what about when you are not at work?
Summary ☐	So to summarise, you don't feel yourself, lacking in energy and low; you have felt this way since moving for your job and had problems with low mood during your school years. You felt happier beforehand when you were with your family. You have had upsetting thoughts of how you could end your life but have made no plans to do this as you do not want to upset your mum. Is that correct?
Impression ☐	It sounds like you have depression.
Experience ☐	Do you know anything about the causes of depression? Or the options for treatment?
Explanation ☐	Causes can include new challenges in your life or a chemical imbalance in the brain.
Empathy ☐	It is very hard to move away from those you love and it sounds like this has been hard for both you and your mum.
Options ☐	Depression can prevent you from looking after yourself. It sounds as if your mum would like you to go home; have you considered this? That sounds sensible. Going home may provide time to decide together what to do in the longer term. What do you think? When it comes to depression there are things that you can do, such as getting some exercise and eating well, things I can help with, for example prescribe medication, and other people, such as your parents or counsellors, can give you support. You may find that returning to a happy and caring environment is enough to help you feel better, but it may be that you need a little more help. It seems you are suffering significantly at the moment so we need to work out a plan which is best for you. What are your thoughts regarding antidepressants or talking therapies? Okay, shall we see how you get on at home and if things aren't improving in the next couple of weeks think about medication? I can issue a work note. Would you like the number of a counsellor? Would you be interested in some online help?
Empower ☐	What exercise could you do? Is there anyone else who could help you?
Future ☐	Can you arrange to see a GP in a couple of weeks? Would you like me to talk to your mum? We need to make sure you are safe and so if your mum is aware of what thoughts you have had she can help you … would it be okay if I explained to her what you have told me? If you decide to stay with your mum, can you call me again to discuss the ongoing plan? Avoid alcohol as it lowers mood.
Safety net ☐	If you feel your mood is dropping or you ever have thoughts of hurting yourself, call a GP, me if available, but there is always a GP on call here. If the surgery is closed there is 111 or the Samaritans. You could even go to A&E. Here are all the contact numbers.

Mental Health – 2

Patient's Story

Depression

Doctor's notes Jessica Miller, 24 years. PMH: No medical history. Medications: None.

How to act Quite short sentences, occasional eye contact. Not smiling. Your depression makes it hard work for the doctor to retrieve information from you.

Often initially answering, *'I don't know.'*

PC After a pause … *'I don't know what's wrong with me.'*

History You started to feel this way when you moved for your job about 6 months ago.

No physical symptoms but you have no energy. No psychotic features.

Anhedonia and hopelessness.

You felt like this in the past, whilst doing your GCSEs, and were seen by the school counsellor – you found this helpful.

Risk: You have had occasional thoughts of not wanting to be alive. You sometimes think it would be good if you didn't wake up in the morning.

You drink some alcohol. You take no drugs. No thoughts of hurting others.

Never self-harmed. You have never made a plan to harm yourself.

Thoughts have included jumping off a bridge or taking an overdose.

If the doctor asks whether you intend to do this say, *'I don't know,'* and if they ask if you would tell someone say, *'I don't know.'*

Protective factor:

You are very close to your mum and you would hate to upset her by committing suicide.

Social You work in marketing. You have been late for work as you struggle to get out of bed, despite being awake since 4–5 am. Your boss is nice and told you to come to the GP. You have fallen out with your flat mates over bills. You moved here for work 6 months ago.

You are eating less. You can't think about cooking.

You spend your days in your room watching TV.

You don't see your friends. You have no hobbies.

You do not exercise. You confide in your mum.

Your parents live 4 hours away. You miss them. They want you to go home.

Your mum is worried. She speaks to you on the phone every night.

ICE You are not sure why you feel like this. You are not worried about anything.

You don't know what to expect today.

You accept a work note but decline antidepressants.

You will go on walks with your mum. You will also see your local vicar.

If offered, accept a referral to counselling services.

You give consent for the GP to speak to your mum if the GP offers this.

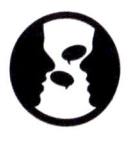

Mental Health – 2

Learning Points — Depression

Recommend a few suggestions tailored to their needs and capacity. Provide a list of the suggestions and contact numbers for organisations. You may have a collection of books you can lend. Structure your management plan: you can do, I (GP) can do, others can do and other resources. Depending on how much the patient can absorb.

'Things that you can do: a healthy sleep and meal regime to give you energy, avoid alcohol which lowers mood, and exercise every day will make you feel better. I can help with providing suggestions, monitoring and prescribing medication if needed. Other people who can help may include family, friends or professionals. You could contact MIND who will advise on local support groups. I suggest arranging counselling if you feel there are emotions or experiences you want to talk about. There are other useful resources, websites such as MoodGym or Mindfulness. There are helpful books also, such as Living in the Moment: with Mindfulness Meditations by Anna Black. (Less helpful if struggling with concentration.) I have a list of all of these suggestions and here are the contact numbers.'

> See the **Link Hub at CompleteCSA.co.uk** for a useful links to **How to Switch Antidepressants** and **An article – Combining Antidepressants**

NICE Guidance – The stepped care model for the management of depression.[1]

Step 1 'Assessment, support, psychoeducation, active monitoring and referral for further assessment and interventions.'[1]

Step 2 'Low-intensity psychosocial interventions (self-help CBT or structured group physical activity programme), psychological interventions, medication and referral for further assessment and interventions.'[1]

Step 3 'Medication, high-intensity psychological interventions (e.g. CBT or behavioural couples therapy), combined treatments, collaborative care ("Only for depression where the person also has a chronic physical health problem and associated functional impairment"[1]) and referral for further assessment and interventions.'[1]

Step 4 'Medication, high-intensity psychological interventions, electroconvulsive therapy, crisis service, combined treatments, multi-professional and inpatient care.'[1]

Duration of treatment of medication therapy

First episode of depression: continue for 6 months after the depression has improved.

Second episode: continue for at least 2 years.[1]

Combining drug medication in the patient resistant to first-line therapy needs careful consideration and 'should only normally be started in primary care in consultation with a consultant psychiatrist'.[1]

Be aware of:

Serotonin syndrome – see http://patient.info/doctor/Serotonin-Syndrome

Malignant neuroleptic syndrome – see http://patient.info/doctor/Neuroleptic-Malignant-Syndrome.

Doctor's Notes

Patient Andrea Lockwood   F   36 years

PMH 15 years old – under Child and Adolescent Mental Health Services for depression.

17–20 years old – under secondary care for major depression and self-harm.

Discharged by mental health services for repeated failure to attend.

Mid-20s – managed by GP for moderate depression and superficial wrist cutting.

Overdose of paracetamol aged 27 years, seen by Crisis Team and discharged.

Termination of pregnancy 29 years old, referred to counselling team. Disclosed a history of sexual abuse as a child (by stepfather), declined to inform police.

Further episode of severe depression in early 30s, suicidal ideation but not attempts, wrist cutting, referred to secondary care but repeatedly failed to attend appointment. Discharged back to primary care.

Medications No current medications.

Several courses of antidepressants in the past including fluoxetine, sertraline, mirtazapine.

Allergies No information.

Consultations GP appointment 4 weeks ago:

'Becoming depressed again, feeling low. Not sleeping or eating well. Got into trouble at work. Only had the job for 4 weeks when got into an argument with a colleague, resulting in her quitting the job on the spur of the moment. Feels colleague was out to get her. Worried about money. Lives alone, no local family. Finds it hard to keep friends, says no close friends. Has a nice neighbour who looks in on her occasionally. Having fleeting thoughts of suicide, no plans or attempts. Has been cutting wrists again, superficial wrist wounds seen.

Plan: Restart sertraline, TCI 3–4 weeks for review. Crisis team number given to patient and worsening advice given.'

Investigations No information

Household No household contacts

Example Consultation — Personality Disorder

Open ☐ — Can you tell me a bit more about how you feel? Tell me your story. That sounds tough (pause). How have you been since you last saw the GP?

Impact ☐ — Has the way you are feeling caused you any difficulties in life recently?

History ☐ — I'm sorry you are feeling so low. Is your mood affecting how you sleep? Or eat? Are you able to go out and enjoy yourself? I can see that you have had problems with your mood in the past; do you feel that you are always battling with low mood? Can you tell me more about what contact you have had with health professionals? Do you think your mood affects how you develop or keep relationships? Who is in your life? How do you get on? Has anyone in the family suffered with mood problems? Have you ever been in trouble with the police? Do you drink alcohol? Or smoke? Have you ever taken illegal drugs? Do you find that sometimes you act without thinking things through? Has this had any bad consequences for you? Do you ever feel paranoid? Do you ever hear or see things which other people cannot?

Flags ☐ — You told the GP last time that you had been harming yourself; is this still the case? How often? Is it possible to explain what drives you to cut yourself? Does it make you feel better afterwards? Have you ever felt so bad that you have wanted to end your life? Have you ever made plans to end your life? What would stop you from ending your life? Do you know where you can get help if you do feel suicidal?

Sense ☐ — I sense that life can be very complex for you at times, would you agree?

ICE ☐ — Do you have any thoughts about what could be causing all these problems for you? Are you worried about anything specific? Was there anything specific you hoped we would achieve today or anything in particular that you wanted?

Summary ☐ — So you feel you have had problems with your mood since you were a teenager. This may have begun as a result of abuse you sadly suffered as a child. You have seen lots of different doctors and you have felt this has been without much success. You find it difficult to maintain relationships and can sometimes act on impulse without thinking of the consequences. You find cutting yourself releases tension and makes you feel better. You do have thoughts that it would be better if you weren't around but haven't made plans to end your life recently. You would like help and for a medical team to stick with you. Is there anything I have missed or you would like to add?

Explanation ☐ — You're clearly suffering with an episode of depression at present, Andrea, but I do wonder if the problem runs a little deeper and if there may be another explanation as to why you have had such complex problems in your life. I wonder if you may have a personality disorder. Have you heard of this? Our personalities are quite complex but in general they are a set of qualities which control how we think, feel and behave. Our personalities develop in a particular way partly due to our genes but also due to our experiences and upbringing. In some people, their personality develops in such a way that it causes them great difficulties in life. These difficulties vary greatly but can be with their mood, their relationships or their behaviour, such as committing crimes. Do you think this could be the case for you?

Options ☐ — I would like to refer you to our complex needs team who can assess you to see if they think you may have a personality disorder. If they do, they can help you by providing a community mental health nurse who will visit you, they can also put you in touch with a support worker and can help you access talking therapies. Sometimes medication can also help but I would like to be guided by their expertise. Is that okay?

Empathy ☐ — I realise this is a lot to take in and may be a bit scary; how do you feel about it?

Future ☐ — Let's continue the sertraline for now as it's helping and I will do the referral.

Safety net ☐ — Can I see you in 3 weeks? If you are worsening in the meantime, please let me know. If you feel suicidal you can phone the Samaritans, but if you feel in danger call the crisis team. Thanks for coming today.

Patient's Story

Personality Disorder

Doctor's notes Andrea Lockwood, 36 years. PMH: see below. Medications: No current medication. Past medication: Fluoxetine, sertraline, mirtazapine.

GP appointment 4 weeks ago: 'Becoming depressed again, feeling low. Not sleeping or eating well. Got into trouble at work. Only had job for 4 weeks when got into an argument with a colleague, resulting in her quitting the job on the spur of the moment. Feels colleague was out to get her. Worried about money. Lives alone, no local family. Finds it hard to keep friends, says no close friends. Has a nice neighbour who looks in on her occasionally. Having fleeting thoughts of suicide, no plans or attempts. Has been cutting wrists again, superficial wrist wounds seen. Plan: Restart sertraline, TCI 3–4 weeks for review. Crisis team number given to patient and worsening advice given.'

How to act Low.

PC *'So, things aren't much better, Doctor.'*

History You had a tough start in life as your natural father was an alcoholic so your home life was chaotic. Your father died following an accident related to alcohol. Your mother was devastated but over time came to terms with what had happened. Your mother suffered with anxiety and depression and was once hospitalised due to her depression. She met a new partner whom you did not like. You disclosed to a counsellor that your stepfather abused you when you were 13 years old but you do not want to go to the police about this now. He and your mother are separated and you do not see him any more. Your relationship with your mother is variable. It's good at the moment. Over the years you have seen many health professionals about low mood. They never help you. You have repeatedly self-harmed and on one occasion took a paracetamol overdose, although you didn't really intend to die. You find that you can make friends easily but often the friendships fail due to arguments; you often feel that the friend doesn't really care about you. You can be impulsive. You have never had a job which lasted more than a few months. You will spend money that you don't have and react to situations without thinking of the consequences. You have once been in trouble with the police due to shoplifting, and you were let off with a caution. At present you feel low and worthless. You have been cutting your wrists as this gives you a sense of relief. You have had thoughts that it would be better if you weren't alive but haven't made plans to end your life. The sertraline has helped a little.

You have no symptoms of psychosis. You want your life to get better and feel you need help from people who *'won't let me down'*. You mean people always give you a tablet then pass you on to someone else. You would like continuity of care. You call the Samaritans regularly. This helps to release anger if you don't want to cut yourself.

Social Currently unemployed, you were given a 'med 3 fit note' by the GP in your last appointment. You drink alcohol occasionally. You smoke 15 cigarettes a day. No illicit drug use. You live alone in a rented flat.

ICE You think you are depressed. You would like to continue sertraline and would like another sick note. You are open to the idea of seeing a specialist if the doctor suggests this.

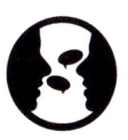

Learning Points

Personality Disorders

Personality disorders can be quite difficult to identify but be suspicious in patients with repeating patterns of behaviour, such as self-harm, emotional instability, criminal activity, problems maintaining relationships or difficulties functioning in day to day life (unable to keeps jobs etc.). Personality disorders are thought to develop due to a combination of genetic factors and 'nurture' factors (early life experiences, abuse). Our personalities have normally formed between our mid-teens to early 20s. Although our personalities cannot be changed (hence personality disorders are often labelled untreatable), intervention can help patients cope with their difficulties and enable them to function better and have a more stable and fulfilling life. NICE recommends a structured approach to assessment and management. Psychotherapy can be effective and drug therapy may help in some cases (e.g. antidepressants to treat depressive symptoms). Antipsychotics or sedatives can be used for short-term crisis management but are not advised long term.[1,2,3]

Below is a summary of the different categories of personality disorder and their typical features. From http://www.rcpsych.ac.uk/healthadvice/problemsdisorders/personalitydisorder.aspx

Cluster A: ('Odd or Eccentric')	Features:
Paranoid	Suspicious, feelings of persecution, feel easily rejected, hold grudges.[4]
Schizoid	Emotionally cold, prefers being alone, 'have a rich fantasy world'.[4]
Schizotypal	'Eccentric behaviour, odd ideas, difficulties with thinking, lack of emotion or inappropriate reactions',[4] visual or auditory hallucinations, may have features of schizophrenia.[4]
Cluster B: ('Dramatic, Emotional and Erratic')	**Features:**
Antisocial or Dissocial	Lack of empathy, easily frustrated, aggressive, criminal activity, difficult to form close relationships, impulsive, lack of guilt, does not learn from unpleasant experiences.[4]
Borderline or Emotionally Unstable	Impulsive, hard to control emotions, features of depression/low mood/low self-worth, self-harm, difficulty maintaining relationships, may feel paranoid, can have auditory hallucinations.[4]
Histrionic	Over-dramatic, self-centred, suggestible, worry about appearance, look for excitement and new things and seductive.[4]
Narcissistic	Overwhelming sense of self-importance, desire success, power and intellectual greatness, crave attention but does not reciprocate, take advantage of others and does not return favours.[4]
Cluster C: ('Anxious and Fearful')	**Features:**
Obsessive-Compulsive (Anankastic)	Worry, doubt, perfectionists, rigid routines, cautious and preoccupied with detail, difficulty adapting, judgemental, sensitive to criticism, obsessional thoughts, high moral standards.[4]
Avoidant (Anxious/Avoidant)	Very anxious/tense, insecure, feels inferior, extremely sensitive to criticism, have to be liked.[4]
Dependent	Passive, can't make decisions, submissive, difficulty coping with daily tasks, feel hopeless and abandoned.[4]

Doctor's Notes

Patient	Chloe Livingstone-Smith 28 years F
PMH	Failed forceps delivery and Emergency Lower Segment Caesarean Section 2 weeks ago
Medications	No current medications
Allergies	No information
Consultations	Midwife visit at home yesterday.
	'Baby doing well, no jaundice, yellow stool nappies. Regained birth weight. Forceps mark fading. Breastfeeding. Up 2 hourly in the night. Mum tired. Not been out, says worried baby will pick up an infection, made an odd comment about the government, seems a little tearful, suggested sees GP, asked husband to make her an appointment tomorrow.'
Investigations	No information
Household	Damian Smith 32 years M
	James Smith 2 weeks M

Example Consultation — Postnatal Psychosis

Open — I see you had a baby 2 weeks ago, congratulations! Is James your baby's name? How has it been going? How are you? How is James? What has been the biggest challenge?

History — How was your delivery? Is this your first child? How are you getting on with feeding? Is James sleeping well? Have you managed to get any rest? Who's at home? What support are you getting?

Sense — You said that you needed to get back to James; is there anything particular making you feel the need to rush?

Flags — Have you been feeling particularly sad or worried since James was born? Why do you think he may be getting an infection? Is there anything that has happened to make you think the government wants to take him away? Do you believe that the government is speaking to you or sending you messages? Do you worry that the government can hear your thoughts or interfere with your thoughts? Do you ever hear or see things which other people cannot? Have you ever had thoughts about harming James? Or harming yourself? Have you done anything to protect James from the government?

Risk — Do you know if any other woman in your family has had problems with their mood after having a baby? Have you ever had problems with your mood before?

ICE — I see that your husband made the appointment for you today, but had you any thoughts about what you would like to happen? You are clearly worried that James may become ill and that the government may take him away; would you like my help with this?

Experience — Have you ever come across a situation where a mother has become unwell with mood problems after having a baby?

Curious — What does your husband think? Is he worried about you or James?

Summary — So you had your baby, James, 2 weeks ago, you had a tough time during the delivery but did recover well. Now, however, you feel unable to take James out of the house due to fear of him becoming unwell or that the government will take him off you as you believe it thinks you are a bad mother. You have been avoiding other people and have been keeping James clean by bathing him 3 times a day and changing his nappy every hour. You have unplugged the TV to stop the government sending you messages and to stop it spying on you. You would like help to protect yourself and James but aren't sure whom you can trust. Is there anything else you would like to tell me?

Explanation — It seems to me, Chloe, that you may be suffering from a condition that can develop after having a baby and causes the mother to have severe mood problems. The condition is called postpartum psychosis. It sounds like your grandmother may have had the same problem. This is what is causing you to feel scared and anxious and worry that James will become ill or be taken away.

Options — I would really like to get you some help with this today. To get the best help, I would like to speak to our specialist colleagues at the hospital and ask them to see you today.

Empathy — I understand this is a scary prospect and it must seem that we are ganging up on you but I would really like to get you some help.

Future — There is a special ward at the hospital where you and James can go until you are feeling better. James will stay with you so you don't need to worry that someone will take him away. How does that sound? Can I call your husband and ask him to meet you here? We can then arrange for you to go up to the hospital.

Safety net — I'll ask a nurse to sit with you until your husband arrives. If you feel worried or change your mind about seeing the hospital doctor, let us know and we can talk it through again. When your husband arrives, may I explain to him what you have told me?

Mental Health – 4

Patient's Story

Postnatal Psychosis

Doctor's notes Chloe Livingstone-Smith, 28 years. PMH: Failed forceps delivery and ELSCS 2 weeks ago. Medications: None. Midwife visit yesterday: 'Baby doing well, no jaundice, yellow stool nappies. Regained birth weight. Forceps mark fading. Breastfeeding. Up 2 hourly in the night. Mum tired. Not been out, says worried baby will pick up an infection, made an odd comment about the government, seems a little tearful, suggested sees GP, asked husband to make her an appointment tomorrow.'

How to act Agitated. You want to reassure the doctor that all is well; however, you open up to the doctor when he/she explores your thoughts.

PC *'Can we make this quick, Doctor, I need to get back to James.'*

History You had your first baby, James, 2 weeks ago. You were induced due to being overdue and had a torrid time in hospital. The induction took a long time and resulted in a failed forceps delivery followed by an emergency caesarean section as James had become distressed in the womb. You were in hospital a couple of days recovering. James needed to be monitored as he had inhaled some meconium and the doctors were worried about infection. Since being discharged, you have become extremely anxious about James becoming unwell, especially that he will get an infection. You change his nappy hourly to keep him clean and bath him three times a day. You worry that the government is trying to take him away from you. You think that it sends messages through the television to you, telling you to give him up as you can't look after him properly and keep him safe and clean. You have unplugged the television and won't allow your husband to watch it. You have left James at home with your husband as you didn't want the government to snatch him whilst you were out. Your husband has told you that you need a check-up after the caesarean so you have come in reluctantly. You remember your mother telling you that her mother went into an 'asylum' after giving birth to her.

Social You are a designer for a large fashion company; previously you have travelled the world through your work. You married a photographer, whom you met whilst working on a fashion show. Your husband was keen to have children as he is a little older than you. You weren't sure at first as you didn't want to take a lot of time off work but were happy when you fell pregnant. Your parents live in Miami so you don't see them often. You are an only child. Your in-laws live fairly locally and have been helping out.

ICE You believe that your baby will be taken from you by the government as it thinks you are an unfit mother. You love your baby and have been doing everything you can to protect him, especially from infection. You believe you have come for a check-up. You expect to be allowed home to your baby straight away. You do not want to go back to hospital. You think the doctor may be on the government's side but, if he/she explains kindly and empathetically, you agree to his/her plan.

Mental Health – 4

Learning Points   Postnatal Psychosis

Mood changes after delivery are common but we must all be on the lookout for women who may be struggling with a mental illness.

'Baby blues' – very common (>50%). Low mood, irritability, anxiety and tearfulness are common symptoms. Usually occurs day 3–4 postnatally and has usually resolved by day 10. Be suspicious if symptoms persist beyond 2 weeks.

Postnatal depression – Occurs in 10–15% of women. Typically begins within the first 8 weeks but can occur several months later. Often there is a history of depression during pregnancy, although this isn't always picked up. More severe and longer lasting than 'baby blues'. Same symptoms as with non-pregnancy related depression, i.e. low mood, tearful, changes in sleep, changes in appetite, anxiety and anhedonia. May be some more specific symptoms related to having a new baby, e.g. difficulty bonding with the baby, lack of emotional connection to the baby, feeling guilty for not loving the baby enough, resenting the baby for the way they feel, thoughts of harming the baby. As with all patients with depression, it is essential to assess any risk posed by the patients to themselves or others. In postnatal depression, be especially alert to risk to the baby or other children in the household.

Screening questions – NICE recommends the following screening questions to help identify PND. *'During the past month, have you often been bothered by feeling down, depressed or hopeless? During the past month, have you often been bothered by having little interest or pleasure in doing things?'* Any positive response should lead to further assessment, possibly using a tool such as the Edinburgh Postnatal Depression Scale. Depending on the severity of the symptoms, the mother may be able to care for herself and her baby without much extra support, but in severe cases the mother may struggle to complete simple tasks. In milder cases, health visitors, community mental health teams etc. can be called upon to help treat the patient in the community setting. In more severe cases, involvement of the perinatal psychiatry team or even admission to a specialist mother and baby unit may be required. Where possible, the mother and baby should be kept together.

Postpartum psychosis (puerperal psychosis) – Much rarer, occurring in 0.1%. Typically begins suddenly within the first 2 weeks following delivery. Symptoms vary but include severe depression, mania, hallucinations and delusions. It may occur in a woman with no history of mental illness, but the risk is increased if there is a personal or family history of mental illness (particularly of postpartum psychosis). There are frequently delusions about the baby: 'the baby is evil'. The patient may demonstrate typical features of psychotic illness e.g. pressure of speech, knight's move thinking, delusions (e.g. paranoia, grandiose thoughts or ideas of persecution) or auditory/visual hallucinations.

Postpartum psychosis is a psychiatric emergency and NICE recommends referral for immediate assessment (within 4 hours) and, where possible, the mother should be treated in a specialist mother and baby unit. Thankfully the prognosis is good with the worst symptoms usually improving around 12 weeks and the majority of cases resolving between 6 and 12 months. However, there is a 50% chance of recurrence in future pregnancies.

> **Antipsychotic induced hyperprolactinaemia**
> See the Link Hub at CompleteCSA.co.uk for helpful advice – when commencing an antipsychotic.

Doctor's Notes

Patient   Eleanor Cartwright   15 years   F
PMH   Constipation aged 4 years
                 Lower respiratory tract infection 11 years
Medications No current medications
Allergies   No known allergies
Consultations No recent consultations
Investigations No information
Household   Faith Cartwright   54 years   F
                 Brian Cartwright   55 years   M

Attends with mother.

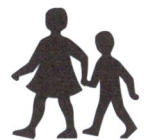

Example Consultation — Eating Disorder

Open ☐ — Hello Ellie. Why have you come to see me today? What have you talked about at home? How do you feel about this? How do you feel about your health? Faith, what are your thoughts please? Have you noticed anything else that has worried you?

Impact ☐ — Ellie, have you noticed a change to your body? Have things at home changed? What about at school? Faith, have you noticed a change in Ellie? Have teachers?

History ☐ — Ellie, have you had any medical problems? Do you take any medicines? Who is at home? May I speak to Ellie alone briefly? It is always helpful, thank you. How are things at home? What is your mum worried about, do you think? What do you like to do when you are not at school? How is school? Have you noticed a change to any parts in your body? Going to the toilet, headaches or periods? Are you pleased or is that a worry?

Curious ☐ — Ellie, your mum says you sometimes get angry. What makes you feel this way?

Risk ☐ — Is anyone at school horrible? Because your periods have stopped, I have to make sure you are not pregnant: do you have a boyfriend? Have you had sex? Has anyone made you feel uncomfortable or hurt you? Do you take drugs or drink alcohol?

Flags ☐ — Do you feel unhappy or tearful? Do you sleep okay? Can you concentrate? Do you ever wish you were not alive? Have you tried to hurt yourself? Do you ever see or hear things that others can't? Or receive instructions that others are not aware of? Thank you for answering my questions. Is there anything else you want to tell me before we invite your mum back in? Okay, let's do that. Does she know about your periods?

Sense ☐ — Hello Faith. Ellie and I have talked about her missed periods. I am not concerned about anything else she has just said. I do sense you are very worried about Ellie.

ICE ☐ — Ellie, do you know why we are concerned? Is there anything you are worried about? When you were in the waiting room, what did you think I might say? Faith, what are your thoughts about what Ellie may be going through? What worries you most? Is there anything else? Is there anything specific you were hoping I would do today?

Examination ☐ — Ellie, I would like to examine you please – check your blood pressure and pulse, your height and weight and feel your tummy and your neck to make sure there is no other reason why you may have lost weight. Is that okay?

Summary ☐ — To summarise, Ellie, you decided to change what foods you eat and exercise more over the past 5 months. Since then, your parents and school teacher have been concerned about you and especially after your mum heard you being sick.

Experience ☐ — Ellie, do you know the risks of losing weight? Faith, you said you have read about problems with eating, can you tell me more about what you have read? Faith, have you come across this before?

Impression ☐ — Ellie, it sounds as if you have decided that controlling your weight is really important to you. However, this needs to be done safely. Sometimes, without realising it, a person can lose too much weight as they continue to focus on avoiding food and start to be sick to avoid absorbing food. This is called an eating disorder and I believe this is why your weight has gone down to a dangerous level.

Explanation ☐ — The body needs nutrition to work. Your periods stopping is an example of your body being affected by the weight loss.

Options ☐ — Ellie, I would like to do a full set of blood tests to check what may be out of balance including your hormones for your periods, thyroid, sugar, liver and kidneys and blood cells and also a heart tracing (ECG). Can you please arrange to see the nurse for this tomorrow? I don't think exercise is safe at present as you may become extremely unwell if you lose more weight. I would also like to write to the team who specialise in helping people when they have lost too much weight, to help you be in control again at a safe and healthy level. This is the children's psychiatry team. Okay? If the bloods are concerning, Mum, I'll call you.

Future ☐ — Can you also arrange to see me again in a week's time, please to see how you are?

Safety net ☐ — If either of you are concerned in the meantime, don't hesitate to speak to a doctor.

Mental Health – 5

Patient's Story

Eating Disorder

Doctor's notes Eleanor Cartwright, 15 years. PMH: Constipation aged 4 years. LRTI aged 11 years. Medications: None.

How to act Eleanor is quiet. Mother (Faith) is initially abrupt but then quiet also.

PC **Faith** *'I want to know what is wrong with Ellie. I'm very worried. She keeps to herself and is getting angry when we try to talk to her. We just want to help you, Ellie!'*

History **Eleanor** You don't know what's wrong and tell the doctor you don't know why you are here. However, you are aware that your mum and dad are watching you eat and don't trust you. You sleep okay. You deny losing your appetite or decreasing your meal size. You just eat healthier food. You are annoyed that your parents have stopped you from exercising when you return home from school. You just want to be healthy. It started when you realised that the other girls at swimming looked 'better' than you. You felt 'fat' so just decided to eat better and exercise – that's what everyone tells you is good for you anyway so you don't see the problem. You eat with your parents but feel annoyed if they try to sneak extra food onto your plate. You hope to lose more weight as you don't think anything has changed since you started being healthier 5 months ago. You do not use laxatives. You do not disclose to the doctor that you have started vomiting. You have always been well and there is no family history. Your periods stopped 4 months ago. You have never had sex. You have no other symptoms.

Faith You heard Ellie vomiting whilst the shower was running yesterday which is why you have made the appointment today. Ellie has lost a lot of weight. Originally you thought this was because her body was changing. When you were at college, a girl died from an eating disorder. Ellie has lost contact with her friends.

Social **Eleanor** You are in all the top sets at the local school. Your mother is a journalist and you don't know what your father does exactly but he is always very busy. You get on 'fine'. You play the piano and the clarinet and have your grade 6 piano exam next month.

You have stopped liking school.

ICE **Eleanor** You don't know why you are here but, if pushed for an answer, your mum is watching what you are eating. You are not worried and expect the doctor will tell you to eat more. You don't like periods and you are thrilled they have stopped.

Faith You believe Ellie is becoming very obsessed with her weight. You do not mention the words anorexia but you do admit to *'looking on the Internet at problems with eating'*. However, you haven't yet come to terms with Ellie having this problem. You are concerned that Ellie has become a recluse and no longer goes out with her friends and her test results have dropped. The school teacher called you to say she was worried about Ellie's weight. Since this call last week, you have been watching Ellie. You feel very guilty and worry what the school will think. You would like the doctor to tell Ellie that she cannot exercise until she puts on more weight and to refer her for counselling. You are aware Ellie's periods have stopped and have talked about this.

Examination BMI 14.7, BP 90/60 HR 58 bpm. Abdomen soft, non-tender with no masses or organomegaly. No lymphadenopathy. HS normal. No palpable thyroid.

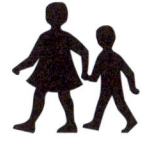

Mental Health – 5

Learning Points

Eating Disorder

Information taken from NICE guidelines CG9. Eating disorders in over 8s: management. 2004.[1] Please refer to full guidance.

As well as a low BMI other factors should raise suspicion[1]

Signs of starvation	Weight concerns and not overweight	Menstrual disturbances
Repeated vomiting	Children with poor growth	Gastrointestinal symptoms

Screening questions

'Do you think you have an eating problem?'[1]

'Do you worry excessively about your weight?'[1]

Diagnosis

Weight and BMI are unreliable indicators and 'attention should be paid to the overall clinical assessment (repeated over time), including rate of weight loss, growth rates in children, objective physical signs and appropriate laboratory tests.'[1]

Assessment should include[1]
- Physical
- Psychological
- Social
- Risk to self and risk of abuse.

Observations/Investigations
- Heart rate, BP, weight.
- Be vigilant for refeeding syndrome, bradycardia and hypotension.
- FBC, U&E, LFT, Calcium, albumin, phosphate, magnesium, glucose ECG.
- NB – continue to monitor the above at regular intervals.

Management
- Refer to and be guided by your local eating disorder team.
- Self-help groups and support groups.[1]
- 'Patients should be advised to gradually reduce laxative use and informed that laxative use does not significantly reduce calorie absorption.'[1]
- Regular dental reviews if vomiting.[1]
- Osteoporosis risk – 'Refrain from physical activities which increase the likelihood of falls.'[1]
- If possible, education and involvement – all household members.
- Regular monitoring of growth, physical symptoms, psychological well-being, social situations, impact and risk.
- At least annual review if stable/remission.

Respect confidentiality
'Children and adolescents with anorexia nervosa should be offered individual appointments with a healthcare professional separate from those with their family members or carers.'[1]

Discuss risk
'People with anorexia nervosa and their carers should be informed if the risk to their physical health is high.'[1]

Mental Health – 5

CHAPTER 13 OVERVIEW
Intellectual Disability (ID)

The term 'Intellectual Disability' (ID) is now used instead of 'Learning Disability' (LD) however, as patients' past diagnoses may include Learning Disability, both terms are used in this chapter.

There are limited CSA resources available elsewhere for this clinical module in the curriculum.

This chapter aims to:

1. Raise awareness of the competencies you need to demonstrate.
2. Provide suggestions of useful communication skills and what potentially can be achieved.
3. Provide examples of how to transfer your knowledge of the above into management plans.
4. Show how to demonstrate understanding and competence of this important curriculum module within the CSA.

Here is a table of example cases so that once you have completed this chapter, you will be able to identify opportunities to demonstrate your awareness of the curriculum and skills in consulting with patients with Intellectual Disability (ID) and prove your competence in this curriculum area within the CSA.

	Cases in this chapter	Within the RCGP curriculum: Care of People with Intellectual Disability RCGP Curriculum Online March 2016[1]	Learning points in the chapter include:
1	Need for Procedure	'Be aware of the concept of diagnostic overshadowing …'	Elderly parents Diagnostic overshadowing
2	Down Syndrome	'The importance of the annual health check …' 'Be aware of the effects intellectual disability has on the aging process … recognition of dementia'	The annual health check, issues specific to the condition/life stage
3	Autism and Transition Process	'Understand the diagnosis and management of patients with autistic spectrum conditions' 'Understand the need to support adolescents …' 'Be aware of the effects intellectual disability has on the life history … particularly at times of transition'	Transition Process Model
4	Mental Health and ID	'Understand the psychiatric disorders prevalent in the adult with intellectual disability and how their diagnosis, detection and management differ' 'Understand the impact of intellectual disability on family dynamics and … carers'	Psychiatric disorders prevalent in the adult with intellectual disability Questions to carers
5	COCP Request	'Recognise the risk to adults with intellectual disability of … abuse'	Risk factors for safeguarding adults

1. http://www.rcgp.org.uk/training-exams/gp-curriculum-overview/online-curriculum/managing-complex-care/3-11-intellectual-disability.aspx

CHAPTER 13 REFERENCES

Need for Procedure
1. Jane Hubert and Sheila Hollins. People with Intellectual Disabilities and their Elderly Carers. http://www.intellectualdisability.info/life-stages/people-with-intellectual-disabilities-and-their-elderly-carers
2. Sandra F. Dowling. Bereavement in The Lives Of People With Intellectual Disabilities. http://www.intellectualdisability.info/life-stages/bereavement-in-the-lives-of-people-with-intellectual-disabilities
3. http://www.rcgp.org.uk/training-exams/gp-curriculum-overview/online-curriculum/managing-complex-care/3-11-intellectual-disability.aspx

Down Syndrome
1. Tony Holland. Ageing and Its Consequences For People With Down Syndrome. http://www.intellectualdisability.info/life-stages/ageing-and-its-consequences-for-people-with-downs-syndrome
2. Stephen Trumble. People with Down's Syndrome at All Ages: Some Tips for Family Physicians. http://www.intellectualdisability.info/life-stages/people-with-downs-syndrome-at-all-age-some-tips-for-family-physicians
3. http://www.rcgp.org.uk/learningdisabilities/~/media/Files/CIRC/CIRC-76-80/CIRCA%20StepbyStepGuideforPracticesOctober%2010.ashx

Transition Process Model
1. http://www.rcgp.org.uk/training-exams/gp-curriculum-overview/online-curriculum/managing-complex-care/3-11-intellectual-disability.aspx
2. Getting it right for young people. Department of Health/Child Health and Maternity Services Branch. 2006.
3. Diana Andrea Barron, Delphine Coyle, Eleni Paliokosta and Angela Hassiotis. Transition for Children with Intellectual Disabilities. http://www.intellectualdisability.info/life-stages/transition-for-children-with-intellectual-disabilities

Mental Health and ID
1. Department of Health. *Valuing People: A New Strategy for Learning Disability for the 21st Century*. 2001.
2. http://www.rcgp.org.uk/training-exams/gp-curriculum-overview/online-curriculum/managing-complex-care/3-11-intellectual-disability.aspx

COCP Request
1. http://www.rcgp.org.uk/training-exams/gp-curriculum-overview/online-curriculum/managing-complex-care/3-11-intellectual-disability.aspx

There are many potential social inequalities for a patient with an intellectual disability, including access to healthcare, financial issues, and educational opportunities. The potential barriers to healthcare include accessing services, communication, using online services, appointment times, patient's fear or a lack of staff training. The responsibilities of the GP include being proactive with setting up a system which provides patients with equal access to healthcare. This may include a patient register, recall system, a team leader, staff education, regular communication with speciality teams and flexible appointment times. The system should ensure clinicians have the time required to gain an understanding of the patient and their carer's challenges, concerns and needs. The GP should be vigilant for atypical presentations of physical conditions, emotional (fear, frustration and loneliness) or psychological concerns and the potential problems which occur within a time of transition in the patient's life. The systemic enquiry should be appropriate to the patient's life stage. An understanding of the patient's social circumstances is essential to effectively screen for isolation, neglect and abuse. Health promotion and when and how to seek help should be discussed. Be aware of local services and provide information which is easy to read. The carer's health and well-being should also be explored. In-practice time and follow-ups are needed for a full assessment. Cutting corners cannot be an option. Remember that the GP may be the only person asking the questions and acting as an advocate for the patient.

Doctor's Notes

Patient	Henry Sutton 60 years M
PMH	Hypoxic Ischaemic Encephalopathy
	Seizures (Seizure-free 30 years)
	Hearing Difficulty. Hearing Aids.
	Myopia
	Learning Difficulties IQ 45
	Attention Deficit Hyperactivity Disorder
	Gastro Oesophageal Reflux Disease.
Medications	Omeprazole 40 mg
Allergies	No known drug allergies.
Consultations	Last consultations: 1 month ago when omeprazole was prescribed.
Investigations	Blood test Helicobacter-pylori negative.
	Hb 105 g/L, otherwise FBC normal.
	U&E, LFT, amylase, CRP, HbA1c, FBG – all normal.
	Weight 65 kg 1 year ago
Household	Rosemary Sutton 88 years F
	Henry attends with mother Rosemary.

Example Consultation — Need for Procedure

Open — Hello. Thank you for coming to see me. Today we will have a chat about how you are, I will ask you some questions and you can ask me questions at any time. If you don't mind, I may need to examine you, then we will have a chat about what happens next. Is that okay? Who have you brought with you today? Henry, can you tell me what has been hurting you? Can you tell me why you had the tests? When does it hurt?

History — Can you point to where you feel the pain? Does it make you sick? Does it make you burp? When you have the pain, what do you do? Does that help? Do you take any other medicines? Who do you live with, Henry? What do you do during the daytime? Who do you tell if you do not feel well?

Risk — Do you smoke? Do you drink alcohol? Do you like coffee or tea? Is there anyone in the family who has a problem in the tummy?

Flags — Have you lost weight, Henry? Do you ever spit your food out because it hasn't gone down into the tummy? Are you coughing lots? Have you felt shivery or hot and cold? Henry, what colour is your poo? Is it ever red like blood or black? Is your poo hard, soft or like water? When you have a wee is that okay or does it hurt? Do you go to the toilet lots to have a wee, or is it the same as always do you think?

Impact — Have you stopped eating as much since this pain started?

ICE — Henry, why do you think you have tummy pain? Are you worried about it? Why are you worried? What did you and your mum think we may decide today? Rosemary, what do you think may be causing this? What are you mostly worried about? What did you hope I might suggest?

Curious — Henry, do you know what your mum means by the 'big C'? Have you talked about what you think?

Summary — To summarise, Henry, you have told me that for a few months you have had pain in the tummy; this has been making you burp but also lose weight. You want some more medicine to make it better.

O/E — Can I ask you to step on the scales, Henry? Now, may I feel your tummy and can you tell me if it hurts when I press? Can I feel your pulse and take your temperature?

Impression — It sounds like this could be a tummy ulcer. Have you had an ulcer in your mouth? This is similar but in the tummy. To give us an answer we need to have a look at different parts of the tummy to see where the problem is. Sometimes an ulcer or pain can be there because of a cancer.

Sense — I can see you are upset.

Experience — Have you seen anyone with cancer? What do you know about it?

Explanation — That can happen but we can also fix it and make it better if we know what it is. The bacteria blood test came back normal but you are anaemic which means your blood count is low.

Empathy — Mentioning the big C can be scary, especially when your gran had it. I have to make sure we've done all the right tests to make sure we know what needs to be done to make you better.

Options — I agree that a jelly scan of your tummy will give us more clues. I also think we should look into the tummy. Henry, we do this by making you sleepy then putting a thin tube with a light into the tummy. Would that be okay? If we see what is causing the pain, we can hopefully make it better. Whatever it is, we can talk about it again.

Empower — If ever you feel hot and shivery please will you tell someone?

Future — You should receive the appointment for the jelly scan and camera test within 2 weeks then I will see you the week after. If you don't receive these tests in that time, please let me know. Is that okay Rosemary?

Safety net — If you have a high temperature or if you see red or black in the toilet, or you are sick or have really bad pain, you need to tell the warden and they need to call a doctor. Rosemary could you pass that on?

Intellectual Disability – 1

Patient's Story

Need for Procedure

Doctor's notes — Henry Sutton, 60 years. (Attends with mother Rosemary.)

PMH: Hypoxic Ischaemic Encephalopathy, Seizures (Seizure-free 30 years), Hearing difficulty. Hearing aids. Myopia, Learning Difficulties IQ 45, Attention Deficit Hyperactivity Disorder, GORD. Medications: Omeprazole 40 mg.

Blood tests: H-pylori negative, Hb 105 g/dL. The rest of the FBC, U&E, LFT, amylase, CRP, HbA1c, FBG – all normal. Weight: 65 kg 1 year ago.

How to act — You are able to answer some questions, but you frequently turn to your mother who either answers for you or repeats the question if the doctor is not being clear.

PC

Mum: *'Henry has come for the results of his blood test.'*

History

Henry: *'I keep getting tummy pain … above the belly button.'* You can't describe a pattern.

No vomiting. If the doctor asks, say: *'My poo is normal.'* No melaena or dysphagia.

Mum: *'I noticed he was losing weight.'*

'He keeps telling me he has pain in his stomach.' This has been the case for months.

Henry came off all his medicines for ADHD in his late teens, followed by his seizure medications. He has been well since. There is no significant family history. He is often belching and he finds this funny. The omeprazole alone doesn't seem to have helped. Henry doesn't drink caffeine or alcohol. He takes no medicines and specifically no ibuprofen. Henry is happy. When the pain is there, you give Henry Gaviscon. It helps a bit, he says.

Social

Henry: You moved to sheltered accommodation 15 years ago where you made friends.

Your mother visits twice a week. You do not smoke or drink alcohol. No tea/coffee.

You do not work but help out in the laundry shop for the residents. There is always a warden on call. You know you can just press the button on the receiver if you need help. You are able to prepare very simple meals such as cereal and sandwiches but have help from staff with hot food.

Mum: He eats a very good diet and enjoys going for walks every day with the staff.

ICE

Henry: You don't know why you have the pain. You just want it to stop.

You think the doctor will give you some more medicine.

Mum: *'I am worried it's something serious.'* If asked to explain *'the big C'.*

You have not told your thoughts to Henry. You would like the doctor to arrange an ultrasound. The other doctor said it might be bacteria, in which case Henry will be given antibiotics. If the doctor starts to talk about the possibility of cancer, Henry becomes distressed. If asked more about this, Henry says, *'People die.'* His granny died in her 80s of lung cancer. If the doctor uses jargon, Henry doesn't want the test. If the doctor empathises and explains why endoscopy is important, Henry agrees.

O/E — Weight 55 kg. Slightly tender epigastrium. Otherwise normal.

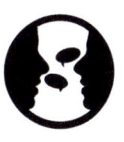

Intellectual Disability – 1

Learning Points

Need for Procedure

When beginning a consultation with a person with intellectual disabilities, it is a good idea to set out what is likely to happen in the consultation. The patient may not be familiar with the consultation process and it can reduce anxiety to explain at the beginning. As with children, address your questions to the patient rather than their carer, be guided by the language the patient and their carer use, to help you use language and terminology that the patient understands. You may need to slow the consultation pace to allow the patient time to absorb what you have said and think of their answer. Be patient; if you aren't understood at first, think of different ways to explain what you mean rather than giving up. Be aware that some patients with intellectual disabilities take what you say very literally so sometimes using similes/metaphors can add to the confusion! Although they are unlikely to be available in the exam, you can get packs of picture cards which help patients explain their symptoms, e.g. happy/sad faces, body parts, toilets, etc.

Points to be aware of

'Elderly parents are often unaware of community support now available to adults with intellectual disabilities.

A mutually dependent relationship may have developed according to their needs and capabilities.

Parents may not ask for help for fear their son or daughter will be taken into care. Elderly parents are often socially isolated.

Elderly parents may be less observant of health changes in their son or daughter.

Comorbid medical conditions are common, but easily overlooked unless actively screened for.

Planning for the future should include recognising inevitable separation by death, and the need to anticipate emotional as well as practical needs.

When people with intellectual disabilities have moved to a home of their own, sustained effort by the new carers is needed to support continuing contact with elderly parents.'[1]

'When a person with intellectual disabilities loses a parent through death, it is not only a loss of someone who is loved, but is also the loss of the person most familiar with their needs, their likes and dislikes, and with whom they had a trusting relationship.'[2]

Diagnostic overshadowing

'Be aware of the concept of diagnostic overshadowing when a person's presenting symptoms are put down to the disability, rather than the doctor seeking another, potentially treatable cause.'[3]

What are the reasons for this?	Time: 10-minute consultations, doctor uncertainty, communication barriers, atypical presentations, lack of continuity – the doctor and patient do not know each other.
How can this be prevented?	GP and healthcare education: early screening for physical and mental health problems. Annual reviews.
	Carer and family education: vigilance for a change in the person and involving the carers in safety netting advice.
	Time (a recurrent theme) and longer appointments.

Doctor's Notes

Patient	Matthew Dalton 24 years M
PMH	Down syndrome
	Closure ASD
	Sensorineural deafness. Hearing aids.
Medications	No current medications
Allergies	No known drug allergies
Consultations	No recent consultations
Investigations	No recent investigations
Household	No household members registered

Example Consultation — Down Syndrome

Open ☐	How are you Matthew? What is going well for you? What has been difficult this year?
Empathy ☐	I'm sorry to hear that. … Do you miss her? Do you cry when you think of her?
Sense ☐	You mentioned your mum told you to see me … is your mum worried about anything?
Curious ☐	Why don't you like going to the doctor? What can you remember? That must have been horrible. Today I would just like to talk and examine you. That's it for today. If either of us is worried about anything we can talk about it and decide together. We won't do anything without your permission. Is that okay?
Sense ☐	Is your ear okay? Why do you keep touching it? Can you hear okay with your hearing aid?
History ☐	Can you remember what health problems you have had in the past? Are you feeling well or is something not right? Can we go through the body to see if you have had any problems? Let's start at the top – do you have any headaches? Can you see everything okay? When did you last have your eyes checked? Can you hear okay? How often do you feel out of breath? Do you have any other strange feelings in your chest? Does your back hurt? Do your arms and legs feel okay? How often do you go for a wee? Does it ever hurt? How often do you have a poo? Is the poo hard like stones, soft or runny? Does anywhere hurt? Have you seen the dentist this year? Who do you live with? What do you do during the day? You have a job: that's great! Do you enjoy it? Do you have friends who live nearby? Are you in a relationship? Is it going well? What do you enjoy doing on your own? It sounds like you are very independent.
Flags ☐	Are you happy or sad most of the time? Do you worry about anything?
ICE ☐	What did you think we might talk about today? Why do you think your ear is hurting? Is there anything you would like me to help with?
Summary ☐	So it sounds as if you have had an upsetting time with losing your gran but Laura has made you feel happy. Your hearing aid is rubbing and you would like a new one.
O/E ☐	Every year we offer an examination so we can check your health. I would like to check your weight and height, look in your ears, listen to your heart and lungs, take your blood pressure, feel your neck, feel your tummy and check your testicles. Do you know where the testicles are? These are the two round parts that are under the penis. This would involve removing your underpants but it is important so I can check there are no lumps or bumps. Would that be okay? I need a chaperone so I will ask Suzie, our nurse, to come in whilst I examine you. Is that okay?
Impression ☐	Your ear is infected. There is also a little lump on the testicle.
Explanation ☐	We commonly find lumps, most are nothing to worry about, but we need to check it with a scan. The scan is in the hospital. It won't hurt and all you will feel is cold jelly. It is important to make sure that the lump is not a cancer, usually it isn't.
Options ☐	Can I arrange this for you? For the ear, please use the spray called Otomize three times a day for a week and let me know if it is still hurting in a week. I will write to the hearing aid team to request they see you to talk about a new one.
Empower ☐	Matthew, your weight is a little high. Do you do any exercise? What exercise would you most like to do? Who cooks your meals? Do you know which foods can be bad for you? Would you like to lose weight? Do you think you could cut out some crisps, biscuits and cakes? I will ask our nurse to see you to discuss diet in more detail.
Future ☐	It would also be helpful to do your annual blood test. Oh dear, do you not like blood tests? It is important to monitor your blood to make sure you're healthy. If I ask the nurse to use a small needle would that help? I can give you some cream to make your skin numb so you won't feel it, if you like? It is a good idea to do exercise together with Laura. Would you like me to write down what we have decided to do next? Shall we see you in 3 months to see how you are getting on? If the scan or blood tests show anything more urgent we will let you know.
Safety net ☐	If you don't receive the appointment for your scan in the next two weeks, please speak to me. If you're worried about anything or feel unwell, please let me know.

Intellectual Disability – 2

Patient's Story

Down Syndrome

Doctor's notes Matthew Dalton, 24 years.

PMH: Down syndrome, closure ASD, sensorineural deafness. Hearing aids.

Medication: None.

How to act Pleasant but quiet. Keep touching your ear.

PC *'My mum said I have to have my yearly check-up.'*

History *'I don't like coming to the doctors.'*

If asked why say: *'Because I always had to go to the doctors.'*

If asked why say: *'I remember being in pain after my operation.'*

Only if asked about your ear, *'It hurts.'* No other ear symptoms.

No other symptoms on systemic enquiry.

You saw the dentist and optician a month ago.

Social You live with your mum. You do not know your dad.

You do not smoke or drink alcohol. You work in the hardware store.

You have been saving money and hope to buy a house one day.

Your girlfriend's name is Laura. Laura has Down syndrome.

You met at a party 3 months ago and you look pleased when you tell the doctor this.

Your gran died earlier in the year. You cried a lot but not since you met Laura.

Your mum makes your meals. You eat an unhealthy diet. You do not exercise.

If encouraged to think about how you could be healthier, suggest going swimming with Laura and say you will tell your mum what the doctor said.

You would be interested in losing weight.

ICE If the doctor mentions any new medical conditions, say you don't know.

Have no understanding of any medical problems.

However, if the doctor says you need tests say: *'I don't want a blood test.'*

If the doctor explains in simple language why you need tests, agree.

You are worried that your hearing aid is rubbing. You would like a new one.

You don't know what the doctor will want to talk to you about.

Your mum said the doctor will do a blood test. (Wrinkle your nose at this.)

Examination The ear canal is eczematous and discharging. The tympanic membrane is normal. No surrounding swelling or lymphadenopathy. Apyrexial. HR 82 bpm. BP 116/62.

BMI is 31. The skin is normal. HS normal. Chest clear.

There is a <1 cm lump on the lower pole of the left testicle.

Intellectual Disability – 2

Learning Points

Down syndrome

Practices are encouraged to have a 'Learning Disability register'. This helps ensure that all patients with intellectual disabilities have an annual review. It is a good idea to send out a questionnaire before the appointment for the patient to complete with their carer. If your practice adopts this approach, make sure you ask to see the questionnaire at the appointment!

The annual health check should include:

- Health screening: observations, weight, height, urine dip, discussion about smoking, alcohol, drugs, diet and exercise, breast or testicular awareness, cervical screening, CVD screening (BMI, BP and blood tests).
- Social assessment: dependence and independence. Discussion regarding social skills.
- Vulnerability assessment: risk of abuse (neglect, physical, sexual, emotional).
- Advice regarding check-ups: vision (e.g. for cataracts), hearing (e.g. for SNHL) and dental.
- Systemic enquiry looking for undiagnosed problems (see below).
- Full physical examination: top to toe approach including ears, neck, chest, abdomen, genitalia, skin, nails etc.
- Mental health assessment.

Discussion of potential issues specific to the condition and life stage, e.g. with Down syndrome:[1,2]

Congenital: Heart disease, hypothyroidism, dislocation of the hip and cataracts.

Childhood: Signs of developmental delay, duodenal atresia, pyloric stenosis, Hirschsprung's disease.

Constipation and tracheo-oesophageal fistulae.

Hearing and visual impairment.

Symptoms of hypothyroidism (may be congenital or acquired). Ongoing cardiac conditions.

Atlantoaxial instability: Have they had X-rays? Once diagnosed – neurological assessments.

Ask about schooling.

Adolescence: Growth and obesity. Dental care.

Menstruation may be slightly delayed. Annual TFTs. Skin and hair.

Late adult: Glaucoma and dementia screening.

Ongoing: Recurrent URTIs – Urine dip and MSU if signs of infection.

Create a Health Action Plan at the end of the annual review. This may be fairly simple such as changes to diet/exercise, coming for blood tests or booking a dental review. It is a good idea to write this down for the patient and some may even have a Health Action Plan booklet which you can write this in. The RCGP provides an example of the questionnaires and action plans that can be used, in its document *A Step by Step Guide for GP Practices: Annual Health Checks for People with a Learning Disability* by Dr Matt Hoghton and the RCGP Learning Disabilities Group.[3]

'Ageing and the problems of old age are particularly relevant to people with Down syndrome as some of these age-related problems develop earlier in life than would normally be the case.'[1]

'The astute GP will remember that the child with Down syndrome is susceptible to the same range of childhood problems as any other and that not all symptoms will be due to the syndrome.'[2]

Doctor's Notes

Patient	Justin Walton 17 years M
PMH	Autistic Spectrum Disorder
	Behavioural concerns 3 years ago
	Lower respiratory tract infection
Medications	Nil
Allergies	No known drug allergies.
Consultations	Letter – Discharged from CAMHS 2 months ago.
Investigations	Nil
Household	Nil recorded

Example Consultation — Autism and Transition Process

Open ☐	Thank you for coming into see me today. Why did you see CAMHS? What did they say was causing you to feel like that? Did they give you a name of a diagnosis? Everyone with autism can struggle with different things … what do you struggle with? What is better now? Are you well at the moment? Is anything causing you worry? What do you think we should talk about? What does your mum think?
Sense ☐	Do you feel quite anxious about all the changes that are happening?
History ☐	Have you had any medical problems? What about people in your family? Do you take tablets? Drugs? Alcohol? How do you spend your day? Do you have any qualifications? Very good. Were you pleased? What would you like to do next? Who is at home? Are you in a relationship?
Empower ☐	Would you like to earn money? What are you good at? What do you enjoy? Can you think of a job you could try? Would you like to live on your own? What do you do by yourself? When might you be at risk? Does anyone say or do hurtful things to you? Who could you tell if this happened? Yes, your family or the GP.
Flags ☐	When you feel angry do you have thoughts of hurting yourself or anyone else?
Curious ☐	Do you get on with your family? Do you feel life is harder for you than for your sister?
ICE ☐	What have you been thinking about recently? Are there any other thoughts that upset you? Or make you feel angry? What do you do when you feel angry? What did you think we may decide today? Is there anything else you were hoping for?
Summary ☐	It sounds as if you have had a difficult few years but there are things you are good at: you have gained GCSEs and have, in your words, calmed down. But recent changes have been stressful. Finishing school, being discharged from CAMHS and thinking about what your mum said about finding work and moving out has made you anxious. You have been spending more time alone. You would like to find a girlfriend and feel this would make you happy.
Impression ☐	You are going through a difficult time of change. You mentioned you have autism.
Experience ☐	What do you know about autism? What do you mean by not good at school?
Explanation ☐	Recent changes in your life have put all of the challenges of having autism together: having to speak to new people, having to think about finding work when you don't find it easy learning new skills and having to make changes in your life, like finding work with the aim of becoming independent.
Empathy ☐	Often people feel angry when they are hurt and upset. Your mum has encouraged you to make changes and this is particularly difficult and worrying for you. I can understand why you feel upset and stressed. Have you spoken to your mum about this? I suspect she wants you to have a fulfilling life, and finding work and your own place in the world can help with this.
Options ☐	There is an organisation called Restore for people just like you who find adapting to work hard. They help build your confidence with areas you are good at. You could tell them you prefer not to work in groups and you are good with your hands. Would you be interested in this? I wonder: how about I give you a work note for the next month, in the short term, and meanwhile we work together to help to achieve your goals of meeting someone and using your current skills in an environment where you are comfortable? You could speak to the Job Centre about your skills and hopes for the future to see what they can suggest too.
Future ☐	Does this sound okay? Shall we meet again in a month? In the meantime, could you call Restore to see how they may be able to help you? You could also contact MIND who may point you in the direction of small social events – you may be able to meet a girlfriend.
Safety net ☐	Please come and see a doctor if your anger increases or you are very upset.

Intellectual Disability – 3

Patient's Story

Autism and Transition Process

Doctor's notes Justin Walton, 17 years.

PMH: Autistic Spectrum Disorder, behavioural concerns 3 years ago and lower respiratory tract infection. Medication: None. Documents: Discharged from CAMHS 2 months ago.

How to act Nervous. Your mother told you to see the doctor alone. She is in the waiting room.

PC *'The CAMHS team said I needed to start seeing you now.'*

History Your mother made the appointment following instructions from CAMHS.

You are physically well and have no current illnesses. No significant family history.

'I have autism. I have learning problems.'

You originally saw the CAMHS team 3 years ago because you were shouting a lot and you were not getting on with your mum. You remember at the time feeling very frustrated that you were struggling at school with friends and the work.

Your mood is okay. You have no thoughts of wanting to hurt yourself or others.

Social You now get on okay with your mum as you have 'calmed down', but you don't get on well with your father or younger sister. *'She is good at everything.'* There is no violence or abuse in the home or in your past. You left school 2 months ago after gaining 3 GCSEs in Technology, IT and Geography. You did not make friends easily and became happy being alone. If the doctor mentions a relationship, say you would like a girlfriend to make you happy. You think you would prefer to live with a girlfriend. This is your main aim. You are not sure where to find a girlfriend. You would like money but you don't like being around new people. However, you do feel you have skills, you are good at mending things. There is an old scrapyard near your home and you enjoy restoring broken things. Your dad lets you keep these in the garage. You think you could do a paper-round on your bike.

ICE You would like a work note. Your mum has said you can live there for 2 more years but thinks you should start earning your own money and then find a place to live. This has made you feel angry and is always on your mind. Since she said this you stay in your room. The thought of going to work is making you feel very 'angry' (stressed) and you think your family will force you out the house, but you struggle to verbalise how you are feeling. You expect the doctor will give you a work note. If the doctor makes other suggestions, follow his or her advice if explained well and if the doctor is supportive. However, you push for a work note if he or she has not explored your skills or do not understand your situation.

You know that *'Autism is where you are not good at school.'* If asked to expand, you mean *'not got lots of friends, not clever, don't notice how people feel which can make them angry'*.

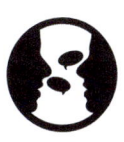

Intellectual Disability – 3

Learning Points — Autism and Transition Processes Model

'Understand the need to support adolescents with intellectual disability as they become adults and no longer have the multidisciplinary support.'[1]

'*Transitions occur throughout life … from childhood through puberty and adolescence to adulthood; from immaturity to maturity and from dependence to independence … extra transitions as a result of other life events for example, bereavement, separation of parents, and being placed in care.*'[2,3]

Complete CSA's Transition Processes Model – grouped into the elements below. First, a few tips …

1. You are not expected to complete the whole model in 10 minutes! If, however, you spend time practising, you are more likely to be able to ask the questions in the CSA exam that demonstrate your ability to practise holistically.
2. Keep the questions in a logical order. Even better … signpost! *'I'm interested to hear about changes at school … now questions about what you can do for yourself'* … An excellent way to feel and appear organised.
3. You can also signpost the elements you would like to discuss in a further consultation.

General health	What is their perception of their current health? How could they improve their health?
Health checks	Dental checks, breast awareness, smears or testicular checks.
Physical health	Any current issues? Any ongoing management required? Health awareness?
Mental health	Do they suffer with anxiety, depression or any mental illness?
Life changes	Have they had a change in environment: school, job or home? How did they cope?
Emotional adaptations	How do they feel about the change: Excited? Scared? Isolated?
Challenges	What has been difficult or upsetting? Changes, stress or bereavements?
Strengths	Have they developed skills and strengths? Are they proud of their achievements?
Achievements	Finishing school, leaving home, finding a job, getting married and parenting.
School changes	Are they managing the workload? Future plans? How is the interaction with friends?
Independence	What do they do alone? What do they rely on others for?
Levels of responsibility	What are they currently responsible for? How do they manage this? Current stress?
Logistical challenges	How do they manage money and legal obligations?
Relationships	How are relationships with parents, siblings, friends, sexual partners?
Sexual health	Experiences, contraception and infection prevention? Are they considering a family?
Personal care	Hygiene, managing periods, toileting and cooking?
Ethnic background	Is their religion/background important to them at their current life stage?
'Perception of risk'[2]	Risk of abuse: what is their experience of risk? When are they most at risk? How do they reduce risk? Risk of neglect? Is there vulnerability to exploitation? Social setting: alcohol and drug use? Avoiding dangerous situations.
Needs	What is causing them worry? What are their hopes? What do they need?
Transition services	GPs have a role in providing additional support and bridging the transition between child to adult social services (through a Connexions worker) and health services.

Demonstrate you are being proactive by:
1. Understanding who is currently involved in the patient's care.
2. Offering to liaise with the current/new teams.
3. Providing follow up and an ongoing point of contact.

Intellectual Disability – 3

Doctor's Notes

Patient	Janine Paton 33 years F
PMH	Cerebral Palsy
	Severe Learning Disability
	Constipation
	Urinary Tract Infections
	Epilepsy – no seizure for 2 years
Medications	Laxido, sodium valproate and carbamazepine
Allergies	No known drug allergies
Consultations	No recent consultations
Investigations	No recent investigations
Household	No household members registered

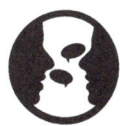

Example Consultation

Mental Health and ID

Open ☐ — Hello Janine, I'm Dr Blount. It is a pleasure to meet you. Who have you brought with you today? (looking to the carer). Can you tell me why you have come to see me today? Let's ask Ruth. Oh dear, what have you noticed? Anything else that has changed? Or changes in behaviour? Or communication? I'm wondering what Janine is like when she is feeling herself?

Curious ☐ — Do you use any special ways of communicating?

History ☐ — Janine, are you in pain? Does it hurt when you wee? Or in your tummy? Have you been for a poo today? Ruth, have her bowels been normal? How often is Janine opening her bowels? Have either of you noticed a change in going to the toilet? A smell or going more frequently?

Flags ☐ — I'm wondering whether you have lost weight Janine? Ruth – how much, do you think? Over how long? Has Janine had a temperature? May I see Janine alone for a moment? Janine – do you like Ruth? Is anyone who lives or works at the home making you feel sad or upset? Thank you. Let's bring Janine back into the room.

ICE ☐ — Ruth, what do you think may be causing Janine to not feel herself? You have mentioned pain; have you had any other thoughts? Is there anything you are worried may be going on? What did you expect we may arrange or decide today?

Sense ☐ — Janine, I am wondering if you are normally a quiet person like today or if you are normally smiling and chatty. Ruth, what would you say? Janine, are you feeling happy or sad? Okay, if I draw a picture of a smiling face and a sad face, can you tell me if you are this one … or this one? I'm sorry you are feeling sad.

Summary ☐ — To summarise what we have said so far: Janine, your carers have been worried about you. You have not had the same energy, you have stayed in your room and not been interested in what you usually enjoy. You tell me you are not in pain but it is not clear what may be wrong. You are feeling sad.

O/E ☐ — Janine, may I listen to your chest, feel your tummy, take your blood pressure and temperature and have a look at your throat, ears and neck please? I will also test your wee. I would like to weigh you please. Can we look at all your joints – arms and legs?

Impression ☐ — I am not sure what is going on. I agree we should do so some tests. It seems you are feeling sad at the moment. It could be that there is a physical problem causing you to change or it could be a mental health problem like depression. We will talk about how to help you feel happier, but I need to make sure this is not because you are feeling unwell.

Empathy ☐ — It must be very hard, Janine, when you don't feel yourself but we will try to find out why.

Options ☐ — I would like to arrange a blood test. Janine, I will arrange for the teams specialising in seeing patients who, like you, need more time, to perform eye and dental checks. This is to check that it isn't pain from your teeth, or problems with seeing clearly, that are making you feel like this.

Empower ☐ — Janine, you can help us in the meantime. Each day, can you tell Ruth or another carer if you are this face or this face? Also, if Ruth points to different parts of your body can you clap your hands if that part doesn't feel okay? For example, if you had a headache and I pointed to your head what would you do?

Future ☐ — So we will arrange a few blood tests to look at your blood count, liver, kidney and thyroid, and ask specialists to check your mouth and eyes. I will send your wee sample to the lab to check for any infection. Shall we catch up again in 3–4 weeks to review the blood tests and see how you are? I will also ask a nurse from the learning disability team to see you at home.

Safety net ☐ — Ruth, please let me know if you do not receive an appointment in the next 4 weeks to see the specialists. If any new symptoms develop or Janine seems worse, please let me know.

Patient's Story

Mental Health and ID

Doctor's notes — Janine Paton, 33 years.

PMH: Cerebral Palsy, Severe LD, Constipation, UTIs and Epilepsy – no seizure for 2 years. Medications: Laxido, sodium valproate and carbamazepine.

How to act — Attends with carer, Ruth, who does all the talking.

Janine looks at the floor unless spoken to and only says yes/no to some questions but not all.

PC — *'We are worried something is wrong. We don't know if she is in pain.'*

History — She usually enjoys sitting in the lounge and watching television shows. Janine also likes it when the music is on. However, over the past 2 months, she has not looked interested and stays in her room. She seems 'weaker' because she has not got the same energy. She does not cry but sometimes makes a wailing sound. You are not sure if this is because she is in pain.

Her urine does not smell abnormal. She is not vomiting. She has required more encouragement to eat her food and she often leaves a lot of it. She has lost some weight over the month. Janine is opening her bowels once daily with Laxido. No rectal bleeding.

Janine has regular periods, the last one being 2 weeks ago. They are not heavy.

Janine does not repeatedly touch her head or ears. She has not had a cough, cold or fever. Janine does not walk and transfers with the help of 2 carers between the bed and wheelchair. The carers have no information on Janine's family.

Social — Janine lives in a home with several other residents cared for by the staff.

ICE — Ruth is worried it may be another water infection.

Ruth also wants to check that there is no abnormality in the stomach causing pain and loss of appetite. Ruth expects she will be given more antibiotics but would like her to have a scan.

Janine only says 'no' when asked about pain. Janine cannot answer about her mood. However, if the doctor asks how best to communicate with Janine, she likes pictures and can respond to pictures with yes or no. Pictures usually used include food, the weather and faces. Janine also likes to clap as another way of saying yes.

O/E — Janine has lost 4 kg in weight since she was last weighed 6 months ago.

HS normal, chest clear, abdomen soft, non-tender, no masses and there is no swelling in any joint. Janine is moving all joints without pain. No lymphadenopathy. ENT normal.

Ruth has brought a sample of urine. Urine dipstick is negative.

Observations are normal.

Intellectual Disability – 4

Learning Points

Mental Health and ID

In 'Valuing People' (2001) a 'learning disability (LD)' is described as a: 'significantly reduced ability to understand new or complex information, to learn new skills, reduced ability to cope independently, which starts before adulthood with lasting effects on development.'[1]

Other suggestions/tips to demonstrate the RCGP curriculum …

'Understand the psychiatric disorders prevalent in the adult with intellectual disability and how their diagnosis, detection and management differ …'[2]

The patient may struggle to express or verbalise their emotions. Helpful questions to consider:
- Has there been a change in behaviour?
- Do they feel angry?
- Are there any changes to their routine – sleep or eating?
- Is there concern among family members?
- Can a collateral history be obtained?

'Psychiatric and physical illness may present atypically in patients with intellectual disability. … Understand the need to use additional enquiry, appropriate tests and careful examination in patients unable to describe or verbalise symptoms.'[2] Use language without jargon, seek a collateral history; however, also screen for risk of neglect and this includes seeing the patient alone.

Have a low threshold for suspicion of mental health problems and be *proactive* to enquire about subtle changes and atypical presentations.

'Be aware of residential situations and daytime activities available locally to adults with intellectual disability, including those provided by the voluntary sector.'[2] Demonstrate your awareness of this by signposting where the patient can go to seek more information.

'Demonstrate the necessary skills to conduct a physical and mental state assessment in a patient with LD with regard to the higher prevalence of some problems, such as respiratory conditions and epilepsy.'[2] Tailor the examination to the condition and life stage. A complete assessment should also be performed in the annual health check.

'Be aware of the atypical presentation of acute and chronic physical and psychiatric disorders.'[2] Use open screening questions for physical and mental health problems and social challenges. Have vigilance and a low level of suspicion for atypical presentations of conditions.

'Be aware of the additional skills of diagnosis and examination needed in patients unable to describe or verbalise symptoms and where to obtain specialist advice and help.'[2] Signpost that, following your initial thorough examination and once you have received investigation results, you may consider involving the Learning Disability Team.

'Understand the impact of intellectual disability on family dynamics and the implications for physical, psychological and social morbidity in the patient's carers.'[2] Always ask about those who support or care for the patient. How are the relationships? Ask about the carer's health and concerns.

Doctor's Notes

Patient	Lilly Young	24 years	F
PMH	Moderate learning disability		
	Constipation		
	Recurrent urinary tract infections		
Medications	No current medications		
Allergies	No known drug allergies		
Consultations	No recent consultations		
Investigations	No recent investigations		
Household	Nil recorded		

Example Consultation   COCP Request

Open ☐	Okay. Why would you like to go on the pill? Do you have a boyfriend? How do you know Karl?
Sense ☐	It sounds like you are quite excited about this relationship. Would you like to have sex?
Experience ☐	What do you know about how to have sex? Do you know anything about infections you can catch through sex? What do you know about the pill?
Curious ☐	Do you want to take the pill? What do you think about having a baby?
History ☐	I see you used to have problems going to the toilet; can you tell me more about that? Are you well now, or not? When was your last period? What are your periods like? Do you have bad headaches? Do you take medicines? Has your mum or your grandparents ever had a health problem? Do you have a dad? Who do you live with? Do you have a job? Do you have a hobby? Who does Karl live with?
Flags ☐	Is Karl making you have sex? Does he ever hurt or upset you? Have you had sex?
ICE ☐	Do you know any other ways to stop you from getting pregnant? Do you know how you can avoid getting infections? Is there anything you are worried about? What would you like to take away with you today? Would you remember to take a tablet every day?
Curious ☐	Have you talked to anyone about having sex? What does Julie say? Did she say anything else? Would you like to ask me any questions? Do you get on well with your mum? Can you talk to her about having sex? What does she say? Did she say anything else? Might you have sex before your birthday?
O/E ☐	May I check your blood pressure Lilly? I would need to put this around your arm and it will swell up like a balloon and feel tight for a minute – is that okay? Can I ask you to step onto the scales please? Thank you.
Impression ☐	Lilly, you would like to have sex and you have decided not to have a baby yet.
Summary ☐	You don't think you will remember a tablet. You don't like having periods. You have decided to talk to your mum again before you decide. You feel excited but Julie has said sex hurts and this worries you.
Explanation ☐	You should only have sex if you want to. You can always say no. Sex should not hurt.
Safety net ☐	If it did hurt, you should tell Karl and tell a doctor too. Do you think you could do this?
Options ☐	The pill is a tablet to stop you having a baby. If you don't think you can remember it every day, there are other options too – an injection every three months or a little stick under the arm which is just one injection and lasts three years. What do you think? Okay, there is also a special plaster that you can put on your arm. You leave it there for a week and change it after every week. What do you think to that idea? Do you think your mum would help you with it? The plaster has a medicine inside which goes into your skin. This medicine can make some people very unwell, the risk is small but you would have to remember that if ever your leg hurt or got bigger one day, or if you had a bad headache, you must let a doctor know straight away. This can be a sign that something is wrong. Could you remember this? Would you like to try this plaster? The real name for the plaster is the patch. Do you have any questions?
Empower ☐	After having sex, go to the toilet to have a wee. This stops those wee infections returning. Have you heard of condoms, Lilly? Condoms are important to stop any bugs or infections from Karl going to you. They also help prevent pregnancy too.
Empathy ☐	It is a lot to remember, so are you happy to talk it through with your mum first? I will give you leaflets about the pill, the patch and the implant so you can talk about the choices with your mum.
Future ☐	Will you see me next week with your mum? Next time we can also talk about ladies' check-ups.
Safety net ☐	Can you remember where in the body you may have pain if the patch is causing you harm?

Intellectual Disability – 5

Patient's Story

COCP Request

Doctor's notes Lilly Young, 24 years.

PMH: Moderate learning disability. Recurrent urinary tract infections. Medications: None.

How to act You respond well if the doctor uses language which is easy to follow.

PC *'I have come for the pill.'*

History *'My mum told me I had to, otherwise I can't go camping.'*

Mum is collecting you after going to Asda.

You have known Karl, who is the same age as you, for many years.

You were in the same class at Rose Hill Special School. *'Karl is like me.'*

Karl asked you to the cinema a month ago. Now you see each other every evening.

Karl lives with his parents and younger sister. They are all family friends.

He wants to take you camping for your 25th birthday.

You've not had sex but would like to when you go camping (not before).

Karl says you will only have sex if you want to.

You are well. No contraindications to the pill. You have light periods 3/28.

No IMB.

'I don't like periods.'

'Going for a poo and wee is okay now.' You take no medicines.

Your mum has told you the doctor will want to know if there are any problems in the family and there are none. If the doctor wants to know what your mum thinks, say your mum said you will talk about what the doctor says at home. You forget this if the doctor does not ask.

Social You live with your mum. You do not know your dad. You have a friend, Julie.

You like going to the cinema and going out to eat pizza. You do not drink or smoke.

You work in the local garden centre café serving the tea and coffee.

ICE *'We talked about sex in class.'*

You don't know anything about the pill or any other contraception.

You are vaguely aware that you can become ill from having sex, i.e. STIs.

Your mum is happy for you to have sex; you have talked about it but promised her you would take the pill. You hate having periods.

You don't think you will remember a tablet every day.

You feel *'scared but excited'*. Julie has had sex and tells you sex hurts.

You don't want any procedure or needles. You would like a baby. But your mum told you not yet. Your mum said she would have to help you look after a baby and she can't do this until she retires.

Examination BP 110/60. BMI 23.

Intellectual Disability – 5

Learning Points

COCP Request

Risk factors for safeguarding concerns:
Dependence on others: learning or physical disability.

Lack of family support/confidantes.

Social isolation.

At risk of neglect.

Partner dominance/unequal relationships.

The impact of multiple negative events.

How do we pick up on risk?
Sensing: behavioural changes, low mood, annual reviews, MDT, awareness of DNAs or the opposite – multiple attendances. Building the relationship.

How to demonstrate the RCGP curriculum, which includes:
'Understand the emotional and sexual needs of adults with intellectual disability and how they can be expressed.'[1]

You can demonstrate this by respecting the patient's request and providing education, an opportunity to ask questions and choices. Do not make assumptions but check their understanding. Support them by offering safe options and helping the patient to consider different scenarios which may guide them to a decision they feel comfortable with.

The common pitfall with this consultation may be forgetting the routine medical checks, e.g. common contraindications, missed pill rules and safety netting advice. Do not avoid this conversation but instead adjust your language to ensure the patient understands and to allow him/her to reach an informed decision.

'Understand how health promotion can be overlooked in the care of patients with intellectual disability and the importance of tailoring health promotion to the needs of this special group particularly with regard to the difficulties of routine screening, such as cervical cytology, mammography, abdominal aortic aneurysm and bowel cancer screening.'[1]

Always remember to 'Empower' the patient and take every opportunity to provide health promotion advice: in this case UTI prevention, STI prevention and signposting the discussion about cervical screening.

Find out if your area has an Intellectual/Learning Disability team or specialist nurse you can ask for advice. These teams/nurses should have awareness of local services available and may be able to help with capacity assessments and challenging behaviour. They can often support patients and provide advice to practices about improving access for those with ID. Sometimes they can also provide tips on encouraging patients to attend for blood tests etc.

Intellectual Disability – 5

CHAPTER 14 OVERVIEW
Cardiovascular Health

	Cases in this chapter	Within the RCGP curriculum: Cardiovascular Health RCGP Curriculum Online March 2016[1]	Learning points in the chapter include:
1	Antiplatelets	'Identify your patient's health beliefs regarding cardiovascular problems and either reinforce, modify or challenge these beliefs as appropriate' 'Communicate the patient's risk of cardiovascular problems clearly and effectively in a non-biased manner'	Indications for aspirin Initiating aspirin PPI cover Dyspepsia and antiplatelets Clopidogrel
2	Atrial Fibrillation	'Manage primary contact with patients who have a cardiovascular problem' 'Be able to manage cardiovascular conditions'	NICE Guidance CG180. Atrial fibrillation: management. June 2014
3	Angina	'Demonstrate an understanding of the importance of risk factors, including chronic kidney disease, in the diagnosis and management of cardiovascular problems'	NICE Guidance CG126. Stable angina: management. July 2011
4	Heart Failure	'Demonstrate a reasoned approach to the diagnosis of cardiovascular symptoms (e.g. chest pain) using history, examination, incremental investigations and referral'	NICE Guidance CG187. Heart failure: diagnoses and management. October 2014
5	Hypertension	'Consider involving the patient in self-monitoring and self-management' 'Advise your patients appropriately regarding lifestyle interventions'	NICE Guidance CG127. Hypertension: diagnosis and management. August 2011
	Extra Notes AF and NOACs		CHA_2DS_2-VASc HAS-BLED NOACs

1. http://www.rcgp.org.uk/training-exams/gp-curriculum-overview/online-curriculum/applying-clinical-knowledge-section-1/3-12-cardiovascular-health.aspx

CHAPTER 14 REFERENCES

Antiplatelets
1. NICE Guidelines. CG126. Stable angina: management. Jul 2011.
2. NICE. http://cks.nice.org.uk/antiplatelet-treatment#!scenario. Revised Oct 2015
3. NICE. http://cks.nice.org.uk/stroke-and-tia#!scenariorecommendation:3. Revised Dec 2013.

Atrial Fibrillation
1. NICE Guidelines. CG180. Atrial fibrillation: management. Jun 2014.
2. http://patient.info/doctor/atrial-fibrillation-pro
3. http://www.mdcalc.com/has-bled-score-for-major-bleeding-risk/
4. NICE. http://cks.nice.org.uk/atrial-fibrillation#!scenario. Revised Oct 2015.

Angina
1. NICE Guidelines. CG126. Stable angina: management. Jul 2011.
2. http://patient.info/doctor/stable-angina-pro
3. NICE Guidelines. CG94. Unstable angina and NSTEMI: early management. Mar 2010.
4. Bosch J., et al. Long-term effects of ramipril on cardiovascular events and on diabetes: results of the HOPE study extension. *Circulation.* 2005 Aug 30; 112(9): 1339–40.

Heart Failure
1. NICE Guidelines. CG187. Acute heart failure – diagnoses and management. Oct 2014.
2. NICE Guidelines. CG108. Chronic heart failure in adults: management. Aug 2010.

Hypertension
1. NICE Guidelines. CG127. Hypertension: diagnosis and management. Aug 2011.
2. NICE Guidelines. NG28 Type 2 Diabetes in adults: management. Dec 2015.
3. NICE Guidelines. CG 182. Chronic kidney disease in adults: assessment and management. Updated 2015.
4. Beckett N., Peters R., et al. Treatment of hypertension in patients 80 years of age or older. *N Engl J Med.* 2008; 358: 1887–98.
5. He F.J., Li J., MacGregor G. Effect of longer term modest salt reduction on blood pressure. Cochrane systematic review and meta analysis of randomised trials. *BMJ.* 2013; 346: f1325.

AF and NOACs
1. http://www.chadsvasc.org/
2. NICE. http://cks.nice.org.uk/atrial-fibrillation#!scenario. Revised Oct 2015.
3. NICE Guidelines. CG180. Atrial fibrillation: management. Jun 2014.
4. Connolly S., Yusuf S., Camm J., et al. ACTIVE W. *Lancet.* 2006; 367: 1903–12.

Doctor's Notes

Patient	Hilda Fisher	52 years	F
PMH	Hypertension, Smoker 20/day		
Medications	Ramipril 2.5 mg		
	Omeprazole 20 mg		
Allergies	No information		
Consultations	BP 130/72 – 2 months ago with the nurse		
Investigations	No information		
Household	Jack Fisher	53 years	M

Example Consultation — Antiplatelets

Open ☐	Mrs Fisher, it's a good question. Let's work out if aspirin is right for you.
Experience ☐	Please tell me more about what you have read.
ICE ☐	Is developing cancer a worry that you think about often? Do you have any other worries that keep creeping into your mind? Is there anything else you were hoping we would do today?
Sense ☐	I sense you feel strongly about starting aspirin.
Curious ☐	What is your experience of cancer? I am sorry, that must have been a shock. How is she?
Impact ☐	In what way has your sister-in-law's diagnosis changed you?
History ☐	Can you tell me in your own words about any medical conditions you have had in the past please? Tell me about the tablets you take. Have you taken any aspirin? I'm interested to know more about you.
Risk ☐	Do you have any other family members who have suffered with cancer? Have there been any heart problems or strokes in the family? Do you smoke?
Flags ☐	How is your stomach? What do you think may be making it worse at present?
Summary ☐	So to summarise what we have discussed so far, as research has found that aspirin can protect against colon cancer, as well as protecting the vessels, you feel that starting aspirin is right for you. Your sister-in-law has recently been diagnosed with colon cancer. You have no blood relatives who have had cancer. You have high blood pressure and also need your omeprazole. Have I understood you correctly?
Empathy ☐	Hearing your sister-in-law's history, I now understand your concerns and I appreciate that we should try to minimise your risk.
Impression ☐	I can help by providing you with the information you need to help you make a decision.
Explanation ☐	Some studies have found that taking aspirin does seem to prevent some cancers. However, there is uncertainty about the dose and number of years that makes the greatest difference. From a heart disease perspective, the evidence for aspirin is inconclusive. It may reduce the risk of heart disease and stroke but there is a significantly increased risk of bleeding from the stomach which seems to outweigh these benefits. For this reason, we now tend to reserve aspirin for those who, like your husband, have heart or blood vessel disease, i.e. where the benefit has been proven. In your case, due to your previous gastritis, your risk of bleeding may outweigh the potential benefits. What are your thoughts now?
Options ☐	We should do everything we can to reduce the risk to your vessels; monitoring your BP, cholesterol and sugar. The best thing you can do to reduce your risk of cancer and heart disease is stop smoking. I would be happy to refer you to our smoking cessation clinic if you would like.
Empower ☐	I will send you further information from a reliable source. You can buy aspirin fairly cheaply from the chemist if you decide to take it. Remember that coffee adversely affects both the stomach and sleep.
Future ☐	Please will you make an appointment for a blood test, then a further discussion with a GP?
Safety net ☐	If you do decide to start aspirin, let the doctor know straight away if you experience any stomach problems, pain or your stools appear black as this could be a sign of bleeding from the stomach.

This case tests your knowledge of emerging evidence and your ability to discuss uncertainty with patients. Keep a lookout for topical health issues which patients may ask you about.

Cardiovascular Health – 1

Patient's Story

Antiplatelets

Doctor's notes — Mrs Hilda Fisher, 52 years. PMH: Hypertension and gastritis. An endoscopy showed gastritis 2 years ago. Medications: Ramipril 2.5 mg and Omeprazole 20 mg. Smoker 20/day.

How to act — Demanding at first.

PC — *'I was just wondering if I could have a prescription for aspirin. I've been reading the paper and it said an aspirin a day will stop me getting cancer and, of course, there is also the benefit of preventing heart attacks. My husband has been taking aspirin for years, ever since his heart attack.'*

History
- Hypertension for which you take ramipril.
- Reflux and you can't cope without omeprazole.
- An endoscopy showed gastritis only.
- No change in bowels, bleeding or melaena.
- Your stomach has flared up again recently.
- No cardiovascular symptoms.
- You have no family history.

Social — You live with your husband. You are a teacher. You smoke 20 a day.

ICE
- The paper said aspirin may reduce cancers.
- You are also aware it can reduce your risk of heart disease.
- Your sister-in-law was recently diagnosed with colon cancer.
- You feel the doctor is just trying to save the NHS money. You are aware it would be expensive to give everyone 'free aspirin'.
- You drink a lot of coffee as you have not been sleeping since your sister-in-law's diagnosis.

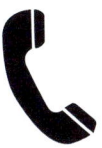

Cardiovascular Health – 1

Learning Points   Antiplatelets

Indications for aspirin (75 mg daily)

Secondary prevention
IHD – secondary prevention[1,2]
2nd line for TIA (off-label use)[3]
    if intolerant of clopidogrel[2]
    in combination with dipyridamole[2]
    unless requiring anticoagulation for AF
Post stent – follow cardiology advice as it depends on the stent

Primary prevention
Off licence and evidence limited ... some specialists recommend aspirin if:
HTN + >50 years + CV risk >20%[2]
    (150/90 – but wait until BP is treated and below this)
HTN + eGFR <45 ml/min/1.73 m^2

Initiating aspirin
Control BP to <150/90 before starting antiplatelets[2]
However, if CVD risk is high consider risk/benefit
Discuss risk/benefit and evidence with the patient[2]
Review medications*, avoid NSAID, alcohol and smoking cessation advice[2]

PPI cover
High-dose aspirin[2] 'Do not prescribe enteric coated aspirin'[2,4]
Elderly (no age stated)[2]
History of ulcer/bleed/perforation[2]
Serious comorbidity (CV, renal, hepatic, DM or HTN)[2]
H. pylori infection[2]
Medication interactions/with an increased risk of bleeding:
*SSRIs, warfarin, steroid, NSAIDs and nicorandil and see full list[2,3]

Dyspepsia and antiplatelet
If red flags then urgent endoscopy[2]
    Seek advice before stopping antiplatelet if high risk of CVD
No red flags
    Co-prescribe an antacid/PPI[2]
    Screen *H. pylori*[2]

If dyspepsia persists despite PPI
Consider clopidogrel instead[2]
Consider an endoscopy as per upper GI guidance
Check haemoglobin for bleeding.

Duration of dual antiplatelet therapy following myocardial infarction will be determined by the discharge team. This may include ticagrelor, prasugrel or clopidogrel in addition to aspirin. Do not stop early without discussion with the specialists.

Cardiovascular Health – 1

Doctor's Notes

Patient	Elizabeth Alderton 65 years F
PMH	Hypertension
Medications	Amlodipine 5 mg
Allergies	No information
Consultations	The nurse has added Elizabeth to your list after a routine ECG for HTN.
Investigations	Blood pressure today 128/72. Recent blood tests normal (U&E, glucose, cholesterol).
Household	Patrick Alderton 67 years M

The ECG shows atrial fibrillation – rate 82 bpm.

Example Consultation — Atrial Fibrillation

Open — Thank you for waiting to see me. Your ECG has found that the rhythm of your heart is irregular.

Impression — This is called atrial fibrillation or AF for short. Your blood pressure may have been a trigger.

Experience — Have you come across atrial fibrillation?

Explanation — Within the heart, an electrical current makes your heart muscles pump. In AF the electrical current is disorganised. Atria, the two muscles at the top of the heart, are where the electrical current starts. As the current is no longer regular this makes the atria fibrillate, which means twitch, and in turn makes the heart beat irregular. You can feel unwell especially if the heart beats fast. AF can also cause complications so we need to manage it.

Sense — I can see this is unexpected news and that you are keen to know what needs to be done. But, in order to make the right decisions for you, can we start at the beginning; take your history, examine you and then make a plan?

Flags — Have you had any pain? Any dizziness? Any breathlessness? Any episodes of losing consciousness? Any changes to your vision? Have you had an episode where your arms or legs felt different or weak?

Risk — How much alcohol and caffeine do you drink? Any recent illness, fever, cough or weight loss?

History — Does amlodipine suit you? Any other tablets? Ibuprofen? Tell me more about you.

O/E — Please may I examine your heart and lungs and take your blood pressure?

Summary — So, to summarise, a routine ECG for HTN has detected AF. You had no symptoms.

Options — The treatment for AF is in two stages. Firstly, a tablet to slow down the heart rate if needed. Your resting rate is normal but we need to get a 24-hour tracing to see if it increases when you walk around. If it does, we need to slow it down with a tablet. Secondly, we need to discuss whether to make your blood less likely to clot. In AF, blood clots can form which can shoot off to the brain to cause a stroke. As high blood pressure also increases stroke risk, I recommend a tablet to reduce clotting. Have you come across warfarin?

Curious — What was your uncle's experience of warfarin? Any questions so far?

Options — Aspirin is no longer recommended as it does not work well; the stroke risk remains high. Any blood thinner increases the risk of bleeding from the stomach, brain, or nose. However, apart from your BP which is controlled, you are well and may feel that the benefits of preventing a stroke outweigh the risks. Warfarin is a drug we know well, including the antidote should you bleed. The downsides are that regular blood tests are needed. There is another option. Apixaban is a relatively new drug. Antidotes are being made. It may be more protective against strokes but only if you remember to take this pill regularly. Compared with warfarin, it is more risky if you forget it. There are no blood tests required with apixaban. This is a lot of information. What are your thoughts?

Empathy — It sounds as if you prefer a plan that doesn't interfere with your lifestyle ... understandable!

Future — So shall we try apixaban? It is taken twice a day. If you experience any persistent nausea with this tablet, let me know. If we find we need to slow the heart, we could consider swapping your amlodipine to diltiazem, a cousin tablet of amlodipine, which slows the heart rate and may continue to control your BP. Or we could introduce a beta-blocker, which slows the heart, in addition to the amlodipine which is already working well for you. Can I clarify anything for you?

Empower — Other things that you can do include decreasing caffeine and alcohol intake.

Safety net — The apixaban is very protective, but I must still advise you as follows. If you ever notice your vision changes or arms or legs feel different or weak, you must call an ambulance as these may be signs of a stroke. If you ever feel lightheaded, breathless or have pain in the chest, this may be because of a fast irregular rhythm so see a doctor straight away.

Patient's Story

Atrial Fibrillation

Doctor's notes	Elizabeth Alderton, 65 years. PMH: Hypertension. Medication: Amlodipine 5 mg. Blood pressure today 128/72 and a routine ECG.
How to act	Very pleasant.
PC	*'I had an ECG with the nurse and he said I had to wait to see you. Is something wrong?'*
History	After a series of home BP readings you were recently diagnosed with HTN.
	You were told to get an ECG but you have been on holiday.
	You feel very well and are very active.
	You have had no symptoms.
	Your father suffered with high blood pressure but you have no other FH.
	You feel well on the amlodipine 5 mg.
Social	You are a librarian. You live with your husband and you have two dogs.
	You walk the dogs daily and enjoy swimming.
	You have never smoked and you drink 14 units of alcohol a week.
	You enjoy coffee.
	You often go on holiday.
ICE	After being informed you have AF you are keen to know the plan.
	'What does that mean … is it dangerous?' Then *'So what needs to happen?'*
	You have never heard of atrial fibrillation.
	If the doctor talks about warfarin, say: *'My uncle was on it. You need blood tests. Can't I take aspirin?'*
	Your uncle had lots of nose bleeds where his nose would need packing.
	You will not take warfarin under any circumstances due to the blood tests.
	You hate needles and have another holiday planned.
	Once aware of the risks/benefits of a NOAC, this is your preferred option.
Examination	HS normal HR 80 bpm irregular. Chest clear. BP 120/70.

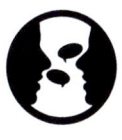

Learning Points — Atrial Fibrillation

Cause[1,2]
- Idiopathic.
- Heart: hypertension, ischaemia, valve disease and other cardiac conditions.
- Metabolic: hyperthyroid or diabetes.
- Acute changes: Infection or electrolyte imbalance.
- Respiratory: PE or lung cancer.
- Drug/food: alcohol, caffeine, salbutamol or thyroxine.

Correct any underlying cause then manage the heart rate or rhythm.

Symptoms — Asymptomatic, SOB, palpitations, syncope, dizziness, chest pain, stroke, TIA.

Complications — Stroke, TIA, heart failure, cardiomyopathy or ischaemia.

Investigations[1]
- ECG to make the diagnosis and for possible signs of old ischaemia.
- Check FBC, TSH and electrolytes for reversible causes.
- U&E and LFT are needed for the HAS-BLED[3] score and medication choice.
- CXR if a lung cause suspected.
- 24-hour tape if daily palpitations or event recorder if infrequent palpitations.

Echocardiogram — If concern of underlying structural disease (murmur) or functional heart disease – which influences medication.[1,4]

AF can be managed in primary care but see reasons for referral below*

Rate control[1] — Beta blocker (bisoprolol) if not contraindicated.
(Do not prescribe sotalol in primary care due to risks.)

OR — Rate-limiting calcium channel blocker (diltiazem) if not contraindicated.
If still not effective may add digoxin to either of above.

OR — Digoxin monotherapy for non-paroxysmal AF only if they are sedentary.[1]

***Consider referral to cardiology**:
- Symptoms continue after the heart rate has been controlled.[1]
- New onset AF with heart failure or 2° to reversible causes.[4]
- For possible amiodarone or catheter ablation if heart failure present.[1]
- For cardioversion following 3 weeks' anticoagulation unless there is good evidence to suggest this is a new AF within <48 hours.
- Amiodarone may be prescribed (by specialist) prior to DC cardioversion.[1]
- Lone AF and in the young.

Left atrial appendage occlusion may be considered by specialists if anticoagulation is CI or not tolerated or there is a high bleed risk.[1]

Acute admission to the medics

Unwell/unstable — E.g. HR >150, SBP <90 mmHg, LOC, chest pain, increasing SOB, dizziness.[4]
Use clinical judgement.

See Extra Notes at the end of this chapter for CHA_2DS_2-VASc and HAS-BLED score and NOACs.

Cardiovascular Health – 2

Doctor's Notes

Patient   Hibiki Hayashi   75 years   M
PMH   Hypertension
Medications Ramipril 5 mg
                 Bendroflumethiazide 2.5 mg
Allergies   NKDA
Consultations
Investigations Last BP 132/78 (1 month ago)
Household   No household members registered

Example Consultation — Angina

Open ☐	Tell me about this pain, perhaps from when it first began.
History ☐	How frequently does it happen? Have you noticed anything that brings it on? What takes it away? Do you have any other symptoms with the pain?
Flags ☐	Have you had a pain that has lasted more than 10 minutes? Do you have pain when you are sitting or lying down? Is this pain becoming more frequent?
Risk ☐	Apart from HTN, do you have any other medical problems? Has anyone in your family had heart problems or a stroke? Do you smoke? Do you get any pain in the lower legs when you are walking?
Sense ☐	You seem very quiet … Are you very worried?
ICE ☐	When you have had this pain, what has gone through your mind? What do you think is causing the pain? What did you think I might say we should do about this pain?
Impact ☐	Has it stopped you from doing anything?
Curious ☐	I'm sorry to hear you lost Maho and Hisae. That must have been devastating. You sound very low just now. Sometimes when people feel so low, they don't want to be alive. Do you feel like this? Have you had thoughts about ending your life?
Summary ☐	So you have also been feeling lonely and, since Maho died, you have had chest pains which you thought may be a heart attack. You thought I might say you need an operation, but you don't want this. Is that right?
O/E ☐	May I have a listen to your heart, feel your pulse and take your blood pressure?
Empathy ☐	The past two years have been life changing for you.
Impression ☐	Mr Hayashi, I think you may be suffering with angina. It is unlikely that you have had a heart attack. If pain goes away when you stop, this is called angina. Angina and depression are very common together, as angina can affect a person's daily life.
Experience ☐	Have you come across angina? Do you know anyone with it?
Explanation ☐	Angina is where the blood flow to the heart is not as good as it could be due to furring of the vessels – a bit like clogged drains. A heart attack is different; this is when the pipe becomes completely blocked.
Options ☐	I would like to give you a spray to use once under the tongue if you have pain. It widens the vessels to your heart. If the pain is still there after 5 minutes, take a second spray. If you feel unwell, or the pain is present 5 minutes later, call an ambulance. You may notice a headache and, if dizziness occurs, sit for a few minutes. Please also use this spray before exercise. Are you happy to try it? Please repeat back to me how and when you would use it. Are you happy to take aspirin to thin your blood to help the blood flow through the vessels? Have you had tummy ulcers as aspirin can make stomach problems worse? We should also start bisoprolol, every morning, to slow the heart and prevent pain when you are walking. If it makes you feel tired or lightheaded let me know. May I prescribe all three medications? I would like to send you to our chest pain clinic where you will be seen within a couple of weeks to confirm the diagnosis. Any concerns from what I have said? I will write it all down for you as there is a lot to remember. Yes, you can drive, unless angina happens during driving, in which case stop driving until the angina is controlled.
Empower ☐	You've mentioned getting another dog to go for walks and for company. When your angina is under control, this is an excellent idea to help both your mood and heart. Have you ever wondered about stopping smoking? We can help you with this.
Future ☐	I will book you in for a heart tracing and blood tests to check your cholesterol and sugar, then a double appointment with me next week so we can talk about your results, your angina and have a longer talk about your mood. I would like to refer you to the heart doctors who may confirm the diagnosis with an exercise test. Is that okay? Have a think about whether you might be interested in talking to someone about your loss and if information on community groups would be of interest. We'll soon get you back to feeling yourself again.
Safety net ☐	If the pain becomes more frequent or occurs at a shorter distance let a GP know immediately. If pain occurs at rest or has been present for 10 minutes, call 999.

Patient's Story

Angina

Doctor's notes	Hibiki Hayashi, 70 years. PMH: Hypertension. Medications: Ramipril 5 mg, Bendroflumethiazide 2.5 mg. NKDA. Last BP 132/78
How to act	You are subdued.
PC	*'Doctor, I keep getting these chest pains.'*
History	It started 3 months ago when you were walking to get the paper.
	Since then it has happened a few times a week, usually after about 500 yards, particularly if you are in a hurry.
	The pain makes you stop. The pain is then gone after about 2 minutes.
	You have not had pain before this distance and no rest pain.
	The pain is in the centre of your chest and feels very heavy.
	There is no radiation. There are no associated cardiac symptoms.
	You have not felt the pain after eating, only when walking.
	No claudication pain.
	You take two tablets for blood pressure. You have no FH.
Social	You live in a bungalow. You have not had pain when at home.
	You lost your wife, Hisae, 2 years ago. Since then your dog, Maho, kept you going.
	You used to walk Maho 2 miles a day but she died 4 months ago.
	You feel very lonely and low.
	You have stopped going to get the paper.
	You don't go out any more. You don't see anybody. Your son lives 2 hours away.
	You think about getting another dog. You smoke 20/day. You do not drink alcohol.
	You moved from Japan to the UK 40 years ago.
ICE	You are not worried. You think you have probably had a heart attack.
	You don't want to die and have had no thoughts about ending your life.
	But you do sometimes think it would be nice to be with Hisae and Maho.
	You expect the doctor will tell you that you need an operation. You don't want this.
	You believe angina is a small heart attack.
Ask the doctor	*'Am I allowed to drive?'*
Examination	HR 66 bpm, regular. BP 130/70. HS normal.

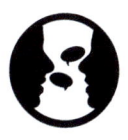

Cardiovascular Health – 3

Learning Points   Angina

NICE Guidelines. CG126. Stable angina: management. July 2011

Investigations	ECG.
	Consider CXR if lung cancer/infection possible.
	FBC for anaemia.
Referral	To confirm diagnosis – rapid access chest pain clinic.
	Re-refer if symptomatic despite medical therapy.
Classification	
Stable angina	May be **typical** (3/3) or **atypical** (2/3) of:
	Constricting pain
	Precipitated by exertion
	Relieved by rest.[1,2]
Unstable angina	Deterioration or angina at rest. Requires immediate admission.[3]
Medications in angina	GTN before exercise and during angina (unless taken Viagra).
	β-blocker or CCB.

CCB   Diltiazem is rate limiting.

However, if HF or needing to combine a CCB with either a β-blocker or ivabradine, CCB should be amlodipine, nifedipine, or felodipine.

Others: Nitrate (ISMN), nicorandil.

Ivabradine – specialist only prescribed.

Secondary prevention drugs: Aspirin 75 mg OD. Continue clopidogrel if on this for another reason.

Statin.

ACEI if: HTN, HF, LVD, CKD, IHD, DM.[4]

Cardiac Syndrome X Consider in ongoing symptoms and normal angiography. Continue antianginal if effective. No evidence of benefit with secondary prevention treatment.

It is possible to have a complex case in the CSA where you may need to manage multiple problems. In this example we suggest completing a risk assessment for depression, then focusing on the chest pain and finally signposting the need to manage the depression at a later date.

See the **Link Hub at CompleteCSA.co.uk** or a helpful guide to **DVLA guidance for medical conditions**

Cardiovascular Health – 3

Doctor's Notes

Patient	Brendon Phillips	74 years	M

PMH Irritable bowel syndrome
Barrett's oesophagus

Medications No regular medication

Allergies NKDA

Consultations 3 weeks ago with GP – SOB on exertion.

Investigations Bloods   FBC, U&E, LFT, TFT, HbA1c, Lipids – all normal.
Chest X-ray   Mild pulmonary congestion, cardiomegaly.
Echo: Ejection fraction 65%
          Severe mitral valve regurgitation
ECG: Sinus rhythm 70 bpm

Household No household members registered.

Example Consultation — Heart Failure

Open ☐   We can certainly go through all your test results today. To enable me to interpret these results in the context of your medical history, and make sure I'm not missing anything, may I go back to the beginning to assess the problem myself? How did the problem start? Anything else you have noticed? When does this affect you? When do you notice the symptoms? How quickly has there been a change in your breathing?

Flags ☐   Any chest pain? Coughing? Phlegm or blood? Whistling? Swelling or pain in the legs? Weight loss? Temperatures or drenching sweats? How many pillows do you sleep with? Have you noticed the feeling of suddenly needing air whilst lying down?

Risk ☐   Has a parent or sibling had any similar problem or any blood clots? Have you smoked? Or drank much alcohol? Have you been immobile; for example, sitting on a long flight? Any travel to other countries? Any exposure to asbestos, animals or birds?

History ☐   What do you know about your medical history? Do you take medicines? Tell me more about you and how you spend your days. Is anyone else at home?

Impact ☐   How is this impacting on your life? What other changes have you had to make?

Sense ☐   I sense you feel quite concerned about this change in health.

ICE ☐   What do you think may be causing the problem? Is there anything you have been worried about? What did you think I may suggest today? Is there anything else that you were hoping I might say or suggest?

Curious ☐   What made you question angina? What made you think about the heart valves? Tell me more about what you have read. That is useful information, thank you.

O/E ☐   I would like to examine you please: your hands, blood pressure, pulse, oxygen level, breathing rate, temperature, listen to your heart and lungs, the veins in your neck, feel your neck, feel your tummy and look at your legs if I may?

Summary ☐   To summarise, over 9 months your breathing has gradually worsened with fatigue and you can no longer go on long walks. You have been informed there is a problem with the valve in the heart and made the connection with previous rheumatic fever. Being told the heart is not right instantly gives you a feeling of doom and fear.

Impression ☐   I think you have a valve problem with your heart, called mitral regurgitation.

Explanation ☐   The mitral valve is in the left side of the heart, which receives blood from the lungs and pumps blood to the body. In your case, the mitral valve does not close fully, causing blood to leak in the wrong direction. Therefore, there is backpressure in the lungs, resulting in fluid collecting in the lungs. After listening to your detailed description, I think this is the only cause for your breathing problems. You may hear the term heart failure or pulmonary oedema. When the heart does not pump out all the blood which goes into the heart, the heart is not 100% effective so it is given the frightening term heart failure. Pulmonary oedema means fluid in the lungs. Any questions?

Empathy ☐   I will provide information to read. Understandably, this is very concerning for you, being told that your heart is not functioning optimally. What is going through your mind? It is important we get an opinion from a cardiologist as soon as possible.

Future ☐   I expect the cardiologist will talk about surgery. If you have not received a date for an appointment within 2 weeks, please let me know. Surgery has good success rates.

Options ☐   I would like to start you on a water tablet called furosemide, taken in the morning. It will make you pee out the extra water which is sitting in your lungs. This should help your breathing. It can drop your BP so, if you feel lightheaded, please let a doctor know. We need to check your kidneys are okay on this tablet. Can you book a blood test in 2 weeks please? I'll see you after the blood test. Are you happy to start the tablet? It is likely that the heart specialist will want to start other tablets, but we will await his opinion first.

Safety net ☐   I do not expect this to happen but, if you ever suddenly feel very breathless or get pain in the chest, you need to seek urgent help, which may mean calling 999.

Cardiovascular Health – 4

Patient's Story

Heart Failure

Doctor's notes	Brendon Phillips, 74 years. PMH: IBS, Barrett's oesophagus. Consultation with GP 3 weeks ago: SOBOE. Medications: None. Investigations: routine bloods normal. CXR: mild pulmonary congestion, cardiomegaly.
	Echo: Ejection fraction 65%. Severe MR. ECG: sinus rhythm 70 bpm.
How to act	Interested in your health.
PC	*'I've come for my echo results please.'*
History	You enjoy hiking and, 9 months ago, you noticed you could not manage the same strenuous walks. You have gradually noticed that it is more difficult to go about your normal life due to your breathing. This has gradually got worse. You had to give up on hiking but still manage to walk the dog around the block. You have no ankle or leg swelling. You feel generally tired. You have never had any pain in the chest.
	You have noticed it is easier to sleep with three pillows but have had no PND.
	You have had no cough or wheeze. You have been well with no temperature.
	You have no weight loss.
	You have no RFs for CVD or VTE.
	You have never smoked or had any exposure to asbestos or animals/birds.
	No recent travel. No drenching sweats.
	You were born in India where your parents worked until you were 14 years, then your family moved back to the UK.
Social	You retired 3 years ago from your job as a surveyor.
	Divorced 10 years ago and have since lived alone.
	You have a good network of friends who share your interests: kayaking and walking.
ICE	You imagine this is due to age, but worry what has caused this sudden decline.
	You wonder if it is angina, although you get no pain.
	You have also done some reading since the ultrasonographer mentioned your valve is slightly affected. You keep quiet about looking into the diagnosis yourself but hint to the doctor *'Maybe the heart valves have been damaged.'* If asked more about this thought, explain you remember your mother telling you that you had rheumatic fever as a child and you have read that this can affect the valves.
	The prospect of a problem with the heart has given you a sense of doom which you can't explain.
	Your mood is good but you worry about being isolated now that you are less active.
Examination	Pansystolic murmur heard at the apex.
	Chest: bi-basal crackles in lower zones.
	HR 72 regular, RR 15, Sats 96%, apyrexial, BP 132/74
	No hepatomegaly.
	No ankle swelling.
	JVP 4 cm. No palpable thyroid. No lymphadenopathy.
	No clubbing.

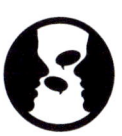

Cardiovascular Health – 4

Learning Points — Heart Failure

Refer to full guidance NICE Guidance. CG108. Heart failure in adults: management. Aug 2010.

History	Dyspnoea, exercise tolerance for NYHA class, PND. Alcohol, nutrition and mood.
Bloods	FBC (Anaemia), U&E and LFTs (baseline /reliability of BNP)
	TFTs (2° cause), lipids and glucose (2° prevention).
	BNP if no previous MI.
Other tests	Urinalysis (protein), ECG (ischaemia/LV hypertrophy). CXR (HF and malignancy).
	Consider spirometry if diagnosis uncertain.
Echo	Systolic and diastolic function, intracardiac shunts and valve disease.[2]
BNP	BNP <100 pg/ml = NTproBNP <400 pg/ml diagnosis of HF 'unlikely'.[2]
	BNP >400 pg/ml = NTproBNP >2000 pg/ml diagnosis of HF 'likely'.[2]
Reduced BNP in:	Obesity, β-blockers, ACEI, ARB and aldosterone antagonists.[2]
Increased BNP in:	Hypoxaemia/PE, eGFR <60 ml/min/1.73 m^2, sepsis, DM, liver cirrhosis, >70 years, LVH, HR>100 bpm.[2]
2-week echo if	Previous MI + suspected HF or BNP >400 pg/ml.[2]
6-week echo	For initial diagnosis and BNP between 100 and 400 pg/ml.

If valve disease present, follow cardiology advice.

Refer back if	NYHA class IV, not responding to treatment[2] and admit if can't be managed at home.
Health advice	Smoking, alcohol, salt, cardiac rehabilitation, flu and pneumococcal vaccine.[2]
	Weight – report if 2 kg ↑ in 2 days.
	Consider referral to a rehabilitation programme.[2]

Medication for left ventricular systolic dysfunction

For each medication check licensing (for indication), contraindications and interactions.

	Diuretics	Titrate up or down according to congestion symptoms.[2]
	ACEI	Titrate to maximum tolerated dose. If intolerant consider an ARB.
		Measure creatinine, U&E (e.g. 2 weeks) after each dose increment.[2]
		Caution includes valve disease – await cardiology advice.
	β-blockers	'Start low, go slow'[2] and check HR and BP after each increment.
		Consider even if elderly, diabetic, COPD, PVD and ED.
		Switch previous β-blockers to one licensed for HF.[2]
	ARB	If intolerant of ACEI and monitor creatinine/U&E.[2]
	Hydralazine with nitrate – seek specialist advice. An option if intolerant of ACEI/ARB[2]	
	Spironolactone	E.g. if NYHA class III–IV.
		Following an MI – initiated within 3–14 days preferably after ACEI.[2]
		Monitor creatinine/U&E – for hyperkalaemia and ↓ renal function.[2]
	Digoxin – if worsening HF despite 1st and 2nd line Rx and seek specialist advice.	
	Aspirin 75 mg	if indicated for vascular disease.
	CCBs	Amlodipine may be considered if coexistent HTN or angina.[2]
HFPEF	Heart failure with preserved ejection fracture (e.g. due to diastolic dysfunction).	
	Diagnosis	Symptomatic, ↑ BNP (other causes excluded) and normal ejection fraction on echo.
	Symptomatic Rx	Diuretics for congestion. Treat comorbidities and seek advice.

Doctor's Notes

Patient   Richard Turner   57 years   M
PMH   No medical history
Medications   No current medications
Allergies   No known drug allergies
Consultations   BP 162/102 at a check with the nurse
Investigations Average ambulatory blood pressure reading 151/96
Household   Gillian Turner   56 years   F

Example Consultation — Hypertension

Open ☐ — What led you to have this tested? Do you know your readings?

ICE ☐ — When you saw the 151/96 figure what went through your mind? Is this a worry for you? What did you think I was going to say?

History ☐ — Do you have any medical conditions?

Risk ☐ — Has a family member had a heart problem, high blood pressure or a stroke?

Sense ☐ — So this has come out of the blue? How do you feel about being told your BP is raised?

Flags ☐ — When talking about blood pressure, I usually check you haven't suffered with any headaches? Or any chest or calf pains? Does your heart ever feel like it is beating too fast?

Curious ☐ — You mentioned your wife was helping you test it and she wanted you to have a check; what does she think? Why do you think she is worried?

Summary ☐ — So to summarise, you've been very well therefore you were surprised when your blood pressure was high. You were hoping that I'd say we'll keep an eye on it but your wife wants you to take tablets, especially with her father's experience. Is that right?

O/E ☐ — I would like to check your BP again in both arms and examine the back of your eyes if I may. Sometimes we can see changes in the eye due to high blood pressure.

Empathy ☐ — I can see you take this seriously and your wife is concerned as her father had high BP.

Impression ☐ — Your eyes look normal. Your diagnosis is Stage 2 hypertension, which is the medical word for high blood pressure. It is Stage 2 because the top number is >150 and the bottom >95.

Experience ☐ — What do you understand about why we treat high blood pressure?

Explanation ☐ — High blood pressure can increase your risk of a stroke, angina or a heart attack which is why it is important to control it. It can also harm your kidneys and eyes. Stage 2 hypertension is not dangerous; however, it does suggest that we should be treating the blood pressure with tablets as well as lifestyle advice.

Options ☐ — Whether to start treatment is your decision. My recommendation would be to start a tablet called amlodipine 5 mg each morning. This helps to relax the blood vessels to decrease the pressure. Like any tablet there may be side effects, such as the possibility of ankle swelling, tummy upset or headaches, in which case we could consider a different tablet. How do you feel about taking the tablet?

Empower ☐ — Things you can do to help include exercising more, reducing alcohol and restricting salt in your diet. A 6 g reduction in salt each day reduces your blood pressure number by 10.[5] Do you feel these suggestions will be possible?

Future ☐ — Thinking ahead, we need to do some routine tests with the nurse to check your general health including an ECG, which is a heart tracing, a urine test and blood tests including cholesterol and to check your kidneys. Is this okay? So to summarise, you will start a morning tablet, make an appointment with the nurse for a heart tracing, blood test and urine test, then see me in 1 month. If you're having a problem with the tablet or have any concerns, please let me know.

Patient's Story

Hypertension

Doctor's notes	Richard Turner, 57 years. PMH: None. Medications: None.
	Last consultation: BP 162/102 (practice nurse)
	Average ambulatory blood pressure reading 151/96
How to act	Interested in your health.
PC	*'I've come to find out what I need to do about my blood pressure.'*
History	You feel well. No PMH or FH.
	You were at a friend's house for dinner and they had purchased a BP machine, so you checked yours.
	'My wife wanted me to go to the nurse to check it again.'
	The nurse found that your BP was raised and gave you a machine to check it at home.
	You discussed the average BP, 151/96, with the nurse and have been sent to the doctor.
Social	Very healthy. You enjoy squash and consider yourself to be a healthy eater.
	You drink very little alcohol and have never smoked.
	You work as a gardener so are active during the day.
	You enjoy your work, and do not find it stressful.
	You have a good relationship with your wife.
ICE	You thought 151/96 was high but thought you'd be told to keep an eye on it. You are worried the doctor will want to start a tablet. You are not keen as this will make you feel old but it won't otherwise impact on your life.
	You thought you had no CV risk factors, so you were quite shocked.
	You understand that it was your father-in-law's BP that led to his stroke.
	You are happy to take the tablet, once its importance has been explained
	You are also interested in other ways to decrease your blood pressure.
	Do not tell the doctor your wife is worried unless the doctor asks.
	You have mentioned your wife twice already. It is your wife who is worried.
	Her father was always talking about his blood pressure before his stroke.
	She would like you to take tablets.
Examination	Fundi normal. BP left arm 155/88, right arm 152/90.

Learning Points — Hypertension

NICE Guidance CG127. Hypertension: diagnosis and management. August 2011 – refer to full guidance.

Investigations[1] Bloods: Lipids (for QRISK) and HbA1c (comorbidity), U&E, eGFR (baseline for Rx), FBC (anaemia) and TFT (cause).
ECG (ventricular hypertrophy, arrhythmia), ACR (microalbuminuria/CKD) and fundi (retinopathy).

Diagnosis[1] Check BP in both arms, if difference >20 mmHg persists use the arm with ↑ readings
Ambulatory monitoring (best)   2 measurements/hour during waking hours.
Home BP monitoring   Twice/day (2 readings 1 min apart) for 4–7 days. Discard 1st day's reading and average remaining.

Stage 1 HTN Clinic BP ≥140/90 and home BP ≥ 135/85   Treat if *(see below).
Stage 2 HTN Clinic BP ≥160/100 and home BP ≥150/95 Start treatment.
Stage 3/severe HTN Clinic SBP ≥180 or DBP ≥ 110   Treat immediately.
Accelerated HTN Papilloedema or retinal haemorrhage   Admission.
Suspected phaeochromocytoma   Admission.
White coat HTN >20/10 mmHg between home and clinic Monitor only home readings.

*Treat Stage 1 HTN if <80 years of age and:
   CVD comorbidity   CVD or CKD or DM or ≥20% CVD risk
   or sign of end organ damage from ACR/ECG/fundi

If symptoms/signs of secondary causes speak to specialists for further investigations.
If Stage 1 HTN <40 years and no sign of CVD comorbidity, consider specialist referral for 2° causes.

Aims of clinic BP <140/90 if <80 years or <150/90 if >80 years with treated HTN[1]
<140/80 if DM[2]
<130/80 if DM and either CKD or retinopathy or cerebrovascular disease[2,3]

Treating hypertension[1] (Check you have stopped the OCP!)
A = ACE inhibitor   B = β-blocker   C = calcium channel blocker   D = thiazide-like diuretic
If <55 years start with ACEI. If required A + C + D (thiazide last as risk of DM).
If >55 years or black people of African/Caribbean descent start with CCB. If required C + A + D.

Resistant HTN HTN persists despite three drugs
4th line. If K ≤4.5 mmol/L and eGFR >60 ml/min/1.73 m^2 consider spironolactone.
Caution ↓ eGFR = ↑ risk of hyperkalaemia.[1]
If K >4.5 mmol/L then consider a 'higher-dose thiazide-like diuretic treatment' and repeat eGFR/U&E in 1/12.[1]
Other options include alpha or beta blockers.[1]
If oedema, HF or risk of HF, caution with C.[1]
If diabetic, caution with B and D and consider A first for microalbuminuria.
'Black people of African or Caribbean family origin, consider an ARB in preference to an ACEI.'[1]
If >80 years, consider starting with D. If required D + A (HYVET study).[4]
We suggest U&E at baseline and 2 weeks after initiating/increasing ACEI or ARB or spironolactone.
Refer if BP remains uncontrolled on four agents[1] or earlier if concerned.
NB: Also be aware of sodium content in drugs (e.g. effervescent).

Secondary (2°) causes of HTN: Primary hyperaldosteronism, phaeochromocytoma, CKD and sleep apnoea. Ask about UTIs as a child. Investigations: urinary normetadrenalines, USS kidneys + referral to exclude fibromuscular dysplasia of the renal artery.

Extra Notes

AF and NOACs

Managing the stroke risk

Warfarin reduces stroke risk by 65% and aspirin by 22%.[1]

CHA$_2$DS$_2$-VASc score[2]	Consider anticoagulation for ♂ with a score of ≥1 or ♀ with a score of ≥2.[3,4]
	After taking into account the HAS-BLED score.
HAS-BLED score[2]	Do not withhold anticoagulation solely because of risk of falls.[3]
	The greater the HAS-BLED score the greater the risk of ICH.
Anticoagulation	Determine person's time in therapeutic range using Rosendaal method.[3]
Aspirin	No longer advised.
	If used, prescribe aspirin with clopidogrel (and PPI cover).[3]

NOACs

Who for	Patient's with AF (**non-valve disease**) and CHA$_2$DS$_2$-VASc ≥1 in ♂ and ≥2 in ♀.
	With poor compliance to warfarin or patient preference.
Benefits	Reduced ICH and haemorrhagic stroke risk[3] and no blood tests.
Limitations	Reversal agents are not widely available.
Interactions	Antiplatelets, ketoconazole, itraconazole, HIV protease inhibitors and more.
Education	Must be compliant. Seek help immediately if bleeding occurs.

> See the **Link Hub at CompleteCSA.co.uk** for helpful information on
> **Which NOAC to use**
> **Comparing NOACs to Warfarin**
> **Switching between Warfarin/NOACs**
> **CHA$_2$DS$_2$-VASc flow chart**

Cardiovascular Health

CHAPTER 15 OVERVIEW
Digestive Health

	Cases in this chapter	Within the RCGP curriculum: Digestive Health RCGP Curriculum Online March 2016[1]	Learning points in the chapter include:
1	Dyspepsia	'Demonstrate a systematic approach to investigating common digestive symptoms, taking into account the prevalence of these symptoms in primary care and the likelihood of conditions such as peptic ulcer, oesophageal varices, hepatitis, gastrointestinal cancers and post-operative complications'	NICE guidelines. CG184. Gastro-oesophageal reflux disease and dyspepsia in adults: investigation and management. September 2014 Gallbladder polyp
2	Irritable Bowel Syndrome	'Understand that digestive symptoms are often multiple and imprecise, and frequently linked to emotional factors' 'Understand the many cultural and social factors which can influence the way patients interpret symptoms and the manner in which this influences their expectations of medical management'	NICE guidelines. CG61. Irritable bowel syndrome in adults: diagnosis and management. February 2008. Last updated: February 2015 Faecal calprotectin
3	Change in Bowel Habit	'Understand the risks associated with various symptoms which may indicate GI cancer, and refer with appropriate levels of urgency'	Colorectal cancer red flags NICE Guideline. NG12. Suspected cancer: recognition and referral. June 2015
4	Inflammatory Bowel Disease	'Have a good understanding of the impact of GI symptoms and illness on patients, their families and their wider networks'	Assessing severity Drug monitoring
5	Abnormal LFTs (Liver Function Tests)	'Understand dietary factors associated with various GI conditions and offer appropriate dietary advice (e.g. in weight loss, irritable bowel syndrome and primary cancer prevention)'	NAFLD Differential diagnosis with abnormal LFTs

1. http://www.rcgp.org.uk/training-exams/gp-curriculum-overview/online-curriculum/applying-clinical-knowledge-section-1/3-13-digestive-health.aspx

CHAPTER 15 REFERENCES

Dyspepsia
1. NICE Guidelines NG12. Suspected cancer: recognition and referral. Jun 2015.
2. NICE Guidelines. CG184. Gastro-oesophageal reflux disease and dyspepsia in adults: investigation and management. Sep 2014.
3. http://www.nhs.uk/news/2010/05May/Pages/ppi-stomach-drugs-harm-vs-good.aspx

IBS
1. NICE Guidelines. CG61. Irritable bowel syndrome in adults: diagnosis and management. Feb 2008. Last updated: Feb 2015.
2. http://www.bsg.org.uk/patients/general/irritable-bowel-syndrome.html
3. NICE Diagnostics Guidance. DG11. Faecal calprotectin diagnostic tests for inflammatory diseases of the bowel. Oct 2013.
4. Van Rheenen P., Van de Vijver E. Faecal calprotectin for screening of patients with suspected inflammatory bowel disease: diagnostic meta-analysis. *BMJ*. 2010; 341: c3369.
5. Spiller R., Aziz Q., Creed F. Guidelines on the irritable bowel syndrome: mechanisms and practical management. *Gut*. 2007; 56: 1770–98. doi: 10.1136/gut.2007.11944.

Change in Bowel Habit/Colorectal Cancer
1. NICE Guidelines. NG12. Suspected cancer: recognition and referral. Jun 2015.

IBD
1. Ford A., Moayyedi P., et al. Ulcerative colitis. *BMJ*. 2013; 346: f432.
2. NICE Guidelines. CG 166. Ulcerative colitis: management. Jun 2013.
3. Truelove S C, Witts L. Cortisone in ulcerative colitis: final report on a therapeutic trial. *BMJ*. 1955; 2: 1041–8.
4. NICE Guidelines. CG152. Crohn's disease: management. Oct 2012.

Abnormal LFTs
1. http://www.nhs.uk/Conditions/fatty-liver-disease/Pages/Introduction.aspx
2. Collier J., Bassendine M. How to respond to abnormal liver function tests. *Clin Med JRCPL*. 2002; 2: 406–9.

Doctor's Notes

Patient	Daniel Hernandez 38 years M
PMH	None
Medications	No current medications
Allergies	No information
Consultations	New patient check last week with HCA:
	Smoker 15/day. Alcohol 25 units/week. BP 124/75. BMI 32. Mentioned abdominal pain, advised to see GP.
Investigations	No investigations
Household	No household members registered

Example Consultation

Dyspepsia

Open ☐	Can you tell me more about this pain? When did you first notice it? Is there a pattern?
History ☐	What brings it on? Does anything make it worse? Or better? Where do you feel the pain? Does it go anywhere else? How have your bowels and waterworks been? Tell me a little about yourself; where do you work? Who's at home? A food magazine – do you eat a healthy diet, would you say? Have you noticed any particular meals which make the pain worse? Have you noticed a cough at night or first thing in the morning?
Risk ☐	Do you smoke? Drink any alcohol? Is there a family history of stomach problems? Have you been taking any painkillers, for example ibuprofen, for anything?
Flags ☐	Have you lost weight? Vomited blood? Passed black stools? Does it cause any other symptoms like nausea, sweating or breathlessness? Have you had any difficulty swallowing?
ICE ☐	You've had this pain a while now; have you had any thoughts what it could be? What worries have crossed your mind? Was there anything specific you were expecting me to do today?
Sense ☐	I sense you are anxious about what happened to your mum; is there anything specific that concerns you?
Curious ☐	Tell me more about your mum's experience. Have you been worried that you may need an operation?
Impact ☐	How has this pain affected you? Has it stopped you doing anything?
O/E ☐	I would like to examine you: I'd like to examine your tummy and check your heart rate. Would that be okay? I can see your blood pressure and BMI have been checked last week.
Summary ☐	So, you have been getting pain in your lower chest and upper tummy for 2 months, it is worse at night and after large meals or alcohol. It can spread upwards to your throat. You thought it could be due to gallstones as your mum had this problem. You are worried about needing an operation or blood tests.
Impression ☐	From listening to your symptoms and examining you it seems that you have acid reflux rather than gallstones. Thankfully there are no worrying symptoms.
Experience ☐	Have you heard of reflux? Do you know anything about it?
Explanation ☐	Reflux is when stomach acid comes out of the stomach and into the food pipe. This causes pain as the acid irritates the food pipe. It can go all the way up to your throat and cause soreness there too.
Empathy ☐	Reflux is very common but can be quite uncomfortable and I can see it has affected your enjoyment of food.
Options ☐	Thankfully, reflux is treatable. Would you like to start a medication called omeprazole which reduces stomach acid and usually makes the symptoms better? You would take it each morning for a month then come back for a review.
Future ☐	In most cases the symptoms will settle but, if not, there are other investigations we can do. For example, some people have a bacterial bug in their stomach which can cause this. If your pain is still there after the treatment, I would like to test for this with a stool or breath test.
Empower ☐	So, meanwhile, there are some things that you can do to help. Avoiding large meals at the end of the day, reducing alcohol and caffeine, avoiding spicy food, raising the head of your bed and losing a bit of weight can all help. I recommend stopping smoking altogether. Would you like to see our nurse for support and help with this?
Safety net ☐	I would like to see you in 4 weeks to see how you are but if you start vomiting, the pain worsens or you pass blood or black stool, please come back to see me straight away. If the pain has gone and all is well, you can cancel the appointment, but let me know if it flares up again.

Digestive Health – 1

Patient's Story

Dyspepsia

Doctor's notes	Daniel Hernandez, 38 years. PMH: New patient, BP 124/75, smoker 15/day, alcohol 25 units/week. BMI 32. New patient HCA consultation last week. Mentioned abdominal pains, advised to see GP. No investigations. No household members registered.
How to act	Relaxed but anxious if tests are mentioned.
PC	*'Doctor, I have a pain in the stomach.'*
History	For the last 2 months you have been getting stomach pains intermittently.
	The pain can be sharp or burning and is located in your upper abdomen/lower chest.
	The pain starts in the lower chest but radiates up, sometimes to your throat.
	You feel you have been belching more too.
	The pain is worse at night after a large meal. It tends to be worse at the weekends when you have been out with your friends.
	You have not been sick, you have normal bowel motions and no black stools. You have not lost any weight, although you have been trying to.
	You have tried Gaviscon which did help a bit. You have since been trying to avoid foods you would normally enjoy. You have taken no other medicines.
Social	You came to the UK from Spain 20 years ago to study at university.
	You got a good job as a graduate journalist so decided to stay. You write for a food magazine and enjoy going out for meals.
	You will often have a few glasses of wine with your meals. When you saw the nurse she told you that you were drinking too much, so you have tried to cut down.
	You do smoke but know you should stop! You're thinking about trying an e-cigarette.
	You live alone but have some good friends and colleagues with whom you socialise.
ICE	You are worried about gallstones. Your mother had an operation to remove her gallbladder and you remember her getting abdominal pains when eating. She still lives in Spain so you haven't had chance to ask her more about her symptoms.
	You have a needle phobia so worry you may need blood tests or surgery.
	You expect the doctor to examine you and possibly order blood tests.
Examination	Abdomen soft and non-tender. Observations normal.

Digestive Health – 1

Learning Points   Dyspepsia

The decision about how to manage these conditions is based upon the presence or absence of 'red flag' symptoms and whether the patient has had an endoscopy before.

NICE criteria for 2WW referral for urgent direct access gastrointestinal endoscopy[1]
Either – Dysphagia.

Or – Age ≥55 years with weight loss AND one of: upper abdominal pain or reflux or dyspepsia.

NICE criteria for non-urgent direct access upper gastrointestinal endoscopy[1]
Either – Haematemesis (if, however, it is an acute presentation or the patient is haemodynamically unstable, then admit to hospital).

Or – Age ≥55 years with either:

    Treatment-resistant dyspepsia

    Upper abdominal pain + low haemoglobin

Raised platelet count + one of	nausea or vomiting or weight loss or reflux or dyspepsia or upper abdominal pain.
Nausea or vomiting + one of	weight loss or reflux or dyspepsia or upper abdominal pain.

If no red flags are present
Has the patient had upper GI endoscopy before?

YES – be pragmatic – if the endoscopy was recent or the symptoms have not changed since the endoscopy you may decide to follow conservative Rx as indicated on the endoscopy.

NO – termed 'uninvestigated dyspepsia' give a trial of treatment.

Dyspepsia treatment[2]	1st PPI for 4–8 weeks.
	2nd H_2 receptor antagonist (H_2RA) therapy.
Lifestyle factors	Always remember to modify lifestyle factors: caffeine, alcohol, spices.
Check drug history	E.g. NSAID, SSRI.

Helicobacter pylori testing
NICE advise 'offer' the test.[2]

If dyspepsia is likely to be secondary to a reversible lifestyle factor – consider avoidance of the precipitant and a treatment trial first.

Either a carbon-13 urea breath test, a stool antigen test or validated laboratory serology testing.[2]

If retesting, only use the breath test.[2]

Return of symptoms	Consider a low-dose maintenance dose as required.[2]
	However, continue to review PPIs. Long-term risks include bone fracture, vitamin B12 deficiency or Clostridium difficile.[3]

Remember PPIs must be stopped 2 weeks before *H. pylori* testing and endoscopy.[2]

Differential diagnosis	Biliary, pancreatic and cardiac disease.
Gallbladder polyp	Single gallbladder polyp <1 cm – repeat USS in 6/12 then yearly surveillance.
	>1 cm refer for cholecystectomy.

Digestive Health – 1

Doctor's Notes

Patient	Rebecca Short 23 years F
PMH	Anxiety
Medications	Sertraline 50 mg OD
Allergies	No information
Consultations	No recent consultations
Investigations	No investigations
Household	No household members registered

Example Consultation — Irritable Bowel Syndrome

Open ☐ — Can you tell me about your symptoms from the beginning? Can you describe your bowels? Do you have any pain? Where do you feel the pain?

History ☐ — Does anything make it better? Does anything make it worse? Do any particular foods make the symptoms worse? Do you feel bloated? Is that persistent or intermittent? Do you have any other symptoms such as vomiting? Tell me more about yourself.

Risk ☐ — Do you have a family history of bowel problems? Any bowel or ovarian cancer in the family? Do you smoke? Do you drink alcohol? Any foreign travel? Do any foods make it worse?

Flags ☐ — Have you lost any weight? Have you passed any blood? Have you passed any black stools? Do you need to open your bowels at night? Have you had any incontinence of stools? That must have been upsetting; tell me more about what happened.

ICE ☐ — You have had these symptoms for a while; have you had any thoughts about what is causing them? Is there anything which has been troubling you? Were you hoping I would do anything specific today?

Sense ☐ — I sense that you have been a bit stressed recently. Is there anything which is causing you stress? How is life at home? How is life at work?

Curious ☐ — You mentioned your mother told you to come. Did she have any particular worries?

Impact ☐ — How have these symptoms affected you at home and at work?

O/E ☐ — Would you mind if I examined you? I would like you to lie on the couch so I can check your tummy, your pulse and temperature, then measure your BP and weight. Is that okay?

Summary ☐ — So, you have been having a mixture of loose and hard stools and you get abdominal cramps which improve when you open your bowels. The symptoms tend to be worse when you are most anxious. You haven't lost weight, passed blood or black stools. You are worried that you may have Crohn's as your cousin has it, and you are concerned you may need time off work which will be financially difficult.

Impression ☐ — From listening to your symptoms and examining you, it seems most likely that you have irritable bowel syndrome rather than Crohn's disease.

Experience ☐ — Have you heard of irritable bowel? Do you know anyone with it?

Explanation ☐ — Irritable bowel syndrome is a condition where the bowel becomes oversensitive and can cause pain, wind, diarrhoea or constipation, and often a mixture of all of these.

Empathy ☐ — It is harmless but can be uncomfortable, embarrassing and a real nuisance.

Options ☐ — Firstly, I think we should do some tests to rule out any other causes of your symptoms. We can check blood tests for coeliac disease (wheat allergy), thyroid, kidney and liver abnormalities, inflammatory markers to help rule out conditions like Crohn's disease. How does that sound?

Empower ☐ — If these tests are all normal, we can be fairly confident that you have IBS. There are several treatment options including medication and a special diet. The diet is related to avoiding the foods which are high in FODMAPs, which are a type of carbohydrate which is poorly absorbed by the intestines. FODMAPs can make you feel full of gas. I will print off a list of all the foods to avoid.

Future ☐ — Can we arrange the tests then meet up again, about a week later, to go through the results?

Safety net ☐ — In the meantime if the symptoms get worse, you pass blood or black stools, or you have any concerns please call the surgery. If you ever have severe stomach pain, see a doctor at the time.

Patient's Story

Irritable Bowel Syndrome

Doctor's notes Rebecca Short, 23 years. PMH: Anxiety. Medication: Sertraline.

How to act Anxious.

PC *'I have been having a lot of diarrhoea recently, Doctor.'*

History You have been having intermittent loose stools for around 9 months. You get cramping abdominal pain which is relieved by opening your bowels and an intermittent feeling of bloating. You sometimes pass mucus. At other times you feel that you get bunged up. You have not lost any weight; you have not passed any blood. No vomiting. No black stools. The symptoms do seem to be worse when you are stressed or worried. At times you have had to rush to the toilet at work which has caused you to get in trouble for leaving your phone. No foreign travel. No pattern with foods.

You have not needed to open your bowels in the night.

You are ashamed to say that once you were caught short and had some faecal incontinence. Only disclose this if the doctor asks.

Social You work in telephone sales. You have been put under a lot of pressure recently by your manager. You have targets to meet all the time and this has been difficult. If you don't meet your targets you get paid less and sometimes struggle to pay your rent. You have had some time off recently with anxiety but went back to work when your job was threatened. You don't get sick pay. The sertraline does seem to help. You live with your boyfriend. Your parents are local. Your mum encouraged you to 'get checked out' as your cousin has Crohn's disease.

Non-smoker. Social drinker.

ICE You are worried that you may have Crohn's disease too. You worry you will need to take time off work which may lead to you being sacked.

Examination Abdomen soft, generalised mild tenderness.

BMI 21.

HR 88 bpm. BP 110/70. Temperature 36.8°C.

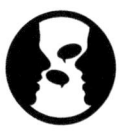

Learning Points   Irritable Bowel Syndrome

Diagnosis (symptoms must be present for at least 6 months)[1]
'Abdominal pain or discomfort that is either relieved by defaecation or associated with altered bowel frequency or stool form.'[1]

+ 2 of: Bloating, distention, tension or hardness.
Altered stool passage (straining, urgency, incomplete evacuation).
Passage of mucus.
Symptoms made worse by eating.

Extra features which make IBS more likely:[1,2] 'Lethargy, nausea, backache and bladder symptoms.'[1]

Red flags
PR bleeding[1,2]   Change in bowel habit
FH of bowel or ovarian cancer[1]   Unintentional and unexplained weight loss[1]
Fever[2]   Diarrhoea waking the patient from sleep[2]
Rectal or abdominal mass[1]   Abnormal blood tests – anaemia, raised inflammatory
                                                markers or CA 125 (Cancer Antigen 125).[1]

Refer to NICE Guidance Suspected cancer: recognition and referral. Jun 2015 to determine whether the patient meets the 2WW referral criteria.

Social history
Travel, mood, stress, diet and alcohol.

Investigations to rule out other causes
FBC (suspicious if raised platelet count or anaemia), ESR and CRP (IBD), coeliac screen and consider CA 125 +/– pelvic USS if raised.[1] If recent antibiotic use or long-term PPI use, consider a Clostridium difficile screen.

NICE state NO need to do: USS, sigmoidoscopy, colonoscopy, barium enema, TSH, faecal ova/parasites, FOB, hydrogen breath tests, unless appropriate to rule out another condition.[1]

Faecal calprotectin
When to test? After ruling out red flags, to differentiate between IBS and IBD, if specialist assessment is being considered.[3]
What is it? A protein secreted from inflammatory cells in the gut.[4]

Differential diagnosis of IBS where the main symptom is diarrhoea (IBS-D)
'Microscopic colitis, coeliac disease, giardiasis, lactose malabsorption, tropical sprue, small bowel bacterial overgrowth, bile salt malabsorption, colon cancer.'[5]

Management[1]
Relaxation and physical activity.

Dietary changes	Regular meals, restricting caffeine, fizzy drinks and alcohol, avoid insoluble fibre and artificial sweeteners, a trial of probiotics for 4 weeks.
Low FODMAP diet	Fermentable oligosaccharides, disaccharides, monosaccharides and polyols.
Pain	Trial of antispasmodics (e.g. mebeverine, hyoscine).
Constipation	Laxatives but avoid lactulose.
Diarrhoea	Loperamide.
Others	Low dose TCA, SSRIs, linaclotide (constipated patients) – See NICE guidance. Irritable bowel syndrome with constipation in adults: linaclotide. April 2013.

Classification[5]
IBS-D (diarrhoea predominant)   IBS-C (constipation predominant)
IBS-M (mixed)   Alternators (switch subtype over time)

Digestive Health – 2

Doctor's Notes

Patient	Emmanuel Adebayo 71 years M
PMH	Osteoarthritis of right knee
	Hypertension
	GORD
Medications	Co-codamol 30/500 PRN
	Amlodipine 10 mg OD
	Ramipril 5 mg OD
	Lansoprazole 15 mg OD
Allergies	No information
Consultations	No recent consultations
Investigations	No investigations
Household	No household members registered

Example Consultation — Change in Bowel Habit

Open ☐	Could you tell me a little bit more about your bowels? How long have they been playing up? Anything else you have noticed? How do you feel in yourself?
Flags ☐	Have you lost weight? Passed any blood? Any fevers?
History ☐	Are your bowels currently either hard or watery? Have you had any other symptoms like pain? Where do you feel the pain? How long does it last? Does anything make it worse? Or better? Have you felt sick? Have you actually vomited? Have you had trouble with your bowels in the past? As we've not met before, could I just clarify your past health problems and which medications you take? Does anyone live with you at home? I'm sorry to hear that. Do you have any other family or friends around you?
Risk ☐	Do you have a family history of bowel problems? Do you smoke? Or drink? Have you travelled abroad recently? Have you taken any antibiotics?
ICE ☐	Have you had any thoughts about what could be causing these symptoms? Have you been worrying about anything in particular? You've mentioned that you would like some laxatives; was there anything else that you were hoping for today?
Sense ☐	I sense that you haven't been particularly concerned about these symptoms but that they have become a bit of a nuisance, is that correct?
O/E ☐	It would be really helpful if I could examine your tummy, check your weight but also perform an examination inside your bottom. This would involve putting one finger into your bottom to feel for any lumps or bumps and to check for blood. How do you feel about that? Could I ask for a chaperone to be present?
Summary ☐	So, you have had erratic bowel movements for around 8 weeks and have passed some blood and lost a little weight. You thought you may have constipation and piles and would like some laxatives.
Impression ☐	Although constipation and piles may explain some of your symptoms, there may be something more serious going on which we need to rule out. As you have noticed this change in bowel habit, lost weight and noticed blood in your stools, I think it's really important that we rule out bowel cancer. I sense this has come as a bit of a shock to you. How do you feel about this? Would you like me to discuss the next steps?
Explanation ☐	When we need to rule out a condition like bowel cancer, we refer patients to the hospital urgently so they can be seen within 2 weeks. The hospital doctor will talk to you, examine you and offer you a test where a thin flexible tube with a light is passed through the back passage to look for any abnormal areas of bowel.
Empathy ☐	I understand this must be a surprise and worrying, especially after your wife's experience. What is going through your mind?
Options ☐	My recommendation would be to see the hospital specialists urgently. Hopefully they will reassure us or they may give us another diagnosis which can help us choose effective treatment. For example, another possibility is diverticular disease – which is not a cancer. Diverticulae are little pouches in the bowel which can become infected. It is also possible the codeine has made you constipated with intermittent overflow where only loose motions can get around the hard stools. Bleeding can occur when you are constipated. However neither of these possibilities explains the weight loss.
Empower ☐	What would you like to do?
Future ☐	I will do the referral straight away and you will be seen by the specialist within 2 weeks. I would also like to do a couple of blood tests to check your blood count, kidney and liver function, which will help us and the specialist at the hospital. Would that be okay? I'll let you know the results. Your bowel motions are formed and normal consistency today but if they become watery, we may need a stool sample. I'll give you a pot in case this happens. Sometimes lansoprazole can affect the bowels – could you manage without it?
Safety net ☐	Should you feel unwell, develop severe tummy pain, vomiting or pass a lot of blood, please let me know straight away. Could I see you after your appointment with the hospital? If you are not seen within 2 weeks, please tell me.

Digestive Health – 3

Patient's Story

Change in Bowel Habit

Doctor's notes Emmanuel Adebayo, 71 years. PMH: OA, HTN, GORD. Medications: DH: Co-codamol 30/500, amlodipine 10 mg OD, Ramipril 5 mg OD, lansoprazole 15 mg OD.

How to act Relaxed.

PC *'Good morning Doctor, I was wondering if you could prescribe me some laxatives?'*

History You have been taking co-codamol on and off for a few years for knee pain; recently your bowels have been playing up. For the last 8 weeks or so you have noticed your bowels have been erratic. Some days you have been rushing to the toilet with diarrhoea and other days you have had sluggish bowels. You have been getting abdominal pain on the left side too. You have read the drug leaflet with co-codamol and wonder if you could be constipated. You have lost your appetite and your trousers have become looser. You aren't sure how much weight you have lost. A couple of times you have noticed a bit of dark blood mixed into your stools but wondered whether this was just due to piles, which you had a long time ago.

You feel generally okay, slightly lacking in energy. You have had no fevers. The bowel motion this morning was formed.

Social You originally moved to the UK from Nigeria in the 1970s. You were an engineer and looking for better job prospects. You are retired now and live alone as your wife passed away 3 years ago from breast cancer. You have some good neighbours who take you shopping as you struggle to get about with the knee pain. You have a son who works in London so you don't get to see him much.

You don't smoke, but do drink a couple of whisky and waters in the evening.

You don't know of any family history of health problems.

ICE You don't have any particular concerns, but you would like your symptoms sorted out. The pain is sometimes bad and opening your bowels at night is a nuisance.

If the doctor mentions bowel cancer, seem surprised. This wasn't what you were expecting but, if the doctor offers urgent referral, then accept this.

Examination Normal abdominal and rectal examination.

BMI 24

Learning Points Colorectal Cancer

NICE Guideline. NG12. Suspected cancer: recognition and referral. Jun 2015

Refer via 2WW Colorectal cancer pathway[1]
Aged ≥40 years with unexplained weight loss and abdominal pain.

Aged ≥50 years with unexplained rectal bleeding.

Aged ≥60 years with either: Iron deficiency anaemia

A change in bowel habit.

Positive Faecal Occult Blood test

Consider cancer pathway referral
Rectal or abdominal mass

Anal mass or ulceration

<50 years and rectal bleeding with any of the following unexplained symptoms or findings:
- Abdominal pain
- A change in bowel habit
- Weight loss
- Iron deficiency anaemia

Offer FOB testing in people without rectal bleeding[1]
Aged ≥50 years and have abdominal pain or weight loss

Aged <60 years and have change in bowel habit or iron deficiency anaemia

Aged ≥60 years and have anaemia without iron deficiency

This case challenges you to discuss a cancer pathway referral sensitively with a patient who was not expecting a potentially serious diagnosis. It also checks your ability to look for serious pathology even if the presenting complaint seems minor or the patient minimises their symptoms. By taking a thorough symptom history and checking for risk factors and red flags you should be able to spot these cases. Use pauses and give the patient opportunities to ask questions before continuing, to ensure you are going at the right pace for that patient. Many clinicians use the word 'camera' when describing an endoscope. This can be frightening for patients who understand a camera to mean a large cube-like box. Try 'thin flexible tube with a light' or something similar.

Digestive Health – 3

Doctor's Notes

Patient	Anthony Carlisle 26 years M
PMH	Ulcerative colitis
Medications	Mesalazine SR 500 mg capsules – 2 g OD
Allergies	No information
Consultations	No recent consultations
Investigations	No investigations in the past year
Household	No household members registered

Letter from Gastroenterology Consultant 6 months ago:

RE: Anthony Carlisle

1 Woodland Avenue, Warwickshire

NHS No: 1234567890

Diagnosis: Ulcerative Colitis (in remission) Diagnosed 3 years ago.

I have reviewed Mr Carlisle in clinic today. I was pleased to find that his ulcerative colitis is well controlled on a maintenance dose of Pentasa. He has suffered very little abdominal pain and diarrhoea and has not had PR bleeding for several months. His weight is stable and he has had no systemic complications. Blood tests done before clinic were satisfactory. His full blood count and inflammatory markers were both normal.

I have arranged to see him again in 12 months but would be happy to see him sooner should he run into difficulty.

Yours sincerely,

Dr S. Patel

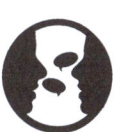

Example Consultation — Inflammatory Bowel Disease

Open ☐ — Could you tell me more about your symptoms? How do you feel in yourself?

History ☐ — Have you had any other symptoms such as vomiting? Are you managing to eat and drink? It seems that your UC has been well controlled recently; have you had many flares in the past? What usually works? Have you needed hospital admission in the past? Have you had any change in your vision? Any joint pains? Have you noticed any rashes?

Flags ☐ — How often are you opening your bowels? Is there any blood in your stools? Do you think that you have had a fever?

Risk ☐ — Have you been taking your medication regularly? Has anyone else had similar symptoms? Do you think you could have got food poisoning or a bug from anywhere? Any recent travel abroad?

ICE ☐ — You feel that you have a flare of UC and wish to have a prescription for mesalazine; was there anything else you have been wondering about? Is there anything in particular that has been worrying you?

Sense ☐ — I sense that you are very keen to get treatment from the surgery; are you concerned that you may need to go to hospital?

O/E ☐ — I'd like to check your heart rate, blood pressure and temperature, and feel your tummy for tenderness. Would it be okay for me to examine you?

Summary ☐ — So, you have been feeling unwell for 3 days and have bloody diarrhoea. You have been opening your bowels around 7 times a day. You are known to have ulcerative colitis and, in the past, enemas have helped settle your symptoms. You need to get better quickly as you have a wedding to go to at the weekend but you don't want to go to hospital as you are looking after the family dog whilst your parents are away.

Impression ☐ — I agree with you that this is probably a flare of ulcerative colitis. However, due to the number of times you are opening your bowels, the presence of blood in your stools and your high temperature and raised pulse rate, I feel it would be better if you are checked out in hospital. What do you think?

Explanation ☐ — There is a scoring system which helps us decide how severe a flare of colitis is. Your symptoms and examination indicate that this is a severe attack of colitis. Severe colitis usually needs intravenous treatment which can only be done in hospital. You may need antibiotics and fluids as well as medication to settle down the colitis.

Empathy ☐ — It must be frustrating and worrying to become ill when you have exciting plans and a dog to care for, but it's likely that the fastest way to get you better is to go into hospital and follow the specialist's recommendations.

Options ☐ — I would advise going into hospital as you could become seriously ill without the right treatment. Could you ask a neighbour, friend or your girlfriend to look after your dog?

Future ☐ — I will phone the on-call medical team to arrange admission and give you a letter to take with you. Do you have someone who could drive you?

Safety net ☐ — If you become more poorly on the way to hospital, stop and phone an ambulance.

Digestive Health – 4

Patient's Story

Inflammatory Bowel Disease

Doctor's notes	Anthony Carlisle, 26 years. PMH: Ulcerative colitis. Medication: Mesalazine SR 2 g daily
	Letter from consultant – all well 6 months ago.
How to act	In discomfort, impatient for a script.
PC	*'Doctor, I'm having a flare-up of my ulcerative colitis. Please can I have some more mesalazine enemas?'*
History	Three days ago you started with some left-sided abdominal pain and your stools became looser. Yesterday you opened your bowels seven times and passed bloody diarrhoea. You are feeling unwell this morning and have already opened your bowels three times. When you have had minor flares in the past, you have responded well to topical treatment (mesalazine liquid enemas).
	You have not been eating well recently and have forgotten a couple of tablets since your mum has been away and not checking up on you.
	You have not been admitted to hospital since the UC was first diagnosed.
Social	You live with your parents as you are saving up for a deposit to buy a house with your girlfriend. Your parents are away on holiday at present; you are looking after the family dog. You work in a restaurant as a barman. You have had to phone in sick for the last couple of days. You are supposed to be attending a family wedding at the weekend so are really keen to get some treatment so you can go.
ICE	You are concerned that you will miss the wedding; you have been looking forward to going for months. You want the doctor to give you a prescription. You are not keen on the idea of going to hospital. You are supposed to be looking after the family dog. If the doctor is helpful, interested and explains her concern to you, accept admission.
Examination	Abdomen very tender on the left side, no peritonism.
	HR 110 bpm. BP 126/74
	Temperature 38.0°C
	RR 16 Sats 99%.

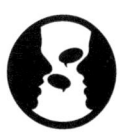

Learning Points — Inflammatory Bowel Disease

Ulcerative colitis (UC)[1,2]

Inflammation/ulceration starts in the rectum and extends proximally to different degrees in different patients.

Incidence	2 peaks of incidence – 15–25 years and 55–65 years.
Common symptoms	Rectal bleeding or bloody diarrhoea, abdominal pain, frequency, urgency and tenesmus.
Associated conditions	Primary sclerosing cholangitis, autoimmune liver disease, seronegative arthritis, ankylosing spondylitis, sacroiliitis, scleritis, episcleritis and anterior uveitis, erythema nodosum and pyoderma gangrenosum.
Investigations	FBC, U&E, LFT, ESR, CRP, stool culture, faecal calprotectin.
	Referral for imaging/endoscopy and biopsy.

The severity of UC in adults. The table is adapted from Truelove & Witts' Severity Index[3]

Feature	Mild–Moderate	Severe
Bowel movements/day	<6	≥6 + a feature of systemic upset
Blood in stool	Small amount or intermittent	Large amount or continuous
Pyrexia	No	Yes
HR >90 bpm	No	Yes
Anaemia	No	Yes
ESR (mm/hour)	≤30	>30
Abdominal tenderness	No	Yes

Crohn's disease[4]

Can affect any part of the GI tract from the mouth to the rectum, most commonly the ileum.

Incidence	Two peaks of incidence: 16–30 years and 60–80 years.
Presenting symptoms	Diarrhoea, blood or mucus in stools, weight loss, lethargy, abdominal pain.

Managing IBD – specialist led

For both Ulcerative Colitis (UC) and Crohn's, most management decisions will be made in secondary care, however see the link below.

Monitoring and shared care protocols

The drugs most frequently used require monitoring. Be aware that shared care protocols for these may exist in your area. We suggest medication review dates should not be reset for more than 3–6 months and, when you are issuing medications, recent blood test results should be checked.

> See the **Link Hub at CompleteCSA.co.uk** for a useful link to: **Monitoring guidance for immunomodulators**
>
> **The management of UC** according to the severity of the acute illness (a useful article which includes a helpful algorithm)

Doctor's Notes

Patient Margaret Simpson 54 years F
PMH No medical history
Medications No current medication
Allergies No information
Consultations 3 months ago. Well woman check with Health Care Assistant. *'Feeling well, no issues, aware needs to lose weight, considering Slimming World. Teetotal. Non-smoker. For routine bloods then review with doctor.'*

1 month ago. Telephone call with the GP. *'Explanation of LFTs given. Agreed repeat tests and then follow up with GP.'*

Investigations BP 135/80 HR 88

BMI 36

Hb 128 g/L   Platelets 300 × 10^9/L   WCC 6 × 10^9/L

Na 140 mmol/L   K 3.8 mmol/L   Urea 7 mmol/L
Creatinine 80 µmol/L

Bilirubin 20 µmol/L   (3–21 µmol/L)
Albumin 35 g/L   (35–50 g/L)
ALP 250 IU/L   (40–150 IU/L)
ALT 75 IU/L   (0–55 IU/L)

HbA1c 42 mmol/mol

Total cholesterol 7.2 mmol/L

Filing comment: 'abnormal LFT, Repeat 4 weeks.'

Repeat bloods: Bilirubin 17 µmol/L, Albumin 36 g/L ALP 237 IU/L ALT 88 IU/L.

Reviewed by locum colleague who arranged an USS:

'Normal sized liver. Bright echo texture of liver parenchyma consistent with fatty infiltration. Normal gallbladder and biliary tree.'

Household Rory Simpson 56 years M

Example Consultation — Abnormal LFTs

Open — I can see that you are keen for your results, but first would you mind telling me what led to these tests being done? Have you been feeling unwell in any way? What did the GP explain to you during your telephone consultation a month ago?

History — Do you have any medical history? It is helpful to know more about your lifestyle. We have been looking more closely at the liver. The USS suggests there is excess fat in the liver which is likely to be the cause of the abnormal results.

ICE — Have you had any thoughts about what could have caused the abnormal test result? Have you been worried about anything in particular? Was there anything specific you hoped I would do today?

Risk — I need to ask quite personal questions; these are necessary to rule out certain conditions. Do you drink any alcohol? Are you taking any medication? Have you ever taken illegal drugs? Is there any family history of liver problems? Do you have any tattoos or piercings? Have you ever taken part in sexual activities which may put you at risk of catching an infection?

Flags — Have you lost any weight recently? Have you had any tummy pain? Any change in your stools? Any swelling of your tummy? Any swelling of your legs?

Sense — I sense you are concerned there is something seriously wrong. Is this because of your uncle?

Summary — So, you came for a routine health check which picked up slightly abnormal liver tests. You are worried that you may develop cirrhosis like your uncle, although you don't understand why as you do not drink alcohol. Is that correct?

O/E — Before we discuss your result further, would it be okay if I examined your tummy, to feel the size of the liver and to look for other signs of liver problems?

Impression — The USS has shown that there is too much fat in your liver. I suspect this is the cause of the abnormal blood tests, rather than it being due to alcohol or infection. Thankfully, you don't have any signs of severe liver disease and your liver is still making protein as it should.

Explanation — The liver is responsible for cleaning toxins out of the blood, storing energy and making proteins, cholesterol and bile for digestion. Sometimes fat is laid down in the liver which irritates it and can cause it to become inflamed. Fat in the liver is very common, particularly in people who are overweight or have high cholesterol or diabetes. In most cases losing weight and lowering cholesterol can help but, sometimes, the liver can develop scar tissue and in a few of these cases cirrhosis, which is irreversible, can develop.

Empathy — I would imagine with your personal experience of cirrhosis this could be quite scary.

Options — Usually the first step would be gradual weight loss (around 1–2 lb/week) and abstinence from alcohol. I would like to do a couple of other blood tests to ensure there is no infection or high iron levels, to check the blood's clotting system is normal and to check for conditions where your body attacks the liver so we can be confident the abnormal bloods are due to fat. Is that okay? I'm sorry, it involves further blood tests.

Empower — Do you have any thoughts about how you could lose some weight? You could see our practice nurse for some advice? I understand that you were hoping to see a specialist but, at present, I don't feel that is necessary unless the test results suggest an alternative diagnosis.

Future — Are you happy to see me after the next set of tests so I can explain the results and answer any further questions you may have after you have had time to think about what we have said today? I will provide reading material on the suspected diagnosis.

Safety net — If you develop any abdominal pain or swelling or feel unwell, please come back sooner.

Patient's Story

Abnormal LFTs

Doctor's notes	Margaret Simpson, 54 years. PMH: None. Medications: None. Recent well woman check, abnormal LFT, cholesterol and USS, suggestive of fatty liver.
How to act	Concerned.
PC	*'I've come to find out what's wrong with my liver.'*
History	You are usually fit and well and try to avoid coming to the doctors. You had put off your 'well woman' health check as you thought you would get lectured about your weight. You are aware that you are overweight and have been thinking about going to Slimming World and joining the gym.
	You were shocked that you needed a repeat liver test because it was abnormal. The last GP said that the tests were probably abnormal due to your weight but decided to arrange an USS to check.
	You have come in today to discuss this.
Social	You are a housewife; you have two children who have both 'flown the nest'. Your husband works for a large manufacturing company in their head office in London. You don't smoke or drink alcohol but you often eat out with your friends or meet up for coffee and cake. Your uncle died of cirrhosis due to alcoholism; he suffered a miserable demise which is partly why you do not drink.
ICE	You are worried that there is something serious wrong with your liver. You are frightened that you will end up dying like your uncle. You are confused as you do not drink alcohol. You wish to be referred to a liver specialist, even if this means being referred privately. However, if the doctor adequately reassures you, then you will accept that this isn't necessary.
Examination	No stigmata of liver disease. Abdomen soft and non-tender, liver and spleen not enlarged. No ascites.

Digestive Health – 5

Learning Points — Abnormal LFTs

Non-alcoholic fatty liver disease[1]
Stage 1: Steatosis (excessive fat laid down in the liver)
Stage 2: Non-alcoholic steatohepatitis (NASH) – inflammation and cell damage due to excess fat
Stage 3: Fibrosis
Stage 4: Cirrhosis

Risk factors for NAFLD — Diabetes, obesity, metabolic syndrome.

Risk factors for liver disease — Drugs, alcohol, viral hepatitis, autoimmune, FH haemochromatosis, Wilson's disease. Iatrogenic (e.g. statins).

Stigmata of liver disease — Ascites, jaundice, spider naevi, palmar erythema, Dupuytren's contracture, finger clubbing.

Liver screen — Hepatitis C antibody, hepatitis B surface antigen, transferrin saturation, anti-nuclear antibody, antimitochondrial antibody, anti-smooth muscle antibody, immunoglobulins, α1-antitrypsin *and others*.[1]

NAFLD suspected — You will need the following: Age, BMI, albumin, AST, ALT, HbA1c and FBC to calculate the NAFLD score – http://www.nafldscore.com/

If there is a raised NAFLD score refer for a fibroscan, or to the liver team for detection of fibrosis if direct referral for a fibroscan is not available.

Disease	Suspect when
Alcoholic liver disease	AST>ALT, macrocytosis, low platelets, raised GGT
Chronic hepatitis B/C	Risk factors: IVDU, blood transfusion, tattoos/piercings especially abroad, unsafe sexual practices or paying for sex. HBsAg positive or HCV antibody positive. Then check HBeAg/eAb, HBV DNA, HCV RNA.
Haemochromatosis	Raised ferritin and transferrin saturation. Low TIBC
Wilson's disease	Neurological signs (e.g. tremor, involuntary movements) Kayser-Fleischer rings caused by raised copper. Low ceruloplasmin
Autoimmune hepatitis	Anti-smooth muscle antibodies and anti-nuclear antibodies are present. Anaemia. Raised: bilirubin, IgG, ESR, ALT and AST and prothrombin time Associated with other autoimmune conditions.
Primary sclerosing cholangitis	Raised ALP, AST and bilirubin. Associated with IBD.
Primary biliary cirrhosis	Consider if high ALP, raised IgM and anti-mitochondrial antibodies. AST/ALT may rise in the later stages.

The above diseases will require referral to the liver team.

See the **Link Hub at CompleteCSA.co.uk** for links to a useful article guiding the GP on **Abnormal LFTs**.

CHAPTER 16 OVERVIEW
Drug and Alcohol Abuse

	Cases in this chapter	Within the RCGP curriculum: Care of People who Misuse Drugs and Alcohol RCGP Curriculum Online March 2016[1]	Learning points in the chapter include:
1	Sleeping Tablets	'Assess each patient's awareness of their drug and alcohol use (including addiction-related problems) and the consequences to them and others'	Benzodiazepines
2	Alcohol and Safeguarding	'Be aware of urgent and important issues of safety including risks to self or others and the need for urgent medical or psychiatric care'	Harmful drinking Hazardous drinking Alcohol dependence Safeguarding
3	Domestic Violence	'Understand the home and family circumstances of the patient and look for hidden harm to children or vulnerable adults'	Domestic violence Child protection
4	Opiate Abuse	'Assess their motivation for seeking help and how they want things to change'	NICE Guidance. Drug misuse in over 16s: psychosocial interventions. Jul 2007
5	Harmful Drinking	'Take an adequate drug and alcohol history including the physical, mental, social and legal aspects' 'Understand the varying degrees of drug and alcohol use and their implications for future management'	NICE Guidance. Alcohol-use disorders: diagnosis, assessment and management of harmful drinking and alcohol dependence. Feb 2011

1. http://www.rcgp.org.uk/training-exams/gp-curriculum-overview/online-curriculum/managing-complex-care/3-14-drugs-and-alcohol-misuse.aspx

CHAPTER 16 REFERENCES

Alcohol and Safeguarding
1. https://www.nice.org.uk/guidance/PH24/chapter/8-Glossary#harmful-drinking

Opiate Abuse
1. NICE Guidelines CG51. Drug misuse in over 16s: psychosocial interventions. Jul 2007.
2. https://www.oxford.gov.uk/directory/3/homlessness_survival_guide/category/35

Harmful Drinking
1. NICE Guidelines. CG115 Alcohol-use disorders: diagnosis, assessment and management of harmful drinking and alcohol dependence. Feb 2011.
2. 'Note that the evidence for acamprosate in the treatment of harmful drinkers and people who are mildly alcohol dependent is less robust than that for naltrexone. At the time of publication (February 2011), acamprosate did not have UK marketing authorisation for this indication. Informed consent should be obtained and documented.'[1]
3. 'At the time of publication (February 2011), oral naltrexone did not have UK marketing authorisation for this indication. Informed consent should be obtained and documented.'[1]
4. 'All prescribers should consult the SPC for a full description of the contraindications and the special considerations of … disulfiram.'[1]
5. Sherwood Forrest Hospitals NHS Foundation Trust. Alcohol: How to reduce your intake safely. Patient information. Jul 2010. http://www.sfh-tr.nhs.uk/images/docs/pil/adlt/piadlt005.pdf

Doctor's Notes

Patient   Ella Jones   42 years   F
PMH   Insomnia
Medications Zopiclone 7.5 mg – 14 tablets last prescribed 3 weeks ago
Allergies   No information
Consultations No recent consultations
Investigations No recent investigations
Household   No household members registered

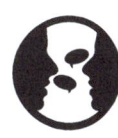

Example Consultation — Sleeping Tablets

Open ☐	Tell me more about your sleep disturbance … and evening routine? What have you tried?
Impact ☐	How does this impact on your life? What do you think about when you can't sleep?
History ☐	Tell me about the pressures you are under. How's life at home? Do you live alone? Are you active? I see that you were given 2 weeks of tablets 3 weeks ago. You are requiring them most days?
Flags ☐	Is your mood okay? Do you suffer with anxiety? Do you drink much alcohol or caffeine? How do you feel in the morning? Do you feel groggy when you need to drive?
ICE ☐	What do you think may be causing the problem with sleeping? Has anything else happened or upset you? What worries you about this sleeping problem? Is there anything else on your mind or anything you have been wondering? Have you had any thoughts regarding what else you could try?
Sense ☐	I hear that you feel you've made an informed decision that this is the right thing for you at present.
Curious ☐	I'm thinking longer term also – what are your thoughts about the future plan for these tablets?
Summary ☐	To summarise, you have always struggled with sleep and, despite trying all the sleep hygiene advice, only the zopiclone 7.5 mg tablet helps. Without it you fear you cannot get through the next few months which will be stressful and require your attention. You are hoping to continue zopiclone on an infrequent basis, as required, as you feel you have no alternative.
Empathy ☐	I appreciate it must be horrible not having any sleep. This is especially difficult when you have your level of responsibility at school. You have also followed all the doctor's advice diligently.
Impression ☐	It sounds as if you suffer with insomnia, exacerbated by recent stress at work.
Experience ☐	Can you please explain to me what you know about the risks of these tablets?
Explanation ☐	If I may explain again the risks of these tablets. Even after a few weeks there is the risk your body becomes tolerant. The sleeping tablets are then no longer effective, only increasing your risk of poor concentration, poor memory, poor coordination and low mood. Although the body has become tolerant, without them you cannot sleep due to the rebound effect of stopping them abruptly. So it seems you cannot be without them. We need to prevent the pattern of tolerance then rebound withdrawal. It may take a few weeks of being free from them before your body finds its natural rhythm. What are your thoughts about this?
Options ☐	We could change the tablet to a longer-acting tablet to avoid withdrawal symptoms; however, side effects may last all day. How do you think longer-acting tablets may affect you at work? An alternative is an antihistamine used for insomnia, promethazine, in the interim.
Future ☐	To safely wean, I suggest zopiclone 3.75 mg for 2 weeks, then use the 3.75 mg tablets then promethazine on alternative nights for a week, then change to promethazine only when required. Is that okay? Do you feel you can try this now? Okay, we could wait until after Ofsted and then try this in 2 months' time.
Empower ☐	Do you think it's reasonable to plan that sleeping tablets are not lifelong? I wonder if you may be interested in CBT … Have you come across this? It is a course designed to help change patterns of thinking and behaviour and can be effective in insomnia. Also avoid strenuous exercise in the few hours before sleep.
Safety net ☐	If you ever feel sleepy, or your coordination does not feel 100%, you must not drive. If you ever feel unwell, for example with palpitations or dizziness, this can be due to the tablets, so please see a doctor. All the best with the next Ofsted meeting.

Drug and Alcohol Abuse – 1

Patient's Story

Sleeping Tablets

Doctor's notes Ella Jones, 42 years. PMH: Insomnia.

Medications: Zopiclone 7.5 mg – 14 tablets last prescribed 3 weeks ago.

How to act Relaxed but pushy.

You are planning to reassure the doctor that you will be safe with the tablets.

PC *'Doctor, I need some more sleeping tablets please. I just need them occasionally.'*

History You have always been a terrible sleeper and over the past year it has become worse.

You were first prescribed sleeping tablets 3 months ago.

You were busy at work and they helped. These days, you do not sleep without them.

You may manage 3 hours between 3 and 6 am. You have a healthy lifestyle and eat well.

You tried the 3.75 mg tablets but these did nothing.

You take the tablet every school night and just put up with the problem at the weekend.

Social You are the headmistress of a school. You have just been given bad ratings by Ofsted and you have further reports to write and further meetings planned in 2 months' time.

You have no children of your own.

You have a female partner and you are both very happy.

You go to yoga and enjoy playing hockey or going for a run in the evening.

You don't drink alcohol or caffeine. You relax, read a book and avoid the computer.

ICE You are concerned that without the tablets you will not be able to function.

You especially need them at the moment due to the stress at work.

You are worried the doctor will stop giving them to you.

You have tried all the sleep hygiene advice GPs have suggested.

You expect the doctor will be concerned …

'I thought you may want to counsel me regarding the risks. I appreciate the risks of addiction but I will only take them when I need them, not every night and it's really important I have them please.'

You are happy to negotiate with the doctor.

Suggest after 2 months you will limit the use to twice weekly.

However, if the doctor explains the risks and understands your situation, agree that you will try to wean off them completely.

You cannot try a long-acting benzodiazepine as you need to drive and function through the day.

Drug and Alcohol Abuse – 1

Learning Points

Benzodiazepines

Negotiate a plan to reach a mutual agreement.

Wean **benzodiazepines** (zopiclone may have similar effects) gradually to prevent: anxiety, panic, depression, palpitations, malaise and seizures.

Withdrawal symptoms may commence up to a week after stopping longer-acting benzodiazepines.

This consultation requires patient education and negotiation after gaining an understanding of the person's individual circumstances.

Converting shorter-acting benzodiazepines (e.g. nitrazepam, temazepam and lorazepam) to longer-acting benzodiazepines (e.g. diazepam) may be required before initiating a gradual weaning process over a period of weeks to months depending on the dose. Note some patients may be concerned with using longer-acting benzodiazepines due to side effects and therefore potential restrictions of driving.

The BNF contains information regarding withdrawing benzodiazepines (hypnotics and anxiolytics chapter) including the approximate equivalent doses when compared to diazepam. Remember you are permitted to take the BNF into the examination to refer to when you need to do so.

> See the **Link Hub at CompleteCSA.co.uk** for a useful link to **Dose conversions of benzodiazepines**

Drug and Alcohol Abuse – 1

Doctor's Notes

Patient	Kirsty West	38 years	F
PMH	No known medical history		
Medications	No current medications		
Allergies	No information		
Consultations	No recent consultations		
Investigations	No recent investigations		
Household	Simeon West	42 years	M
	Rose West	11 years	F
	Toby West	6 years	M

Example Consultation — Alcohol and Safeguarding

Open ☐	(Nod and silence.) … Tell me the story from when this began.
History ☐	How is your husband's health? How is his mood? And how about you? Do you work? Do you have any close family or friends? Are they aware? Do you drink any alcohol? What has made you come today; has something happened?
Flags ☐	Is there any violence in the home? How have the children reacted? Does your husband drive? Does your husband take care of the children alone? Does he ever take drugs?
Impact ☐	What impact has his drinking had on you? Your relationship? The children? How are you coping financially?
Sense ☐	I can see how exhausting this is for you.
ICE ☐	What has been going through your mind? What makes you feel most upset? Did you have any hopes of what we may decide today?
Curious ☐	Why have you not asked your family for help? Are you close to them? How may they react? Do you feel there is risk of violence if your husband knew you were speaking to me?
Summary ☐	To summarise, you are very concerned about the amount your husband is drinking and the impact this is having on your family. You are worried he won't find work and that home life will continue to be stressful. You are aware the children are having to make their own meals and you have felt too embarrassed to inform your parents. You were hoping I could speak to your husband. You don't know what else to do.
Empathy ☐	Kirsty, I can see this is a really difficult situation. You feel the pressure of running the home is on you and you recognise your husband may be depressed and you want to seek help for your family.
Impression ☐	It sounds as if your husband is drinking a harmful amount; he may be depressed too.
Options ☐	To begin with, I could call your husband. You have done the right thing seeking help. There is much that we can do to help your husband: support, medication, counselling and advice. As a couple, you may also wish to go to relationship counselling. I wonder if your children need someone to talk to? I am concerned that the children are having to make their own meals. When any children are involved I have a duty to inform the safeguarding team, social services. I can see you are upset; what is going through your mind?
Experience ☐	What do you know about social services?
Explanation ☐	I appreciate this is not what you were expecting but I believe this would be a positive step toward moving forward. This team will be able to provide you with support during this time of crisis. Social services aim to help families through difficult times and not take children from their parents. Your husband sounds unwell and it seems you would welcome additional help. Do I have your support to inform this team so they can contact you to make their assessment and offer help?
Empower ☐	Would you be able to discuss our conversation with your husband? What do you think he'll say? If he will not come in to see me, I could visit. As well as involving your parents, I wonder if you need a work note so you can either leave work early or have time off work if you feel you need to relieve this pressure. We have identified many options today. Out of these options can you summarise how you would like to proceed? Good!
Future ☐	We should meet again with your husband within the week. Shall we aim to do this?
Safety net ☐	If ever you feel there is a risk to anyone, including your husband, contact the police or your GP.

Drug and Alcohol Abuse – 2

Patient's Story

Alcohol and Safeguarding

Doctor's notes	Kirsty West, 38 years. PMH: None. Medication: None.
How to act	Concerned. Articulate. You are mentally and physically well.
PC	*'Doctor, I want to talk about my husband's drinking.'*
History	He is in good health but has started drinking half a bottle of whisky every night.
	He was made redundant last year and can't find a job. You are worried and angry.
	Your life has changed as he has stopped interacting with the children and you feel the pressure. Your relationship is strained as you are often angry with him.
	There is no violence in the home. You think he is depressed.
	You are looking after the children, running the home as well as bringing in the income.
	You are not depressed, *'just fed up with it'*.
	Last night he fell over. He was not injured but the children started to cry.
Social	You work full time in the pharmacy as an assistant and return home at 7 pm. You drink no alcohol. Your children are 6 and 11 years old. You have no time for hobbies.
	Your family are close by. You've felt too embarrassed to tell your parents about the problem.
ICE	*'I don't know what to do.'*
	You are worried he will never get a job now and you can't see life getting better.
	'Will you come to the house to see him? He may listen to you.'
	If the doctor asks you to bring him in, you tell him or her that you don't think he will come in. However, if the doctor arranges a phone call with your husband, you think this may encourage him to attend. If the doctor asks you to persuade him, you will try.
	If asked, you feel the children are starting to become withdrawn and spending more time in their rooms.
	He is not violent. He is home alone with the children after school and on Saturdays.
	He does not drive. The children return home on the school bus.
	He sometimes makes their tea but often the older child is making them beans on toast.
	If the doctor mentions contacting social services, start to cry. Tell the doctor the children are safe. Then suggest you will inform your parents who can look after the children.
	Plead with the doctor not to inform social services and be angry – you have come for help! If the doctor asks what you are thinking, say: *'We are not bad parents.'*
	If the doctor makes suggestions, a work note for altered hours for you whilst your husband seeks help or explains why he or she is informing social services, agree you need help. You accept any suggestions offered. You believe your husband will accept help when he is aware of how serious this is.

Learning Points   Alcohol and Safeguarding

Harmful drinking   'A pattern of alcohol consumption that is causing mental or physical damage.'[1]

Hazardous drinking   'A pattern of alcohol consumption that increases someone's risk of harm. Some would limit this definition to the physical or mental health consequences (as in harmful use). Others would include the social consequences. The term is currently used by WHO to describe this pattern of alcohol consumption. It is not a diagnostic term.'[1]

Alcohol dependence   'A cluster of behavioural, cognitive and physiological factors that typically include a strong desire to drink alcohol and difficulties in controlling its use. Someone who is alcohol-dependent may persist in drinking, despite harmful consequences. They will also give alcohol a higher priority than other activities and obligations. For further information, please refer to: "Diagnostic and statistical manual of mental disorders" (DSM-IV) (American Psychiatric Association 2000) and "International statistical classification of diseases and related health problems – 10th revision" (ICD-10) (World Health Organization 2007).'[1]

Safeguarding

This case required the doctor to negotiate regarding the home visit and the safeguarding referral.

It can be difficult to decide when social services should be involved. If you are considering it, it is likely that a referral is required and, if safe to do so, make your thoughts known to the patient (and examiner). You may signpost that you will seek advice from your safeguarding lead and be in touch with the patient/relative again.

Safeguarding teams ask that you gain consent from the parent before making the referral. You can also proceed without consent if this is not forthcoming.

Doctor's Notes

Patient   Isabel Forster   33 years   F
PMH   Fracture of thumb 1 year ago
Medications   None
Allergies   No information
Consultations   No recent consultations
Investigations No recent investigations
Household   No household members registered

Example Consultation — Domestic Violence

Open ☐ / **ICE** ☐ — Okay, this is a good time to come in and discuss that. What are your thoughts about this? Have you had thoughts about what may be delaying a pregnancy? Are you worried? What would you like to happen?

Sense ☐ — I am sensing David is more concerned about this than you. Is that right?

Curious ☐ — What discussions have you had as a couple? Do you argue? Do you want to have a baby?

History ☐ — Are you worried about your health? Do you: take any medicines? Work? Have regular periods? How often do you have sex? Have you ever had an STI? When were you last checked? What made you have an STI check? How is your relationship now? What else do you argue about? Is David violent? Tell more about that. Do you have any support from family/friends? Can you confide in them? Do you feel isolated? Do you drink alcohol? Or take drugs? Do you own your house? Do you have your own access to money? What do you enjoy doing? Would you like to investigate your fertility? Thank you for sharing this with me.

Flags ☐ — Questions about David … Does he work? Does he hit you? Has he used objects to hurt you? Does he force himself sexually on you? Is anyone else aware? Does he spend time with children? What is he capable of? Do you feel that your life is at risk? Has he ever been arrested? Has he threatened to kill you or someone else? Does he have any mental health problems? How much alcohol does he drink? What about drugs? Thank you for telling me. I appreciate it must be upsetting to talk about. Is the abuse getting worse? He is in the waiting room; do you feel he is controlling you? How is your mood? Do you ever have thoughts that life if not worth living? Have you ever tried to self-harm or commit suicide? Have you ever made plans to? Do you have any other injuries? Has he harmed himself? Have you tried to leave before?

Impact ☐ — How do the violence and unkind words you receive affect you?

Summary ☐ — To summarise, David is keen for a family but because of the violence in the relationship you are taking the depo injection to give you time to think about your options.

Impression ☐ — It sounds like you do not feel safe in your home.

Explanation ☐ — Violence in the home is just as illegal as violence in the streets.

Empathy ☐ — This must be very difficult for you to talk about. It can also be frightening telling someone.

ICE ☐ — What are your thoughts about your options? What would you like to happen? Are you starting to think about planning to leave? What frightens you? What do you need? Have you thought about telling the police?

Experience ☐ — Have you heard of any support groups? Are there family/friends who may be able to help?

Options ☐ — I am here to inform you of your options and the support available. If you are thinking of leaving there are a lot of people to help: Domestic Violence helpline, Women's Aid, GP, Freedom Programme, Recovery Toolkit, Sanctuary Scheme. Would you like time in our quiet room to read this information before you go back into the waiting room?

Empower ☐ — We need to give you the control back. Have a think about what steps you would like to take.

Future ☐ — Would you like to meet again next week? What will you tell David?

Safety net ☐ — I have a sticker which looks like a barcode which has a crisis number on it – put it on something like a lipstick. If you ever feel you need help you could call this number, your GP, 111 or the police.

Drug and Alcohol Abuse – 3

Patient's Story

Domestic Violence

Doctor's notes	Isabel Forster, 33 years. PMH: Fracture of thumb 1 year ago. Medications: None.
How to act	Very quiet. You have a concern that you have not shared with anyone else.
PC	*'Doctor, we've been trying for a baby for over a year now.'*
History	You are well. Fracture of the thumb after a trip 1 year ago.
	You have regular periods. No STIs and smears are up to date.
	You have had no other sexual relationships since this relationship with David.
	'David thought I should come. He is in the waiting room.'
	If the doctor offers for him to come in decline, saying he is busy with his emails.
	'He thinks something must be wrong.'
Social	You met David 4 years ago. You work in the kitchen of the local primary school.
	David is a building manager for large corporation sites. He has no children.
	You drink no alcohol and take no drugs. David drinks *'too much'* alcohol.
ICE	You tell the doctor it is likely that you haven't fallen pregnant because David is often at work or you have been busy around the time of ovulation.
	'I'm not worried. I know it takes time. I'm not sure now is the right time anyway.'
	'We argue about it.' If asked why, say you feel you should wait until you have bought a house.
	'I thought maybe have some blood tests, that is what David would like.'

If the doctor responds to cues or senses that there is more you want to tell him or her …

David is violent towards you. You have been taking the contraceptive injection every 3 months at family planning since your coil was removed 1 year ago. You would like to leave the relationship but you are waiting for the right time. You have no concerns about your health. You had a GUM check 6 months ago because you were concerned David may have had an affair. It was normal. David drinks large amounts after work. He says hurtful things, e.g. that you are fat and ugly. He has never used a weapon and has never hurt another person or animal. He sometimes apologises and can be very loving. He takes no drugs. He has no access to children. He has never been involved with the police. He doesn't drink and drive. You do not feel he would kill anyone including yourself. You want to start thinking about ending the relationship. You tried before and he got very angry then very remorseful and loving. You were scared and you stayed. He is controlling. He pushes himself on you for sex but you do not resist. You need time to think about how and when to leave. One year ago you broke your thumb after he pushed you into a radiator. Your mood is okay. You have lived with his aggression for years. You have never had suicidal thoughts. You have a best friend whom you may now tell. You have no money. You don't know where you would go or how you would pay for rent if you lost your job. You will lie to him and say you have an appointment next week for blood tests.

Drug and Alcohol Abuse – 3

Learning Points   Domestic Violence

Opportunities to discuss domestic violence

Asking about relationships is part of any social history. The doctor should always be prepared to sensitively ask about DV if there are any concerns or it crosses the doctor's mind.

There are many opportunities to ask about DV: injury, pregnancy, contraception, pain (e.g. abdominal) and repeated minor illness.

Raising DV:
- *'Tell me more about your relationship. Do you often argue?'*
- *'Does he/she ever say or do anything that upsets you?'*
- *'Do you ever feel threatened by anyone at home?'*
- *'Is there any violence in the home?'*

Be aware of your local support groups for domestic violence.

Child protection

Establish whether there was a child protection concern:
- *'Does he/she have any contact with children?'*
- *'Do any children witness the violence?'*
- *'Has a child been hurt?'*
- *'How are the children getting on?'*
- *'How are they getting on at school?'*
- *'Is there any pet abuse?'*

Ensure immediate reporting to the local safeguarding team if another adult or child is at risk.

Suggestions of how to approach a consultation if the person presenting is the perpetrator, not the victim:
- *'You have honestly explained when you feel angry you …'*
- *'And recognise this is serious.'*
- *'It sounds as if you would like to receive help for this?'*
- *'What thoughts have you had?'*
- *'We have local teams … e.g. Give Respect – here is their number.'*
- *'May I ask you to see me again and follow this up …?'*
- *'Could you bring your husband/wife with you next time?'*

Do not collude or offer relationship counselling

Doctor's Notes

Patient	Michaela Butt 32 years F
PMH	2 NVDs – 2 and 3 years ago
	Postnatal depression
	Sciatica
	Referred to the spinal team and now discharged to physiotherapy
	MRI 2 months ago showed minor degenerative changes only
	DNA last physiotherapy appointment
Medications	Morphine Sulphate M/R 30 mg BD. Last issued 60 tablets 20 days ago
	Oramorph 10 mg/5 ml
	Codeine 30 mg
Allergies	No information
Consultations	No recent consultations
Investigations	No recent investigations
Household	Neil Butt 38 years M
	Jasmine Butt 3 years F
	Joseph Butt 2 years M

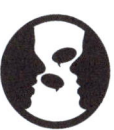

Example Consultation

Opiate Abuse

Open ☐	Tell me more about the pain from when it began. And the nature of the pain? Have you noticed any other symptoms? Tell me please exactly how and when you take each of your medicines.
History ☐	Tell me about any medical problems you have had? I see you had depression …? How is your mood now? How do you spend your days? Who is at home with you? What can you do yourself? Do you drink alcohol?
Flags ☐	Have you injured your back? Does the pain wake you? Is there weakness in your legs? Do you lose control of going to the toilet? Have you lost weight? Are you running any fevers?
Impact ☐	What impact has your pain had on life? What can you no longer do? What makes the pain worse?
ICE ☐	What are your thoughts regarding the cause of your back pain? How can we make progress? What do you think stops your back from recovering? What are you most worried about? What did you think we may decide?
Experience ☐	What is your understanding of what they found on the MRI?
Sense ☐	Do you feel angry? Tell me more about why.
Curious ☐	Do you see things getting better in the future? Did you enjoy being able to do more in the past? Why would going to work make you depressed? Do you fear becoming depressed again? What stress do you have in your life?
Summary ☐	It sounds as if you have made great progress with your mood but your back prevents you from living an active life. You fear that going back to work would make your back worse and make you ill again with depression. You haven't done the exercises and didn't attend your physiotherapy as this all increases the pain.
Impression ☐	You have a small amount of wear and tear in your back, as seen on the MRI.
Explanation ☐	It's a worry how much pain relief you require. We obviously need to change how we help you. You have a responsibility to keep the tablets safe, especially when you have two small children.
Empathy ☐	You are in a lot of pain and have had a difficult couple of years. I want to help you today but also aim to get you better in the long term. Is this something you could work towards with me?
Options ☐	I suggest we set up an agreement to prescribe you 1 month of tablets on repeat but you will not be able to collect the tablets early. In the meantime, if you are in pain take 5 ml of your Oramorph. Please keep a record of when you need extra. Then we may need to change your background pain relief. Does that sound okay? You should take the Oramorph instead of codeine. You should not be on both codeine and morphine. Also I will add paracetamol. I appreciate that paracetamol alone doesn't help but it works with the morphine. Have you tried an anti-inflammatory, ibuprofen or naproxen? Did you try an additional tablet with this called omeprazole? Would you like to try that again but with this additional tablet to prevent acid in the stomach? It may help reduce any inflammation whereas the other pain relief just masks the pain.
Empower ☐	It is important to keep your back moving. What steps could you take towards getting back to your previous activities? Could you try the exercises half an hour after you have taken some Oramorph? They may make you feel stiff at first but then you should start to see an improvement. Do you think you could try yoga or pilates which will help your core muscle strength, flexibility and aid relaxation? Would you be interested in therapy which helps you feel stronger when you have been worried or anxious, called CBT?
Future ☐	May I refer you to the pain team for advice? Will you attend? Can you meet with me in 1 month? Can I refer you back to physiotherapy? Please attend, otherwise this is an appointment which someone else could have.
Safety net ☐	If you ever lose control of the bowels or bladder, you need to see a doctor straight away. With the plan you have made I'm confident we will make progress.

Drug and Alcohol Abuse – 4

Patient's Story

Opiate Abuse

Doctor's notes Michaela Butt, 32 years. PMH: 2 NVDs – 2 and 3 years ago. Postnatal depression. Sciatica. Referred to the spinal team and now discharged to physiotherapy. MRI 2 months ago showed minor degenerative changes only. DNA last physiotherapy appointment. Medications: Morphine sulphate M/R 30 mg BD. Last issued 60 tablets 20 days ago, Oramorph 10 mg/5 ml, Codeine 30 mg.

How to act Demanding.

PC *'I need more tablets. I lost the others.'*

History You stopped working in the local care home when you had children.

During your pregnancy you suffered with sciatica and pelvic pain.

You have had no injuries. There are no back pain red flags.

'Lifting the kids' makes it worse.

You have an uncomfortable bed and can't afford a new one.

You suffered with postnatal depression. You were seen by the postnatal depression team and you were discharged after your medications stopped.

You are feeling mentally well now.

Your sciatica pain was ongoing after the delivery and you have gradually had to increase your pain relief. The pain radiates down both legs.

You have no neurological symptoms.

You're annoyed the MRI scan didn't show anything.

'No one knows what is causing it.'

You had an appointment with the spinal team who discharged you to physiotherapy.

You do not do the exercises at home as they hurt your back.

You take occasional codeine.

You take your Oramorph twice a day and sometimes take an additional morphine tablet.

You missed your last physiotherapy appointment.

Social Your husband doesn't work. He has to look after the 2 children.

You are both on income support. You do not smoke or drink alcohol.

Your husband does the housework. You make the meals.

ICE You would like more morphine tablets.

You believe the doctors don't know what the problem is.

You are not worried, only that the doctor may tell you to stop taking so many tablets.

Refuse any NSAID – they don't work and make you feel sick.

You did not try it with a PPI and agree to this if offered.

You can't see your back getting better.

You will have to spend your life on these tablets.

You can't do anything due to the pain.

If the doctor tells you not to take extra morphine, say: *'I obviously need more.'*

If the doctor asks about work, the thought of going back to work fills you with dread. Having to get up on cold mornings with a painful back.

'If you make me go back to work I will become depressed again.'

Drug and Alcohol Abuse – 4

Learning Points

Opiate Abuse

NICE Guidance. Drug misuse in over 16s: psychosocial interventions. July 2007

During every contact it is important to build a rapport and work together towards set goals. NICE stresses the importance of respecting the patient and offering continuity of support. Also take every opportunity to provide education for the services available.

Using a motivational interview strategy may be helpful. NICE encourages the patient to identify vulnerable situations where they may be at risk of substance misuse and equips the patient with coping strategies for these challenges. Consider Read Coding the patient as a vulnerable adult and enquire if there are safeguarding concerns in the home.

Coping strategies include self-help (which may be from CBT) as well as help from agencies. Make sure ongoing support is available as well as support in times of crisis.

If patients are asking for more tramadol or codeine tablets than the maximum allowed dose try ... *'I cannot prescribe more than eight tablets a day as I would be prescribing an overdose. Instead we need to decide together whether this is the correct medication for you.'*

Consider a different working diagnosis and psychosocial reasons why the amount of pain the patient is experiencing seems disproportionate to the suspected cause. Consider a referral to the pain clinic or the drug and alcohol team if you feel there is drug misuse or abuse. There are some tactics you can employ to help keep control of opiate prescribing in patients where there is a concern regarding opiate abuse (e.g. drug seeking behaviour or PMH of illegal drug use). Prescribe in small quantities, e.g. weekly scripts. This will help you monitor use, reduce the risk of overdose and, when patients claim to have 'lost' a prescription, they will only have to wait a few days before another can be issued – rather than twisting your arm as they can't manage 3 weeks without the medication. Avoid using long-acting opiates in patients who may still be using intravenous drugs. These increase the risk of overdose as a patient may forget they are wearing a patch or have taken MR oral opiates when they use drugs intravenously. Always get help from an experienced drug/alcohol team as such patients are notoriously difficult to manage. Using patient warnings/pop-ups on the electronic record can also highlight risk of opiate misuse to colleagues who may be unfamiliar with the patient.

Know your local services. Mentioning these services in your CSA will help your management plan.

'Ensure that maintaining the service user's engagement with services remains a major focus of the care plan.'[1]

For example, in Oxford services include:[2]

>GPs with training in drug and alcohol management
>Alcoholics Anonymous (AA)
>Evolve for young people
>FRANK
>Narcotic Anonymous (NA)
>Oxfordshire DAAT (Drug and Alcohol Action Team)
>SMART or SMART (DIP)
>SWOP Scheme
>The Women's Service or Women's Initiative on Street Health

Find out if you have social prescribing coordinators locally to help guide patients in the right direction for community and professional support. Ask them to send you their directory of local services for you to peruse at your leisure – an investment in time!

If you do not have this service, are you struggling to think of a QIP (quality improvement project)? Why not research local services and ask your colleagues for services they use, form a directory and email it to local practices and the CCG with a social prescribing proposal for your practice. *Voilà!*

Drug and Alcohol Abuse – 4

Doctor's Notes

Patient	Katherine Knight	68 years	F
PMH	No medical history		
Medications	None		
Allergies	No information		
Consultations	No recent consultations		
Investigations	No recent investigations		
Household	Barry Knight	63 years	M

Example Consultation — Harmful Drinking

Open ☐	What's prompted seeing me today? Tell me about your drinking pattern. How do you feel about it?
History ☐	Do you drink in the morning? Alone? Are you in good health? Any medicines? Any physical symptoms? Tremors? Stomach changes? Sleep problems? What do you do each day? Tell me about home life. Have you ever not done something expected of you due to drinking? Have you ever started drinking and felt you couldn't stop?
Sense ☐	You seem very sad. I'm interested to know why. Are there people you are close to?
Risk ☐	Do you feel isolated? Have you had any mental health problems/depression? Do you take any drugs?
ICE ☐	What do you think has led to this? What else have you been wondering? Have you known anyone else who struggled with alcohol? What worries do you have? What did you think we may decide today?
Flags ☐	Are there any dangers you can see associated with drinking? Any injuries? Are you down? Any thoughts of life not worth living? Have you acted on them? Do you have plans to end your life? Are either of you violent or unkind? Have you had thoughts of hurting another person? Do you eat well and look after yourself? Do you drive?
Impact ☐	How has this affected your life? Or relationships? Or hobbies?
Curious ☐	What does your husband think about the alcohol? And the relationship? Has it had an impact on him?
Empathy ☐	You've taken a big step today. It must seem like a difficult journey ahead.
Empower ☐	We can help. How would life be different without alcohol? Do you think you can stop? What steps could you take? Why might it be difficult? Who could help? What is your aim? When would you like to achieve that by?
O/E ☐	I'd like to check your BP and pulse, look at your hands and feel your tummy if that is okay?
Summary ☐	To summarise, you've been increasing your consumption of alcohol over 6 months. You feel low and this is due to being alone and bored. You hope to cut down and spend more time with your husband.
Impression ☐	It sounds like you have alcohol dependence and depression.
Experience ☐	What do you know about why alcohol is dangerous?
Explanation ☐	Alcohol affects most parts of the body. As well as damage to the liver it can cause problems with the nerves and the functioning in the brain. Sometimes people can suffer with a dementia-like illness because of alcohol. Alcohol keeps you awake at night. Alcohol is a false friend; it makes you more depressed.
Options ☐	There are things that you can do. It is actually dangerous to stop drinking straight away. We should either cut down gradually or provide support through a detox programme. What are your thoughts about these options? Reducing your alcohol intake by 2–3 units (a large glass of wine) per day is a good starting point. Others can help with your recovery. Your husband, the alcohol team, or Turning Point can support you through the process and, afterwards, Relate are relationship counsellors. Would you be interested in seeing these teams? You may also want to attend AA for ongoing support. I can help by guiding you through the process. I would like to give you some vitamin tablets – thiamine and vitamin B compound. These are really important to prevent you becoming confused and unwell. Can I ask you to see the nurse for some blood tests to check your health?
Future ☐	Can you see me again next week? We can discuss your progress, blood results and do a memory test.
Safety net ☐	If you ever feel you are muddled, or start vomiting or feel shaky or generally unwell, or have thoughts of wanting to hurt yourself or anyone else, can you see a doctor straight away? See you again next week.

Drug and Alcohol Abuse – 5

Patient's Story

Harmful Drinking

Doctor's notes	Katherine Knight, 68 years. PMH: None. Medication: None.
How to act	Speak quietly. Look unhappy. Do not be forthcoming with information.
PC	*'My husband thinks I'm drinking too much.'*
History	You started to drink 1 bottle of wine every night about 6 months ago.
	You just enjoyed it and the amount gradually increased.
	You are bored and don't have anything else to do!
	You sometimes also have a brandy or two. You take no drugs.
	You have always had good health and take no medicines.
	You usually start to drink at lunchtime.
	You feel upset when others mention the alcohol.
	You drink alone. Your husband has stopped drinking *'to make me feel guilty'*.
	You have no physical symptoms that you know of. Your bowels are fine.
	You feel shaky if you don't drink. You drink every day.
	Your appetite is reduced. You often wake through the night.
Social	You spend the day watching TV or you may wander to the supermarket.
	You eat quick meals these days. You do not feel like cooking.
	You have never driven a car.
	Your husband is still working as a caretaker. *'He is too busy to notice.'*
	You have lost touch with friends. You missed a catch-up with a friend as you'd been drinking and fell asleep on the sofa.
ICE	Your husband told you to see your GP.
	Your relationship is not good. He is becoming upset.
	He is polite and kind to you but you feel very alone. You regret not having children.
	You wanted to talk to the GP today but are unsure what you want from the meeting.
	You are worried that you rely on the alcohol. You don't know how to cut down.
	You would like to cut down, but boredom may prevent it.
	However, overall you believe you can, and know your husband will help you.
	You think you are depressed but want no medication.
	You have occasional thoughts that life is not worth living but no plans and you would not attempt suicide.
	You would like to get out of the house more. You would like to do more things together. You agree with the doctor's advice about your relationship and self-help measures.
	You understand that alcohol is bad for the liver.
Examination	All the examination is normal.

Drug and Alcohol Abuse – 5

Learning Points   Harmful Drinking

Perform a risk assessment   Self (neglect, harm, suicide, injury)

Others (the public, children/vulnerable adults)

Assess psychological and social problems:

e.g. mental health problems, work issues, housing issues, driving, criminal activity, relationship problems

Investigations   U&E, LFT, GGT ± FBC and clotting

Questionnaires   AUDIT, SADQ and APQ

Divide who can help into self, GP and others (friends, professionals or support groups (AA or SMART recovery)). Involve families and carers in the recovery process with the patient's consent.

Consider the addition of acamprosate[2] or naltrexone[3] to psychological therapy if this therapy alone has not been successful in mild alcohol dependence.[1] In practice, for most GPs, this will require a referral to the local drug and alcohol team.

When to offer community detox programmes

For those who 'drink over 15 units of alcohol per day and/or who score 20 or more on the AUDIT, consider offering: an assessment for and delivery of a community-based assisted withdrawal, **or** assessment and management in specialist alcohol services if there are safety concerns …'[1]

When to consider inpatient or residential assisted withdrawal[1]

15–30 units/day   and 'significant psychiatric or physical comorbidities …

or a significant learning disability or cognitive impairment'[1]

SADQ score   >30

History of   epilepsy

withdrawal-related seizures

delirium tremens

consuming alcohol and benzodiazepines

'Consider a lower threshold for inpatient or residential assisted withdrawal in vulnerable groups, for example, homeless and older people.'[1]

'After a successful withdrawal for people with moderate and severe alcohol dependence consider offering acamprosate[2] or oral naltrexone[3] in combination with an individual psychological intervention.' … or (3rd line) disulfiram[4] after explaining the risks.[1]

Advise patients wanting to cut down that this should be done slowly to prevent withdrawal symptoms and explain the importance of this to patients. If withdrawal symptoms start to develop, the patient can drink 2 units of alcohol and wait 30 minutes to see the response.[5]

CHAPTER 17
ENT, Oral and Facial

	Cases in this chapter	Within the RCGP curriculum: ENT, Oral and Facial RCGP Curriculum Online March 2016[1]	Learning points in the chapter
1	Facial Nerve Palsy	'Demonstrate empathy and compassion towards patients with ENT symptoms that may prove difficult to manage, e.g. tinnitus, facial pain, unsteadiness'	Causes, natural history and management of facial nerve palsy (Bell's palsy)
2	Otitis Media	'Understand when watchful waiting and the use of delayed prescriptions are indicated'	Management of otitis media and externa
3	Snoring	'Understand the significant quality-of-life impairment that may arise from common ENT and oral complaints, e.g. snoring, rhinosinusitis, persistent oral ulceration and dry mouth'	Assessment and treatment of snoring DVLA rules for obstructive sleep apnoea (OSA)
4	Sinusitis	'Manage primary contact with patients who have a common/important ENT, oral or facial problem, e.g. vertigo or tinnitus'	Management of sinusitis
5	BPPV	'Carry out appropriate examination including more detailed tests where indicated, e.g. audiological tests and the Dix–Hallpike test to help diagnose benign paroxysmal positional vertigo (BPPV)'	Causes and management of BPPV Assessment using Dix–Hallpike test Epley manoeuvre
Extra notes	ENT 2WW and Emergencies	'Understand how to recognise rarer but potentially serious conditions such as oral, head and neck cancer' 'Understand when urgent (or semi-urgent) referral to secondary care may be indicated, e.g. in trauma, epistaxis, quinsy (peritonsillar abscess), severe croup or stridor'	Suspected cancer referral criteria Unilateral deafness Epiglottitis

1. http://www.rcgp.org.uk/training-exams/gp-curriculum-overview/online-curriculum/applying-clinical-knowledge-section-2/3-15-ent-oral-and-facial-problems.aspx

The RCGP curriculum states:
- '15% of consultations in GP involve the upper respiratory tract or head and neck.
- Guidelines for appropriate management are widely available but not always used.
- Knowledge of normal anatomy and examination techniques makes diagnosis easier.
- Variable training in ear, nose and throat (ENT) at undergraduate level means that trainees and trainers have to review current knowledge and skills.
- Head and neck cancer rates are increasing and outcomes depend on early diagnosis.'

CHAPTER 17 REFERENCES

Facial Nerve Palsy
1. NICE. http://cks.nice.org.uk/bells-palsy (revised October 2012).
2. http://patient.info/health/bells-palsy
3. Margabanthu G., Brooks J., et al. Facial palsy as a presenting feature of coarctation of aorta. *Interact CardioVasc Thorac Surg.* 2003; 2(1): 91–9.
4. Peitersen, E. The natural history of Bell's palsy. *Am J Otol.* 1982; **4**(2): 107–11.

Otitis Media
1. NICE. http://cks.nice.org.uk/otitis-media-acute (revised July 2015).
   Patient information leaflet: http://patient.info/health/ear-infection-otitis-media

Snoring
1. http://patient.info/doctor/snoring-pro
2. http://www.britishsnoring.co.uk/sleep_apnoea/epworth_sleepiness_scale.php
3. http://patient.info/doctor/obstructive-sleep-apnoea-syndrome-pro
4. https://www.gov.uk/government/publications/assessing-fitness-to-drive-a-guide-for-medical-professionals. Contains public sector information licensed under the Open Government Licence v3.0.
5. https://www.gov.uk/government/uploads/system/uploads/attachment_data/file/503534/INF159_150216.pdf. Contains public sector information licensed under the Open Government Licence v3.0.
   Patient information leaflet: http://patient.info/health/snoring-leaflet

Sinusitis
1. NICE. http://cks.nice.org.uk/sinusitis (revised October 2013).
   Patient information leaflet: http://patient.info/health/acute-sinusitis

BPPV
1. http://cks.nice.org.uk/benign-paroxysmal-positional-vertigo (revised September 2013).
2. http://patient.info/doctor/vertebrobasilar-occlusion-and-vertebral-artery-syndrome
3. http://www.thebsa.org.uk/wp-content/uploads/2014/04/HM.pdf
   Patient information leaflet: http://patient.info/health/benign-paroxysmal-positional-vertigo-leaflet

ENT 2WW and Emergencies
1. https://www.nice.org.uk/guidance/NG12/chapter/1-Recommendations-organised-by-site-of-cancer#head-and-neck-cancers
2. http://patient.info/doctor/labyrinthitis
3. NICE. http://cks.nice.org.uk/sore-throat-acute#!diagnosisadditional:6. July 2015.

Doctor's Notes

Patient   Mike Williams   55 years   M
PMH   Hypertension
Medications   Ramipril 5 mg daily
Allergies   No information
Consultations Recent consultation with PN – BP well controlled.
                  Calculated CVD risk 12% – statins discussed but patient declined.
                  Medication reauthorised for 3 months.
Investigations 3 months ago
                  Normal U&E, total cholesterol 6.1 mmol/L, ratio 2.2
Household   Barbara Williams   55 years   F

Example Consultation — Facial Nerve Palsy

Open ☐	Mr Williams, it's good to meet you. I'm sorry to see you looking so concerned and with this weakness in your face. Tell me how it started. Have you noticed anything else? How is your health generally?
History ☐	Any earache? Any deafness or dizziness? I notice you have high BP. Can I check if you've been taking your medication? And tell me more about you. Do you have family or friends around you? Tell me about your work.
Flags ☐	I need to ensure this problem is confined to the nerve in your face. Are your arms and legs feeling and working normally? Any problems with your vision? Are you able to wrinkle your forehead? Any problems with your speech?
Curious ☐	Have you known this happen to anyone else? Were your father's symptoms the same or different?
Sense ☐	I can see how worried and upset you are and understandably so.
ICE ☐	You are worried this is a stroke. Do you have any other thoughts or worries? Did you have anything in mind you hoped I might be able to do for you today?
Impact ☐	I understand you want this to resolve as quickly as possible. How might this problem affect you?
Summary ☐	To summarise, you woke up this morning with a lopsided face, blinking is difficult and you have been drooling from your mouth. You are worried it might be a stroke due to your BP and your father's history, but also because you don't take medication for cholesterol. You fear how this looks to others and want to do whatever is required to help you return to work as soon as possible. Have I missed anything out?
O/E ☐	I would like to check your BP, examine the nerves in your face, both ears and your mouth and check for lumps around the ear. Is that okay?
Empathy ☐	I appreciate this is distressing. I understand why you questioned a stroke but thankfully it isn't.
Impression ☐	We call this Bell's palsy – it's a temporary weakness of the face nerve.
Experience ☐	Have you heard of Bell's palsy? Do you know anyone who has had it?
Explanation ☐	In Bell's palsy, the facial nerve suddenly stops sending normal electrical impulses to the muscles in the face so they can't work normally. We don't know what causes it, though it may be a virus. Most people make a full recovery over a period of weeks or months and only a few are left with any lasting weakness. If there were 100 people like you, 71 would make a full and complete recovery, 13 would have a little weakness and just 16 would have lasting facial weakness.
Options ☐	We know that taking steroid tablets for about 10 days may help this to get better quicker. How do you feel about that? You are correct – steroids may increase your BP temporarily. Like any treatment, we need to weigh up the benefits against the risks. Your BP is nicely controlled so I am happy for you to take the steroids. What do you think? We also need to protect your eye as the surface of the eye can become too dry. I'm going to prescribe some lubricants and an eye pad to use at night. A good thought, Mr Williams, but unfortunately antivirals don't work.
Empower ☐	I'm going to give you a leaflet to read about Bell's palsy.
Future ☐	Come back and see a GP in a week when you have finished the tablets.
Safety net ☐	If you feel you are getting worse, or if the eye becomes sore or if the other side of your face becomes affected, see the GP the same day or ring 111 if it is out of hours. I don't think this will happen but if your arm, leg or other parts of your body become weak, call 999 straightaway.

Patient's Story

Facial Nerve Palsy

Doctor's notes	Mike Williams, 55. PMH: Hypertension. Medication: Ramipril. All well in the routine check with the nurse 3 months ago. Medication renewed. Statins declined.
How to act	Very worried.
PC	*'I woke up this morning and my face is lopsided. Have I had a stroke?'*
History	You realised you are drooling at the mouth and can't move the left side of your face. You have no other neurological symptoms and you feel well in yourself.
	You were diagnosed with hypertension 5 years ago. You mostly (but not always) remember to take Ramipril. The nurse discussed statins but you had read they cause leg cramps and didn't think you needed them.
	Family history of stroke – father died of this 2 years ago.
Social	You live with your wife. You have no children. You work at a local stately home, showing visitors around. Money is tight as your wife lost her job. Never smoked. Minimal alcohol.
ICE	You believe you have had a stroke. You have no other thoughts of what may be causing this. You are angry at yourself for declining the statin.
	Before your father died you saw a change in him mentally as well as physically, which was upsetting to see.
	You work with the public and you fear what people may think. Whatever is wrong you want to get back to work soon. You don't think you get sick pay.
	If the doctor mentions this might be 'a virus' you will ask for antiviral drugs to get better as quickly as you can. If the doctor mentions steroids, you would be concerned they would push your BP up.
Examination	CN VII – Asymmetry visible. Left side – face drooping and cannot close eye or blink.
	Only if specifically asked, left side of forehead is affected – does not wrinkle when asked to 'screw up face or raise eyebrows'.
	BP 130/70
	Ears and mouth – NAD
	No parotid swelling
Questions	*'Will this get better? Will the other side of my face go the same way?'*

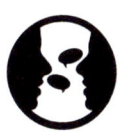

Learning Points — Bell's Palsy

Bell's palsy is the commonest cause of facial weakness.

Aetiology	A problem with facial (VII) nerve at the geniculate ganglion.
	Cause unknown but ? viral ? reactivation (herpes or varicella).
Ramsay-Hunt	A painful vesicular rash of the external ear and vesicles may appear in the palate.[1]
Epidemiology	Age group: 20–50. Men and women equally affected, rarely children.
Risk factors	Diabetes or FH of Bell's palsy.
Symptoms	Rapid onset of a unilateral facial weakness with drooling and excessive tears.
Investigations	Usually none; however, consider serology for herpes simplex/zoster and Lyme disease.
Prognosis	Recovery generally starts in 2 weeks, but may take up to 12 months to fully resolve.[2]
Treatment	If within 48 hours of onset of symptoms, consider 10 days of prednisolone.
	Either 25 mg BD for 10 days **or** 60 mg daily for 5 days then reduce by 10 mg each day.[1]
	Antivirals not recommended. No evidence of effectiveness.[1]
	Corneal protection essential – lubricant drops/ointment at night/eyepatch

Differential diagnosis – rare but serious conditions

Stroke	In an UMN lesion the forehead is generally spared due to dual innervation.
Cholesteatoma	'Hearing impairment, discharge, bleeding, dizziness, vertigo, disorder of balance, pain, headaches, or tinnitus.'[1]
Malignant OE	Malignant otitis externa – signs include polyposis or granulations.
Parotid tumour	'Asymmetry of the oropharynx and ipsilateral tonsils'[1] or palpable tumour
Coarctation	Raised BP, high level of suspicion in children.
	Reports of Bell's palsy + HTN leading to detection of underlying coarctation of aorta.[3]
Lyme disease	If a rash or symptoms of Lyme disease has been present.
Referral	**To neurology if**
	Any doubt about diagnosis.
	Recurrent Bell's palsy.
	Bilateral Bell's palsy.[1]
	To ophthalmology
	If cornea remains exposed when trying to close eyelid (for tarsorrhaphy).
	To ENT
	If no improvement within 1 month or if suspect serious underlying problem such as parotid tumour, malignant otitis externa, cholesteatoma.[1]
	To plastics
	If residual paralysis at 6–9 months.[1]
A study of 1011 patients[1,4]	71% complete recovery
	84% complete or near complete recovery
	16% permanent deficit of facial function

Doctor's Notes

Patient	Sarah Smith	5 years	F
PMH	None		
Medications	No current medications		
Allergies	No information		
Consultations	No recent consultations		
Investigations	No recent investigations		
Household	Natasha Smith	33 years	F
	Darren Smith	34 years	M
	Charlie Smith	9 years	M

Sarah attends the GP with her mum today.

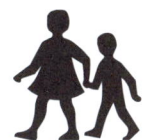

Model Consultation — Otitis Media

Open — Hello Sarah, hello Mrs Smith. Oh, I'm so sorry to hear you've got earache – that's horrid, isn't it? Sarah, tell me how it feels. Mum, can you tell me more about her earache? Anything else that you have noticed?

History — Have you tried any medicine? How is Sarah's health? Any problems at birth? Any concern in the past with hearing or development? Is she fully immunised? Is she allergic to any medicines? Who is at home? What do you both do for a living?

Flags — Is Sarah drinking okay? Any signs that she can't hear so well? Has she had a high temperature? When did this start? Do the fevers go down with pain relief? Is she moving her neck and looking at lights okay? Any concerns with her breathing? Rashes? Good, it sounds like the rest of you is okay, Sarah, but we need to look at your ears!

Risk — Does anyone in the family have any ear problems?

Sense — It's rare that you need to bring Sarah to see us and I sense you must be concerned about her.

ICE — May I ask if you've come across ear infections before? Did anything particularly worry you about Sarah? Did you have anything in mind that you hoped I might be able to prescribe or do for Sarah today?

Impact — Has Sarah needed time off school? Has that been difficult for you, for example with your own work?

Curious — You mentioned that you are not keen at all on antibiotics. May I ask why you prefer to avoid them? I'm sorry to hear about Charlie's experience but I can tell you that allergies don't normally run in families.

Summary — To summarise so far, Sarah is healthy but has had earache for 5 days. You were hoping to avoid antibiotics due to previous experience. You feel this is likely to be a virus but you would like to check there are no complications developing, like mastoiditis which you have read about. Have I understood correctly?

O/E — I'd like to check Sarah's temperature and pulse, look at the throat and ears, check she has no swellings and listen to her chest. Is that okay with you, Sarah? Would you like to sit on Mum's knee while I have a look?

Empathy — The ear drums are red with discharge and look sore. There are no signs of additional complications.

Impression — My impression is that she has a middle ear infection causing a temperature.

Experience — What is your experience of ear infections … or with friends' children?

Explanation — The fact that Sarah has had a cold for 2 weeks and now earache for 5 days with no improvement despite regular pain relief, and the discharge in her ear canal, makes me think it is more likely than not that she has a bacterial infection. Therefore, antibiotics might help. What are your thoughts? Grommets may be inserted with repeated ear infections where the fluid build-up may prevent hearing development.

Options — Like you, I'm keen to only use antibiotics when they are really needed but I do think that Sarah needs them. Research suggests that after 4 days of symptoms antibiotics are more likely to be necessary. A fever and pus also suggests it is not clearing. What are your thoughts now? Okay, I will issue amoxicillin.

Empower — Please give this antibiotic three times a day for 5 days. Here is a leaflet on children's ear infections.

Future — I expect her to start getting better in a couple of days, in which case I don't need to see her again.

Safety net — If, however, she gets worse please bring her back. For example, a fever which does not come down with paracetamol/ibuprofen, ongoing symptoms after completion of the antibiotics, a swelling behind the ear, pain moving the neck, breathing problems suggesting a chest infection or hearing problems.

ENT, Oral and Facial – 2

Patient's Story

Otitis Media

Doctor's notes	Sarah Smith, 5 years. Attending with mum, Natasha Smith, aged 33 years.
	PMH: None. Medications: None.
How to act	Caring, articulate, sure of yourself and going to stand your ground.
PC	*'She's had earache for the past 5 days. I just wanted you to check her out, please.'*
History	Sarah can tell you it hurts but then looks to Mum.
	Sarah has had a cold for a couple of weeks and started with earache about 5 days ago. You thought this might be something she had caught at school. You have been giving her regular paracetamol and ibuprofen but with no real improvement. You noticed some discharge in her ear canal this morning. She has had a fever since last night but it settled with analgesia.
	There are no lower respiratory symptoms.
	She is a little miserable and off food but drinking and passing urine.
	No symptoms of meningitis.
	She seems able to hear normally but keeps pulling at her ears.
Social	Two-parent family. Dad is an accountant and mum is a part-time teacher.
	One older child: Charlie, aged 9 years.
ICE	Most ear infections are viral. Antibiotics should be avoided because they interfere with your immune system. Charlie got a rash with amoxicillin and is now 'allergic' to it. It didn't seem to make him any better.
	Sarah has never had antibiotics and you don't intend her to start now.
	Deep down you believe she is fine, you have experience with children, but when it's your own you doubt your judgement and want an opinion. You looked on the Internet and started reading about the mastoid bone. You would like reassurance this bone is okay.
	If antibiotics are offered, you will refuse them. *'Are you sure? She's never had antibiotics and I don't want her to have them now.'*
Understanding	You have read that it is much better for children to make their own antibodies to infections. You have known some children tell you they have had an operation for grommets.
Ask the doctor	*'When is the grommet operation necessary?'*
Examination	Temp 38.5°C, HR 100 bpm, throat red, both ear drums very red, discharge in left ear canal, chest clear.

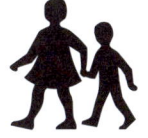

Learning Points   Otitis Media

Otitis media is common and usually viral.

NICE guidelines (revised 2015) suggest:
- Treat pain and fever with **either** paracetamol **or** ibuprofen then try the other if ineffective.
- Do not use together.
- The other analgesia can then be given between doses of the first analgesia if the child remains distressed or becomes distressed on the single agent.[1]

Use antibiotics if[1]
- Systemically unwell but admission not indicated.
- Immunocompromised.
- Serious chronic disease such as heart/lung/liver/neuromuscular.
- Where symptoms have lasted 4 days or more and are not improving.

Consider giving an immediate prescription for children where:
- Discharge in the canal or a perforation is visible.
- Younger than 2 years with bilateral otis media.

Antibiotic of choice: 5-day course of amoxicillin, or erythromycin if allergic to penicillin.[1]

Reasons for admission[1]
- Sign of acute complications: meningitis, facial nerve paralysis or mastoiditis.
- Systemically unwell.
- Under 3 months of age.
- 3–6 months of age with a temperature of >39°C.

If no antibiotics are required, advise the parent that antibiotics are 'not usually needed because they are likely to make little difference to symptoms, may have adverse effects (for example diarrhoea, vomiting, and rash), and can contribute to antibiotic resistance.'[1]

A delayed prescription may be given with the advice to start treatment 'if symptoms are not improving within 4 days of the onset of symptoms or if there is a significant worsening of symptoms at any time.'

However, always 're-consult if the condition worsens or if symptoms are not improving within 4 days of the onset of symptoms'.[1]

It is easy to jump to assumptions; for example, that the mum of a hot poorly child is wanting antibiotics but, as in this case, that is not always the situation. Always keep an open mind and check the patient's thoughts, fears and hopes (ICE) so that you are informed rather than surprised and you can tailor your explanation and shared management plan appropriately.

Doctor's Notes

Name	John Anderson	46 years	M
PMH	No medical history		
Medications	No current medication		
Consultations	No recent consultations		
Investigations	No recent investigations		
Household	Rachel Anderson	46 years	F

Example Consultation   Snoring

Open ☐	I'm really sorry to hear that. Tell me more about what your wife has noticed and let's see what we can do to find out what's wrong and help with the snoring.
History ☐	How long has this been going on? Is it every night? Do you tend to sleep on your back? Any nose problems, e.g. a broken nose in the past? Tell me a bit about yourself. And what do you do at work?
Curious ☐	What do you think she means by 'or else'? Has this been on your mind?
Flags ☐	Does your wife notice you stop breathing at night? Do you have headaches in the morning? Are you sleepy during the day? Any 'near misses' when driving?
Risk ☐	Can I ask whether you smoke? Do you drink alcohol? How much? How about exercise?
Sense ☐	I sense you are quite embarrassed about this and that it was difficult to come in, so well done you! It's important for your health and your relationship and I'm sure we can help.
Impact ☐	How has this affected you over the last few months?
ICE ☐	What thoughts have you had about this? Was there anything particular you were worrying about? Anything specific you were hoping I might be able to do today?
Summary ☐	To summarise, for the last few months your wife has complained about you snoring and now sleeps in another room. You've never felt sleepy in the day and have not had near misses when driving. You are concerned about your marriage and your licence. The impact on your life is so great you have considered an operation but believe I may suggest weight loss, which is difficult with your work. So you are interested to know your options. Have I got it?
O/E ☐	I'd like to weigh and measure you, measure your collar size and thoroughly examine your heart and circulation and your breathing including your nose, throat and lungs. I'd also like to feel your neck for your thyroid gland. Is that okay with you?
Impression ☐	I can help by making some suggestions about what you can do to help.
Experience ☐	Do you know what causes snoring or any treatments that are available?
Explanation ☐	Snoring is from vibrations of the walls of your nose and mouth. Your body mass index is higher than it should be – 39 when the ideal is 25 or less. Your heart and lungs seem fine and your nose is clear and your thyroid gland is not enlarged.
Empathy ☐	It must be miserable being told you have been snoring and keeping your wife awake when you aren't even aware of it because you are fast asleep. I sense your frustration that you have tried to lose weight without success. I appreciate that you were considering an operation to fix this but it is good to avoid the risks of an operation if we can.
Empower ☐	Other things you can try include nasal decongestants and strips to open the nose, from the chemist. Stopping alcohol and smoking and weight loss are usually the key. You are also likely to feel healthier overall.
Options ☐	I would like to refer you to our health trainer. A dentist may be able to supply you with an appliance which sits in the mouth. If, down the line we are still not winning, perhaps a referral to the surgeons then? How do you feel about my suggestions? We need to do a few blood tests to check your blood sugar, cholesterol, kidney and thyroid function and also arrange to get your oxygen levels measured overnight using a simple fingertip sensor whilst you are asleep at home in your own bed.
Future ☐	Please make an appointment for the blood test. I will arrange the overnight oxygen test, then see you back.
Safety net ☐	Please ask your wife again about if you have pauses in your breathing in the night and come back if this happens.

ENT, Oral and Facial – 3

Patient's Story

Snoring

Doctor's notes	Mr John Anderson, 46 years. PMH: None. Medications: None.
How to act	Embarrassed.
PC	*'My wife says I snore badly. She's had to move to the spare room. I need to sort this out or my marriage is on the rocks.'*
History	For the last few months your wife has been increasingly frustrated by your snoring. She is now in the spare room and has told you to sort this out *'or else'*. Your wife says you are noisy but you have never stopped breathing in the night. You have not noticed daytime sleepiness or morning headaches.
Social	You work as a coach driver, long-distance holidays. You eat when you can, often from roadside cafés, and don't take any exercise. You smoke 10/day and drink a couple of pints each night; you are careful not to exceed this because you are worried about losing your driving licence.
ICE	You are worried about your marriage. You have also heard that if you snore you might lose your PSV licence, meaning you could not do your job. You have wondered if an operation may help.
	You think the doctor will tell you to lose weight and stop smoking and that's something you have tried and failed with for years.
Ask the doctor	*'Why do I snore?'*
	'Will an operation help?'
Examination	Height 1 m 90 cm, Weight 142 kg, BMI= 39.3
	Neck circumference – 55 cm
	HS normal BP 124/62 Chest clear
	No palpable thyroid

ENT, Oral and Facial – 3

Learning Points   Snoring

Noisy breathing during sleep affects 40% of population: men > women, usual ages 40–60.

Children: prevalence 1–20%, usually due to adenotonsillar enlargement or craniofacial abnormalities. There is a link with atopy and respiratory infections.

Cause: can be generated in nose, soft palate/uvula, pharyngeal walls/tonsils, base of tongue.

Definitions
- Simple snoring — Snoring but no hypoxia or erratic breathing. May be associated with increased CVD risks.
- Obstructive sleep apnoea (OSA) = erratic breathing at night + daytime symptoms.

Risk factors Overweight/obese; thick neck; large tonsils/adenoids; acromegaly; nasal problems, e.g. deviated septum.

Other factors Alcohol, smoking, sleeping on back, sedative medication.

History How long? How frequent? Disturbing own sleep/partner's sleep; Any reports of 'gaps in breathing' at night? Waking up at night gasping? Daytime sleepiness?

(Use Epworth Sleepiness Scale[2] to assess). Accidents? Poor concentration?

Examination BMI, neck circumference, cardiovascular and respiratory systems, nose, thyroid.

Investigations Arrange pulse oximetry and/or sleep clinic referral, CVD bloods (glucose, lipid fractions, U&E, TSH).

Management[1] Self – Weight loss, stop alcohol, stop smoking, avoid sedatives, increase exercise.

Other[1]
- Pharmacy – OTC: ear plugs for partner, nasal decongestant spray.
- Dentist for oral mandibular advancement appliance.
- Other – nasal strips to flare nares, chin straps to keep mouth closed. CPAP, if pulse oximetry shows dips.
- Surgery – palatal, e.g. soft palate implants, radiofrequency ablation, nasal septoplasty.

OSA The most common sleep-related disorder.

Significantly increases the risk of accidents.

Estimate at least 4/100 men have this.[3]

DVLA

Even in mild OSA, or with any condition or medication which causes excessive sleepiness, the patient should be advised not to drive.[4]

'This requirement also applies for a suspected diagnosis yet to be confirmed.'[4]

For advice regarding when they can return to driving and whether they need to inform the DVLA, see DVLA guidelines.[4]

See the Link Hub at CompleteCSA.co.uk for a link to The 'Tiredness can kill' leaflet (INF159)[5] – and a link to patient information explaining about the sleep study.

Doctor's Notes

Patient	Jennifer Richards 39 years F
PMH	2 normal vaginal deliveries
	Upper respiratory tract infection
Allergies	No known drug allergies
Medications	Rigevidon
Consultations	Routine Pill check with practice nurse 2 months ago – all well
Investigations	BP 2 months ago 102/60
Household	Alan Richards 30 years M
	Louis Richards 10 years M
	Amy Richards 8 years F

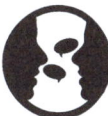

Example Consultation — Sinusitis

Open — Hello Mrs Richards. Oh, I am sorry to hear that. Please tell me more about how your sinusitis started this time and what symptoms you are getting.

History — Tell me about the nasal discharge – clear? Green? Any headaches – whereabouts? Has this happened before? Please tell me about any medical problems in the past. Have you tried any medication for this?

Flags — Does the light bother you? On a scale of 1 to 10, how bad are the headaches? Do you feel ill? Any double vision? Have you had a fever?

Sense — You seem quite tense and upset at the moment. Tell me what's going on in your life as well as the sinus pain?

Impact — How is the sinusitis affecting you at home and work?

Curious — Tell me about school and the pressures at work. What do you teach? How long? Are you busy at home too? Do you have support there?

ICE — You mentioned you had sinusitis before and it didn't get better with a normal antibiotic and you were prescribed a powerful one. Tell me what worries you about the sinusitis? As well as antibiotics, was there anything else you were hoping I could do to help?

Summary — To summarise so far, you had a cold for about a week and now facial pain and discharge for 3 days which is not getting better with paracetamol. There's pressure in your face and pressure in your life too as Ofsted is coming in 3 days and it's important to be at your best and do well.

O/E — I'd like to check your temperature and feel the bones around your face – in your forehead and either side of your nose. I'd also like to feel around the eye sockets. Is that okay?

Empathy — Feeling lousy with facial pain and headaches must be pretty miserable, especially with the stress of an imminent Ofsted visit.

Impression — From what you've told me, I think you are absolutely right – you have sinusitis.

Explanation — To be honest, it's far more likely to be viral than bacterial and there is no evidence that antibiotics make any difference for people like you who are normally fit and well. I suspect that last time you got better despite the antibiotics rather than because of them. Let's talk about how we can have you feeling better as soon as possible.

Options — I will talk you through some self-help measures. I don't want to prescribe antibiotics because all the evidence suggests that they will make no difference and they may give you diarrhoea and contribute to drug resistance.

Empower — I will give you a PIL that describes things you can do that will make a difference: regular fluids and pain relief, warm facial compresses, salt solution for your nose, a decongestant spray. Breathing in steam probably doesn't help. You may wish to try nasal douching. People either love it because it flushes out the sinus passages or hate it because squirting salty water into your nose isn't pleasant.

Future — This should get fully better within 2–3 weeks and, with the treatment, you should start to feel better soon.

Safety net — If you are not fully better in 2–3 weeks or if you get bad headaches or feel really ill, come and see me straight away or phone 111 if it's out of hours.

Patient's Story

Sinusitis

Doctor's notes	Jennifer Richards, 39 years. PMH: 2 pregnancies, URTI. Medications: Rigevidon.
How to act	Anxious, demanding.
PC	*'I won't keep you long, Doctor. It's my sinusitis again – I just need antibiotics.'*
History	Sore throat and runny nose for a week, self-medicated with paracetamol. Last 3 days, increasing nasal discharge (sometimes clear, sometimes green) and facial pain. Some headaches: frontal, worse when you bend your head forwards. You've had headaches for a few weeks anyway and think it is work stress. Paracetamol has been useless.
Social	Married with 2 children. English teacher at local secondary school. Ofsted inspection in 3 days' time – school was 'failing' last time, pressure to do better this time, otherwise the school might close and you could lose your job.
	You rarely drink alcohol and do not smoke.
ICE	You know that doctors are reluctant to prescribe antibiotics but you don't ask for them often and this time you really need them as you believe they will make you better quicker. Last time you had amoxicillin and it didn't do anything and you had to come back for stronger ones (cefalexin) which made the sinusitis better after a week.
Ask the doctor	If refused antibiotics: *'What can I do? I need to be on top of this in 3 days when the inspectors come.'*
	If given antibiotics: *'What do I need to do about contraception? Will they interfere with my pill?'*
	If offered amoxicillin: *'It does not work and I need cefalexin.'*
Examination	Temp 37.2°C, tender in forehead and cheeks, worse when you bend forward.
	No nasal polyps visible.

Learning Points — Sinusitis

Acute sinusitis[1]
>98% are caused by a virus. Self-limiting illness that gets better in 2–3 weeks.

Usual management[1,2]
Paracetamol and/or ibuprofen (relieve symptoms by reducing pain and temperature).
Rest and take plenty of fluids.
Apply warm compresses to the face.
Irrigate nose with saline solution.
Intranasal decongestant, e.g. spray (OTC). [Oral decongestant not recommended.]

No proven benefit[1]
Steam inhalation
Antihistamines
Oral steroids

Antibiotics only indicated if[1]
Serious comorbidities such as immunosuppression, CF, severe heart/lung/liver/kidney problems.
Age >80 + 1 additional risk factor.
Age >65 + 2 additional risk factors.
(Risk factors = diabetes type 1 or 2, taking oral steroids or hospital admission in last 12 months.)

If using antibiotic – amoxicillin or erythromycin if penicillin allergy.
Additional learning point – no need for extra contraception with antibiotics.

Rare but important complications needing admission[1]
Severe systemic infection.
Orbital involvement (double vision, oculomotor nerve paralysis, eyeball displaced, ↓visual acuity).
Intracranial involvement with symptoms/signs of meningitis or frontal bone swelling.

Chronic sinusitis[1]
Consider if nasal blockage/discharge or loss of smell for 12 weeks.
Associated with atopy, chronic dental infection, immunosuppression.
Manage with above measures but also consider 3 months of intranasal corticosteroids.
Consider referral to ENT if 3 months' trial of intranasal corticosteroids + above measures are ineffective.

Doctor's Notes

Patient	Freda White	60 years	F
PMH	Type 2 diabetes.		
Medications	Metformin, gliclazide.		
Allergies	No known allergies		
Consultations	Diabetes check 1 month ago – all well		
Investigations	1 month ago	HbA1c 54 mmol/mol, lipid profile normal, U&E normal	
		BP 130/70	
		No microalbuminuria	
Household	Raymond White	70 years	M

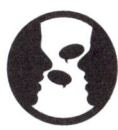

Model Consultation   BPPV

Open ☐	I'm sorry to hear about that. Please tell me more about the dizziness from the beginning. Tell me how and when this started.
History ☐	By dizzy do you mean lightheaded or is the room spinning? Do you still have symptoms now? How long did it last? Have you had this before? Apart from the diabetes, do you have any other significant medical problems?
Flags ☐	Have you had any headaches? Have you vomited? Any deafness or ear problems? Any other symptoms in the chest like pain or palpitations? Any symptoms of the arms or legs not feeling or working normally? Any ringing in your ears?
Risk ☐	How is your diabetes? Blood sugars at home? Has the dizziness made you fall?
Impact ☐	Tell me about work. What do you do? Do you need to drive to get to work? How has the dizziness been affecting things that you normally do at home?
ICE ☐	What thoughts have you had about this? Did you worry it may be from the cruise? Did anything make you worry that there might be something significant going on?
Sense ☐	I sense you are very concerned about this and perhaps, particularly, about whether there is something seriously wrong with you.
Curious ☐	I'm wondering why you think it may be a tumour; have you read something online?
Empathy ☐	That is very sad to hear. It must be very unpleasant feeling dizzy and sick so much. I understand your fears about what this could be and the consequences that not working would bring for your family. No wonder your husband is concerned.
Summary ☐	To summarise, for the last few weeks you have had episodes of the room spinning lasting a minute or so, worse in the mornings. You have felt sick but not been sick. You wondered if it might be a hangover from the cruise or even a brain tumour.
O/E ☐	I would like to examine you and to move your head and neck to see if I can work out what's going on. Do you have any serious neck problems such as bad arthritis or have you injured your neck recently or had a broken neck in the past? May I also check your eye movements side to side while you keep your head still. Now please touch my finger then your nose a few times. Now with the left. Now can I ask you to turn each hand over quickly like this? May I see you walk? May I check your BP sitting and standing please?
Impression ☐	I think your dizziness is coming from the inner ear where there is fluid in three curved tubes called the semicircular canals. The fluid in these canals normally helps you keep your balance but, if the fluid levels become altered, you can get dizziness, particularly when you change position. We call this benign paroxysmal positional vertigo. Benign means it's nothing serious, paroxysmal means it comes and goes, positional means when you move your head and vertigo means spinning dizziness.
Experience ☐	Have you known anyone with vertigo or dizziness when they move their head?
Explanation ☐	I know that your symptoms are distressing but I don't think it's anything serious and it will get better whatever we do. Most people get better within a few weeks.
Options ☐	So we could do nothing and this will most likely settle on its own but we could also try to reposition the fluid in your inner ear by a series of neck movements and this could make you better very quickly. If there were 100 people like you, at least 66 and possibly 89 of them would get better with this treatment.
Empower ☐	I will give you an information leaflet to read about the problem and the treatment which is called the Epley manoeuvre. This is something we could do at the surgery and we would ask you to book a 20-minute appointment with me. Think it over and perhaps talk to your husband. Until then, take care in the mornings and get up slowly. Be careful on stairs. You can drive once you feel safe and the dizziness stops.
Safety net ☐	I would expect the dizziness to start improving – longer intervals between episodes and the dizziness becoming less severe – but, if for any reason you start to feel worse or something new happens, please see the doctor.

ENT, Oral and Facial – 5

Patient's Story

BPPV

Doctor's notes	Mrs Freda White, aged 60. PMH: Type 2 diabetes. Diabetes check 1 month ago, all well. Medications: Metformin, gliclazide. Ix: HbA1c 54 mmol/mol, lipid profile normal, U&E normal, BP 130/70, no microalbuminuria.
How to act	Concerned.
PC	*'I woke up feeling dreadfully dizzy and sick this morning. It isn't the first time.'*
History	For the last few weeks you have had frequent episodes of suddenly feeling dizzy. If asked more about the dizziness – the room is spinning. The episodes last less than a minute each but are unpredictable. Your house has stairs and you nearly fell down them this morning as you were going down to make a cup of tea. You have never had serious problems with your neck. You have always been well.
	You have no cardiac or neurological symptoms. You have not vomited. You have no ear symptoms including pain or discharge.
Social	Cleaner at the local primary school. Husband older and retired factory worker. No alcohol and never smoked.
ICE	You are worried this is a brain tumour. One of the children at school had one and died recently and this was very sad for everyone. You think she had dizziness too.
	Could it also be to do with getting seasick on a recent cruise (your first, to celebrate 40 years of marriage)? Your husband is very worried about you. You want to know what this is and how to make it better. You are not sure you can work like this and you rely on your wage to supplement his pension.
Ask the doctor	*'Is it a brain tumour?'*
	'Will it get better?'
O/E	Dix–Hallpike test positive with nystagmus on turning head in each direction.
	No cerebellar signs.
	BP 128/66 sitting and 130/70 standing.

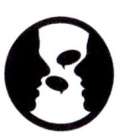

ENT, Oral and Facial – 5

Learning Points　　　　　　　　　　　　　　　　　　　　　　　　　　　　BPPV

Benign paroxysmal positional vertigo (BPPV) is a common cause of recurrent dizziness.

Who?	Middle aged (usually >50 years) and older people. Women:men = 2:1.
Symptoms	Severe dizziness and nausea when head in certain positions (e.g. lying on one side, or face up in bed). Can feel off balance for several hours after the dizziness has gone.
Cause	Otolith particles fall into semicircular canals (esp. posterior canal – 85%) and cause fluid in inner ear to move.
Precipitating factors	Spontaneous; ear surgery; head injury; bed rest; post-viral.
	Children – migraine.
Diagnosis	Confirm symptoms of dizziness that are related to the position of the head.
	Note that attacks last 20–30 seconds but get better if the head is kept still.
Differential	Ménière's, anxiety, postural hypotension, viral labyrinthitis, vestibular neuritis, acoustic neuroma, chronic otitis media, MS, CVA, vertebrobasilar occlusion (patient.co.uk has a useful description for the doctor[2]), brain or nasopharyngeal tumours.
Examine	Tailor the examination to the symptoms. Consider: BP, ears, Dix–Hallpike manoeuvre, cerebellar signs + full neurological assessment to rule out differentials.
Treatment	May resolve with no treatment. Epley manoeuvre, Brandt-Daroff exercises.

Contraindications for Dix–Hallpike manoeuvre, Epley manoeuvre and Brandt-Daroff exercises

Absolute	'Fractured odontoid peg, recent c. spine fracture, atlanto-axial subluxation, cervical disc prolapse, vertebro-basilar insufficiency that is known and verified, recent neck trauma that restricts torsional movement.'[3]
Relative	'Carotid sinus syncope (consider if history of drop attacks or blackouts), severe back pain, recent stroke, cardiac bypass within the last 3 months, severe neck pain, rheumatoid arthritis affecting the neck, recent neck surgery, cervical myelopathy, severe back pain, severe orthopnoea may restrict duration of test.'[3]

Additional learning point

How much can you do in 10 minutes? Taking a history from a patient, using the Dix–Hallpike test as a diagnostic tool and then treating the patient using an Epley manoeuvre is not realistic in a normal 10-minute consultation. Use the opportunity to give the patient a leaflet to read about your proposed treatment and book them in for a separate appointment for treatment sometime soon.

Extra Notes

ENT 2WW and Emergencies

2WW Referral criteria for suspected ENT, oral and facial cancer

Laryngeal[1]   Age >45 with persistent unexplained hoarseness **or** unexplained neck lump.

Oral[1]   Unexplained ulcer in the mouth lasting more than 3 weeks.

Persistent or unexplained lump in neck.

Persistent red or red and white patch in the mouth.

Thyroid[1]   Unexplained thyroid lump.

Emergency ENT problems

Unilateral deafness[2]   Sudden onset of unilateral deafness may be caused by acute ischaemia of brainstem or labyrinth – EMERGENCY: refer within 12 hours as possibility hearing may be restored.

Epiglottitis[3]   Now commoner in adults than children. DO NOT examine the throat – send to hospital 999. Risk of complete airway obstruction.

- Adults: severe sore throat with painful swallowing. Predictors of airway obstruction are sitting upright, stridor and breathlessness.
- Children:
  - Tentative, careful breathing (normal respiratory rate)
  - Tachycardia
  - Cry and voice muffled – reluctance to talk
  - May have inspiratory stridor and hoarseness
  - Drooling

ENT, Oral and Facial

CHAPTER 18 OVERVIEW
Eye Problems

	Cases in this chapter	Within the RCGP curriculum: Care of People with Eye Problems RCGP Online Curriculum 2016[1]	Learning points in the chapter
1	Blepharitis	'Understand the common eye conditions in primary care and manage them appropriately' 'Be able to diagnose and manage common conditions causing red eye and lid problems, such as blepharitis, chalazion and conjunctivitis'	Management of blepharitis and conjunctivitis
2	Squint	'Appreciate the importance of the social and psychological impact of eye problems on the patient'	Causes and management of squint
3	Acute Glaucoma	'Make timely, appropriate referrals on behalf of patients to specialist and community eye services'	Presentation and management of acute glaucoma
4	ARMD and Cataract	'Understand the significant psychological impact of sight loss for the patient and their family' 'Understand the importance of exploring the ideas, concerns and feelings of patients who are threatened with sight loss'	Presentation and management of ARMD and cataract
5	Retinal Detachment	'Recognise ophthalmic emergencies and refer appropriately' 'Understand the significance of visual impairment for a patient's ability to self-manage other chronic illness'	Presentation and management of retinal detachment
Extra notes	The Red Eye	'Manage primary contact with all patients who have an eye problem' 'Manage superficial ocular trauma' 'Be able to diagnose and manage common conditions causing red eye …' 'Recognise ophthalmic emergencies and refer appropriately'	Differential diagnosis of the red eye

1. http://www.rcgp.org.uk/training-exams/gp-curriculum-overview/online-curriculum/applying-clinical-knowledge-section-2/3-16-eye-problems.aspx

CHAPTER 18 REFERENCES

Blepharitis
1. NICE. http://cks.nice.org.uk/blepharitis. Oct 2015.
2. http://patient.info/doctor/blepharitis-pro. Accessed Mar 2016.
   Patient information leaflet:
3. http://www.moorfields.nhs.uk/sites/default/files/uploads/documents/A%26E%20Blepharitis.pdf

Squint
1. http://patient.info/doctor/strabismus-squint
2. http://patient.info/doctor/amblyopia-pro
3. http://www.nhs.uk/conditions/Squint/Pages/Introduction2.aspx – includes a video of an ophthalmologist describing squint and its treatment for patients/carers.

Acute Glaucoma
1. NICE. http://cks.nice.org.uk/glaucoma. Mar 16.
   Patient information leaflet:
   http://patient.info/health/acute-angle-closure-glaucoma
   http://patient.info/health/glaucoma-chronic-open-angle

ARMD and Cataract
1. ARMD http://cks.nice.org.uk/macular-degeneration-age-related.
   http://patient.info/doctor/age-related-macular-degeneration-pro
   Patient information: https://nei.nih.gov/health/maculardegen/armd_facts (available in auditory form and large text).
2. NICE http://cks.nice.org.uk/cataracts. Sep 2015.
   Patient information: http://www.rnib.org.uk/eye-health-eye-conditions-z-eye-conditions/cataracts
3. DVLA https://www.gov.uk/driving-eyesight-rules.
   Contains public sector information licenced under the Open Government License v3.0.

Retinal Detachment
1. NICE – http://cks.nice.org.uk/retinal-detachment. Mar 2015.
   Patient information leaflets:
   http://patient.info/health/retinal-detachment-leaflet
   http://www.rnib.org.uk/eye-health-eye-conditions-z-eye-conditions/retinal-detachment
   http://www.moorfields.nhs.uk/condition/retinal-detachment

Doctor's Notes

Patient	Alison Hughes	50 years	F
PMH	NVD aged 31 and 33 years		
Medications	No current medications		
Allergies	No information		
Consultations	No recent consultations		
Investigations	No recent investigations		
Household	John Hughes	52 years	M
	Sally Hughes	19 years	F
	Louise Hughes	17 years	F

Example Consultation — Blepharitis

Open ☐ I'm very sorry to hear that. Please tell me more about your eyes; how did this start and how long have you had problems?

History ☐ Are your eyes sticky all day or just in the mornings? Do you wake up and find that they are closed shut? Any problems focusing? Have you tried anything so far? Do you wear contact lenses? What sort of lenses are they? Tell me about work. What do you do and where do you work – is it an air-conditioned environment?

Curious ☐ I can see you aren't wearing your contact lenses today; tell me, why that is?

Flags ☐ Are both eyes equally affected? How is your eyesight? Any changes recently? Have you seen your optician for a sight check? Are your eyes sensitive to light?

Risk ☐ Does anyone in the family have eye problems? Any skin problems such as dry, red or flaky skin on your face?

Impact ☐ Tell me how this is affecting you each day so I can fully understand your situation.

Sense ☐ I sense that this is embarrassing, working in the fashion industry where appearances matter.

ICE ☐ You wondered if this was conjunctivitis. Did you have any other concerns? Or worries about your eyesight? You wondered if I could give you antibiotics; was there anything else you thought might help?

Summary ☐ To summarise, for a few weeks you have had recurrent stickiness and discharge from both eyes. You've had to leave your lenses out. Your sight is fine. You tried antibiotics but they did not work. This is important to you, and for you at work. It is uncomfortable and unpleasant to wake up with sticky eyes but, in addition, working in the fashion industry means you need to look your best and resolve this as soon as possible. You would prefer to wear contact lenses if possible.

O/E ☐ I'd like to have a good look at your eyes – at the eyelids and eyes and also check how well you can read the sight chart, if I may?

Empathy ☐ It must be embarrassing and difficult having sticky eyes that you have to clean at work.

Impression ☐ My impression is that you have an inflammation of the eyelid margin, which we call blepharitis. The eyes are fine and, in particular, the white part of your eye is not inflamed or infected so I don't think this is conjunctivitis. Also, conjunctivitis would probably have got better with antibiotic ointment and your symptoms haven't.

Experience ☐ Have you heard of blepharitis or known anyone who has had this?

Explanation ☐ Blepharitis is common and can be managed at home by careful cleaning of the eyelids. You will need to use warm compresses and buy some baby shampoo to use every day. Try to avoid eye makeup, if possible. If you must, please use water-soluble products that you can easily remove. I'm sorry, but you should probably leave your contact lenses out for the moment. Thankfully, this condition does not put your eyesight at risk.

Options ☐ I would like to give you a PIL about blepharitis which gives you advice on how to clean the eyes. I recommend arranging an appointment with your optician to check for dry eyes and for their professional advice about your contact lenses.

Empower ☐ It can be persistent so you will need to continue for a number of weeks or even longer. How do you feel about what I've suggested? Do you have any questions?

Safety net ☐ Please come back in 2–3 weeks if this is not working. If you have any new eye symptoms or are concerned, please come back at any time, or see your optician/contact lens practitioner.

Eye Problems – 1

Patient's Story

Blepharitis

Doctor's notes Alison Hughes, 50 years. PMH: NVD aged 31 and 33 years. Medications: None.

How to act Worried but expecting to be cured with some drops or ointment.

PC *'I keep getting conjunctivitis. My eyelids are stuck together every morning. Do I need antibiotics?'*

History For the last few weeks you have woken up on most days with sticky eyes. You are usually a contact lens wearer but have left them out. This has not helped. You went to the chemist and got ointment (antibiotics) but this did not make much difference. Comments have been made at work both about you wearing glasses and also about the appearance of your eyes.

Social You live with your husband and work as a PA to a fashion editor of a newspaper where it is important to look good at work. It is an air-conditioned office.

ICE You believe this is conjunctivitis which you have had experience with your children and understand it is an infection. Worried about the appearance, you need and expect the doctor to give some stronger antibiotics to sort this out quickly. You are slightly worried about your eyesight long term.

You have not come across blepharitis.

Keen to continue to wear contact lenses, you respond negatively if the doctor suggests leaving them out long term and react with incredulity if doctor suggests baby shampoo.

Examination Wearing glasses. Eyelid margins are red and crusty. No redness of conjunctiva.

Questions *'Will this get better? How quickly will this happen?'*

'Could it affect my sight?'

'Do I have to stop wearing contact lenses?'

Eye Problems – 1

Learning Points   Blepharitis

Common eye problem in General Practice.

Age Typically >40 years, but can be younger.

Symptoms Eyelids stuck together in the morning. Eyelashes sticky, greasy or crusty. Gritty sensation in eyes. Eyelids feel sore. Unable to tolerate contact lenses. Light sensitivity.

Differential diagnosis Conjunctivitis

Two types Anterior blepharitis = the base of eyelashes affected.

Posterior blepharitis = Meibomian glands affected.

… but it can be difficult to distinguish between the two types.[1]

Aetiology Staphylococcus. Can be associated with seborrhoeic dermatitis or rosacea. May be linked to demodex (microscopic mites) – possibly causing sensitivity or irritation to eyelids.[2]

Management Chronic condition, so management rather than cure.

1. Warm compresses to the eyes for 5–10 minutes.
2. Massage the eyelids with a cotton wool bud to loosen oils and crusts.
3. Clean the edge of the eyelids with warm water and a little baby shampoo (1:10 dilution). Diluted sodium bicarbonate solution is not recommended because it is more likely to cause irritation.

Recommend the above steps twice daily at first, then once daily as it improves.

If the above steps do not work, topical antibiotic ointment or cream for 6 weeks can be prescribed.

1st line – Chloramphenicol. 2nd line – fusidic acid. 3rd line – oral tetracycline or doxycycline for 6–12 weeks.[2] There is no clear evidence for steroid drops.

If linked with seborrhoeic dermatitis or dandruff, an antidandruff shampoo for hair and eyebrows may be needed. If linked with dry eyes, lubricant drops or artificial tears may be required.

Advise avoiding contact lenses during acute episodes.

Blepharitis and conjunctivitis are two of the commonest eye conditions in primary care. Be sure that you can distinguish between the two and that you can explain about treatment options.

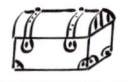

> See the **Link Hub at CompleteCSA.co.uk** for useful links to **Moorfield's Eye Hospital PILs**

Always ask about contact lens wear as those who do are more prone to get Gram negative infections. Do not assume that the patient in front of you always wears glasses!

Remember that a 'minor' problem is not necessarily trivial to the patient.

Eye Problems – 1

Doctor's Notes

Patient   Amena Khalil   4 years   F
PMH   No information
Medications   No current medications
Allergies   No information
Consultations No recent consultations
Investigations No recent investigations
Household   Lilia Khalil   28 years   F
                   Ahmed Khalil   29 years   M

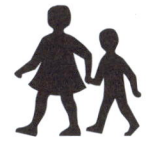

Example Consultation — Squint

Open ☐	How can I help?
History ☐	Oh I see. I'm very sorry to hear that. Please tell me more about her eyes. For example, when did you first notice this?
Flags ☐	Has this stayed much the same or has it got worse? Does she seem to see okay? Can she run around without tripping and falling? Can she look at books with you?
Risk ☐	Has anyone in the family had eye problems? Did Amena injure her eye as a baby?
Sense ☐	I sense you are worried about how she looks, about her eyesight and about whether not being able to get her to a doctor has made things worse.
ICE ☐	Do you know anything about eye problems like this? Is there anything you've been worried might be wrong or that you hoped we might be able to do to help?
Impact ☐	Tell me what's been happening in your life recently.
Curious ☐	I see you've only recently registered with us. How are you getting on in the UK?
Summary ☐	So, to recap, Amena was fine at birth but, quite soon after she had an illness with a temperature, you noticed that her eyes were not straight and this has continued, not getting any better. You are worried about her vision and whether this can be corrected. Do you have any other questions?
Empathy ☐	You must have been through such a lot in the last few months; I can't imagine how difficult it must have been for you.
O/E ☐	I would like to examine you, Amena. I need to look at your eyes to see how they move and shine a small light to see if the light bounces off the back of your eye.
Impression ☐	Mrs Khalil, looking at Amena, the light test is fine but her two eyes don't point the same way, as one turns in. This is called a convergent squint.
Experience ☐	Can I check that you understand this word 'squint'? Have you heard about this before? Squints are very common, about 1 in 20 children have a squint and the good news is that we should be able to help. Convergent means pointing inwards.
Options ☐	Amena, we need to get your eyes tested. You may well need to wear glasses for a while at least. You might also need to wear a patch on one eye to make the weak one stronger. This may well be all you need but it is possible you might need a small operation in the future to straighten the eyes.
Empower ☐	Mrs Khalil, this is not your fault. There's nothing you've done wrong or neglected to do, it's just bad luck. We can sort this out for you and there will be nothing to pay; treatment in the UK is free of charge. You can best help Amena by taking her to her appointment and following the treatment plan, for example by making sure she wears her glasses and uses an eye patch if that's what is recommended for her.
Future ☐	I'm going to make a referral to the eye hospital. You should get an appointment for Amena soon. Remember that NHS treatment is all free; there will be nothing to pay. I would also like to offer the support of a Health Visitor. Every child in the UK has a Health Visitor from birth until they attend school to support the mum and child. Often they weigh the child and answer any questions or concerns you may have. May I ask Julie, our Health Visitor, to make contact with you? Is there anything else you need? There is also a local organisation called Asylum Welcome, which you may be interested in. There are also Children Centres where you can meet other mums with small children. I'll give you contact details for all of these.
Safety net ☐	If for any reason you don't hear from the hospital, let me know. If her eyes change, or her sight seems to get worse, please contact a doctor or an optician. Opticians are available locally, usually at the shopping centres and are also free for children – there is nothing to pay to have your child seen and tested.

Eye Problems – 2

Patient's Story

Squint

Doctor's notes	Amena Khalil, 4 years. New patient. PMH: None. Medications: None.
How to act	[Mum] Worried, ground down, sad.
PC	*'Her eyes are crossed, Doctor; she cannot look straight. Can anything be done?'*
History	Amena is your first child. Quite soon after her birth, your village was overrun by terrorists. You stayed in increasingly bad conditions for some months and then fled with just a few possessions and eventually went to a refugee camp, where you have been for 2 years. There was no medical help. You were one of the first families to be evacuated to the UK. You are very grateful to be safe but conscious of all the family you have lost and left behind in Syria: your parents, brothers, sisters, nephews and nieces. You have a university degree and speak good English.
Social	You, your husband and daughter Amena (the patient) are Syrian refugees. You are staying in temporary housing. A helper there suggested booking a GP appointment.
ICE	Amena appeared normal at birth but developed 'crossed eyes' a few months after birth, after a febrile illness. You knew there was a problem but could not afford medical help and then there were no doctors in the refugee camp. You fear that not being able to feed her properly may have made it worse, especially a lack of vitamins. You are worried you have left it too late – that she will look like this forever and may not see straight. A friend said that, at 4, Amena may be too old to have surgery and may not be able to see properly. You have little money and are unsure whether you will have to pay.
Ask the doctor	*'Can anything be done?'* *'Is it my fault?'* *'Can she see out of that eye?'* *'Will an operation put things right?'* *'Will I need to pay?'*
Examination	PERLA. Convergent Squint.

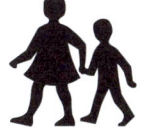

Eye Problems – 2

Learning Points   Squint

Terminology   Strabismus – any misalignment of the eyes. AKA 'Squint'.[1]

Amblyopia – decrease in vision caused by an abnormality of vision during eye development (i.e. first 2–3 years of life). Common causes are strabismus, congenital cataract, and refractive error. AKA 'Lazy Eye'.[2]

Incidence[3]   Squint (strabismus) is common – incidence about 1:20.

Who to refer[3]   It is 'normal' for eyes not to move together for a few weeks after birth but, if persisting longer than the age of 3 months, this needs a referral to a paediatric orthoptist.

Cause[3]   Squint can appear from birth or may be acquired later.

There can be a genetic link.

Sometimes appears after febrile illness; however, would have happened anyway.

Complications[3]   Often associated with refraction problems such as long or short sight.

Convergent squint is linked with long sight.

Treatment objectives[3]
1. Good sight in both eyes.
2. Both eyes working together (3D, stereoscopic vision).
3. Both eyes appear 'straight'.

Children often need glasses, then 'patching' of the good eye to make the weaker one stronger.

Surgery is often needed to straighten the eyes. One or more muscles are tightened or detached/reattached. This is generally very successful day-case surgery and recovery is quick. The eye can feel itchy or sore for a few days afterwards. Treatment is best started as early as possible and, beyond age 6–7 years, it is difficult to achieve optimal results. 3D vision is essential for some occupations such as a fire fighter or airline pilot.

Social prescribing

Social prescribing recognises the positive impact that voluntary services can have on a patient or their family. For example, a patient suffering with depression who is under housing, financial and emotional stress may benefit more from community advice and support than a doctor's pill. Social prescribing is a service becoming increasingly available in GP practices and the GP often refers to a Social Prescribing Coordinator employed by the practice and commissioned by the CCG. It is the concept of recognising the social and psychological needs of the patient and directing patients to the community services available with the aim of increasing quality of life. Local services may include: the Citizen's Advice Bureau, Age UK, Mind, Asylum Services, Children's Centres, Women's Centres and hundreds/thousands more. A GP should be aware of the services available locally (community orientation).

The patient in this case is an asylum seeker who is not well versed in the structure and processes of the NHS. It is worth spelling out what may appear obvious to you but not to the patient – for example, that NHS treatment is free. If the patient is worrying about cost, this may inhibit him or her from attending the specialist appointment.

Doctor's Notes

Name   Abida Khan   70 years   F
PMH   No information
Medications   No information
Consultations Routine elderly person review with nurse – BP 140/90

Recent consultation with viral URTI – advised to get OTC preparations from the chemist.

Investigations None
Household   Rashid Khan   72 years   M

Example Consultation — Acute Glaucoma

Open ☐	Hello Mrs Khan, I'm very sorry to hear that. Please tell me more about your eye and the sickness.
History ☐	Have you had this before? How is your vision just now? Are there haloes around lights? Have you been sick or just felt queasy?
Impact ☐	Tell me a bit about yourself. How has this affected you today, up until coming to see me?
Flags ☐	Has anyone in the family had eye problems?
Risk ☐	Are you long-sighted or short-sighted? Have you taken any medication at all lately?
Sense ☐	You mentioned your father's blindness. Are you worried that might happen to you?
ICE ☐	What thoughts have you had about this? Any other worries? Did you have anything in your mind you thought I might be able to do today?
Curious ☐	You thought you needed antibiotics for your recent cold. Were you annoyed that they weren't prescribed?
Summary ☐	For a few months you have had occasional episodes of pain in the eye and blurred vision. You have recently taken a medicine from the pharmacy. You went to the cinema last night and these symptoms came on really severely. You fear you have an infection which may harm your eyesight.
O/E ☐	I want to have a good look at both eyes. I need to feel the eyes with your lids closed, shine a light in both eyes to check the pupils, test how well you can focus with a chart and look at the back of the eye. This will mean I need to come quite close to you, is that okay?
Empathy ☐	I can understand how worried you are, particularly with your father going blind.
Impression ☐	My impression is that there may be a build-up of fluid pressure in the eye, which we call glaucoma. You wondered if it was an infection but I don't think it is.
Experience ☐	Have you heard of glaucoma or known anyone who has it?
Explanation ☐	In glaucoma, the eye fluid can't circulate as it should and pressure tends to build up, giving you pain and sickness. Left untreated it can be very serious. It's not an infection but it is possible that the decongestant tablets may have contributed to bringing this on. Being long-sighted and from SE Asia are also risk factors. Being in the near darkness of the cinema may have been the final trigger.
Options ☐	It is really important that we get you to the hospital to be seen by a specialist eye doctor as soon as possible. I will phone the emergency eye clinic now to arrange this. Have you got someone who can drive you to the hospital? Whilst you are waiting, you may be more comfortable lying flat on your back on my couch, face up with no pillow. Would you like some painkillers and something to take away the sickly feeling?
Empower ☐	I am going to print off a PIL about glaucoma so that you understand what has happened and what to expect.
Future ☐	I think the doctors at the hospital will give you some eye drops and medicines to reduce the pressure in your eye so that you are more comfortable. It is likely that they will suggest a small operation on your eye with a laser to make a wider passage for the fluids in your eye to move around.
Safety net ☐	If for any reason you are not seen at the hospital, please let me know and I will sort this out. Please call or see me next week to tell me what is happening.

Patient's Story

Acute Glaucoma

Doctor's notes Abida Khan, 70 years. PMH: Routine elderly person review with PN 4 weeks ago – BP 140/90. Recent GP consultation: viral URTI. Advised OTC preparations. Medications: None.

How to act Very worried. In discomfort. Annoyed (you think you should have had antibiotics recently and that you are ill now because you weren't prescribed them).

PC *'I was watching the new James Bond film at the cinema last night when I started to feel sick and my left eye became sore. It's no better today.'*

History You were out at the cinema last night with family for a birthday celebration when you noticed your left eye starting to ache. You were all right when you set out from home but your sight became blurred and there were haloes around the street lights when you went home. You have had a few similar but very mild episodes, but they passed quickly. Things are no better today – you feel sickly and unwell. You have recently had a cold that was troublesome. You came to the doctor for antibiotics but were told you did not need them and that you should go to the chemist. This annoyed you because you are entitled to free prescriptions. Nevertheless, you went to the supermarket and bought some decongestant tablets (Sudafed Blocked Nose).

You have always been long-sighted and wear glasses. You remember that your father had very poor eyesight in later life (though you are not sure why) and he was blind for the last few years. He lived with you and you had to look after him with this disability.

You have no fever or symptoms of a lung infection. Your cold is better but you feel sick and disorientated.

Social Housewife, married to an accountant. Lives with husband. Grown-up children. Never smoked and no alcohol.

ICE What is happening? Why do I feel so ill? Has the cold affected my eye – an infection perhaps? Will I go blind like my father?

Ask the doctor *'What is happening?'*

'Have I got an eye infection because you wouldn't prescribe antibiotics?'

'Am I going blind like my father?'

Examination Right eye normal. Left eye – pupil does not react to light. VA 6/9 right eye, 6/60 left eye. Left eye red.

Eye Problems – 3

Learning Points

Acute Glaucoma

In presentations of acutely red and painful eye suspect acute angle closure glaucoma, particularly when:

- Female, older, long-sighted and Asian.
- History of similar problems – headache, blurred vision, nausea, eye pain, haloes around lights.
- Recent use of antimuscarinic (e.g. amitriptyline) or adrenergic (e.g. phenylephrine).

Symptoms   Headache, nausea and vomiting, blurred vision and haloes.

Signs   Eyeball feels hard to the touch. Pupil fixed and semi-dilated. Reduced VA. Optic disc abnormal – engorged vessels (difficult for non-specialist to detect.)

Management

Medical emergency. Refer immediately to ophthalmologist for admission. If this is not immediately possible:

- First aid – lie patient flat (no pillows) face up – may reduce pressure.
- Give pain relief and antisickness drug.
- If available – pilocarpine 1 drop 2% in blue eyes and 1 drop 4% in brown eyes (evidence based).
- Acetazolamide 500 mg orally if no contraindication.

Secondary care management – topical and IV drugs to reduce pressure then usually laser surgery to iris. The unaffected eye is treated too as it is also at risk.

Always ask about OTC medications and do not assume that they are benign products with few relevant side effects. The product bought by this patient contained phenylephrine which may well have contributed to the sudden onset of acute glaucoma.

Doctor's Notes

Name   Fred Scott   81 years   M
PMH   Hypertension
Medications Atenolol 100 mg daily
Consultations BP check with nurse 2 months ago – all well
Investigations U&E, cholesterol normal 2 months ago
Household   Daisy Scott   84 years   F

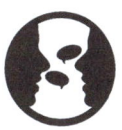

Example Consultation — ARMD and Cataract

Open ☐	Hello Mr Scott – thank you – let me just have a moment to read the note. Did the optician explain to you his concern?
History ☐	Okay, now was this a routine check or had you noticed any problems with your sight? Tell me what problems you had noticed, for example with reading or distance vision.
Risk ☐	Are you driving? How about at night? Have you had any near misses?
Flags ☐	Can I check if you smoke? Do you eat a good diet? Fruit and veg?
Sense ☐	I sense that you have had some concerns yourself about your sight and whether it's safe to drive, even before you saw the optician.
Impact ☐	Tell me about your home situation. How far are you from the shops? Does anyone else drive? Any family nearby? Can you use Internet grocery shopping?
Curious ☐	You mentioned your father went blind; can you tell me about that?
ICE ☐	What thoughts have you had since you saw the optician? Tell me what worries you about your sight or not driving. Was there anything you were hoping I might suggest?
Summary ☐	After the near miss you were worried about your sight and your optician has confirmed your worst fears and told you not to drive, which is a real blow.
O/E ☐	Your blood pressure is reasonably well controlled and your pulse is regular.
Empathy ☐	It must have been a shock for you being told that you had some problems. The car is a lifeline for you and being told not to drive is worrying.
Impression ☐	The optician says you have two problems: one is that you are developing cataracts and the other is age-related macular degeneration or ARMD.
Experience ☐	I know your father had eye problems; have you heard about cataracts or ARMD?
Explanation ☐	Cataracts are a cloudiness of the eye lens so the light can't pass through it so well. The other problem means that the most sensitive and the important area of the back of the eye is becoming worn and less sensitive, so your sight will not be as sharp as it used to be.
Options ☐	You mentioned vitamins. Eating a balanced diet is important but there is some evidence that supplements with vitamin C and antioxidants can slow ARMD. Controlling your BP well may also help and we should recheck that in a couple of weeks. It's good that you don't smoke. Surgery will cure the cataracts and I can refer you for this, if you like. There is no need to wait until the cataracts are worse. It will not help the ARMD but your sight could be reassessed after the operation and it might mean you can drive for a while longer. Your vision may deteriorate with time but this can be quite a steady change.
Empower ☐	How do you feel about this? Would you like me to refer you? I am going to give you a PIL about ARMD; I will print it off in large type so it is easier to read. If your children can help you with the Internet, you can also listen to the leaflet being read out loud.
Future ☐	Come back in 2 weeks to see the nurse for a BP check. We will do some blood tests to make sure everything else is okay, e.g. your blood sugar. You shouldn't drive for now – your insurance would not cover you if you had an accident. Could one of your children help with shopping for now? Could they shop on the Internet for you and get groceries delivered to your home?
Safety net ☐	If your sight deteriorates further whilst waiting for the appointment, please come back and see me.

Patient's Story

ARMD and Cataract

Doctor's notes	Fred Scott, 81 years. PMH: Hypertension. Medication: Atenolol.
How to act	Polite, concerned about your eyesight.
PC	*'I went to the optician this morning and she wrote this for you.'*
History	You went for an eye check today and the optician told you that you are developing cataracts and ARMD. She said your sight was borderline for being able to drive and suggested you stop. She told you to see your GP to discuss this. You had noticed that your sight seemed a bit worse than usual and troublesome 'haloes' around street lights had already made you give up night-time driving. You had a near miss last week when you did not see a car and pulled out of a junction. You have had to stop buying a newspaper as you cannot read the print any more.
Social	You are a retired teacher and live with your wife who is also retired. You live quite a way from the shops and rely on being able to drive to do the shopping and get out and about. The car is your 'lifeline'. Your wife has never driven; you have always been the family 'chauffeur'. There are no family members close by. Your father went blind in later life, when he was about 83. You remember how he struggled and became virtually housebound before he fell over at home, fractured his hip and died shortly afterwards. You have never smoked, and eat a balanced diet. You are a basic computer user, not Internet literate.
ICE	You are now very worried about your sight.
Understanding	You have never heard of ARMD and will react badly to the use of this acronym that means nothing to you (unless described). You saw your father lose his independence once he started to lose his sight and are worried you are going the same way. You are sure you are still safe to drive to the shops – it's not far and you know the way.
Ask the doctor	*'What is ARMD? Is it okay to drive short distances?'*
	'Am I going blind?'
	'Will an operation help?'
	'Why can't I have an operation now?'
Optician's note	'… I have advised him to see you for referral to an ophthalmologist for treatment of his ARMD and cataracts. His sight is below the legal level for driving.'
Examination	BP 150/80. Pulse 60 bpm regular.

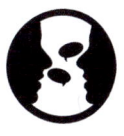

Eye Problems – 4

Learning Points

ARMD and Cataract

Cataract

Epidemiology	Mainly >65. Men and women equal risk.
Aetiology	Changes in proteins that make up lens.
Symptoms	Cloudiness. Especially night vision with haloes around lights.
Risk factors	FH, diabetes, eye surgery or injury, uveitis, prolonged or high-dose steroids.
	Other risk factors: smoking, alcohol, poor diet, sunlight.
Treatment	Surgery. No need to wait 'until cataract is ripe' any more.
	Usually LA, go home same day. Lens removed and replaced with plastic one. May still need glasses for distance or near vision.

ARMD

Epidemiology	Women > men. Commoner in white and Chinese heritage people.
Symptoms	Affects central but not peripheral vision.
	Reading, facial recognition more difficult. Colours become duller.
Risk factors	FH, age (>60), smoking, alcohol, poor diet, sunlight.
Dry AMD	Commonest type, macula cells become damaged by build-up of drusen deposits. Visual loss gradual, over many years.
	Treatment: diet rich in vitamins A, C, E may help.
Wet AMD	10% people with dry ARMD may develop wet ARMD.
	Abnormal blood vessels develop beneath the macula and damage the cells.
	Much more serious than dry ARMD – vision can deteriorate in days.
	Treatment: injections of anti vascular endothelial growth factor; laser treatment.

DVLA driving requirements

Vision at least 6/12 using both eyes

+ adequate field vision

+ read number plate from 20 m

When a patient has sight problems, think about how you can give them accessible patient information, e.g. auditory leaflet or print off in large type. Remember that older people may be highly Internet literate or may have a basic level of skills – don't make assumptions, check it out.

Doctor's Notes

Name Eric Johnson   61 years   M
PMH Type 2 diabetes diagnosed 10 years ago.
Medications Metformin 500 mg tds
Gliclazide 160 mg daily
Blood glucose testing strips
Consultations Annual diabetes review with practice nurse 1 month ago
Investigations HbA1c – 59 mmol/mol
BP 150/80 (recheck booked). Foot check normal.
Diabetic eye check at hospital – mild retinopathy.
Household Kathleen Johnson   61 years   F

Example Consultation — Retinal Detachment

Open ☐	Hello Mr Johnson. I'm very sorry to hear that. Please can you tell me more about the blurred vision, starting from when you first noticed it?
History ☐	Does the vision fluctuate or is it just as bad all the time? Any pain in the eyeball? Any redness? Any other eye symptoms? Has it affected your driving? Tell me about your work.
Flags ☐	Any floaters? Anything that appears to be like a curtain coming across your vision? Any flashes?
Risk ☐	You wear glasses – are you short-sighted or long-sighted? Did you have any eye problems when you were a baby? Has anyone in the family had anything similar? Have you been hit in the eye recently?
Sense ☐	I sense this is very worrying for you and understandably so.
ICE ☐	What thoughts have you had about this? What concerns you most? Tell me, did you have any thoughts yourself about how I might be able to help you best today?
Impact ☐	Your sight is really important and you need to be able to drive safely to do your job. With diabetes, you need to be able to see well to check your blood sugars so that you can monitor your control. Diabetes, as you know, can affect eyesight so it is especially important to get your blood sugars under control.
Curious ☐	You mentioned being stressed; please tell me a bit about that.
Summary ☐	To summarise, for the last couple of weeks your sight seems to have got worse in your right eye but not your left. The vision is blurred and you had a near miss in your car. You have had some understandable stress at work and I understand that it feels very important to fly to the US next week.
O/E ☐	I'd like to thoroughly examine your eyes by checking your sight using a chart, checking your fields of vision and looking at the back of the eye. I will need to be close to you to do this – is that okay?
Empathy ☐	It's very scary noticing that your vision is blurred for no apparent reason.
Impression ☐	I don't think it's likely this is caused by your diabetes but the squash ball may possibly have had a role. Being very short-sighted is another risk factor.
Explanation ☐	I think it is very likely that the membrane at the back of the eye, which we call the retina, has come unstuck and this is why you have had these symptoms.
Experience ☐	This is called a detached retina; is this something you have heard of before?
Options ☐	It's important we get you to an expert as soon as possible as this condition can get worse if left untreated. I would like to ring and speak to the on-call doctor for eye problems at the local hospital. I would expect them to examine you and they may want to treat you today either with laser treatment or by putting a gas or oil bubble into the eye to help hold the retina back in place.
Empower ☐	I'm going to give you a leaflet that will help make more sense of this.
Future ☐	Here is a letter for you to take to the hospital. Please phone me tomorrow to let me know what has happened. I'm sorry but I think it is unlikely that you will be able to fly to the US next week as this could prevent healing of the retinal problem and could be very risky for your eyesight. You must not drive while your vision is a concern. Who can drive you to the hospital?
Safety net ☐	If for any reason you aren't seen and examined at the hospital today, please phone me at the surgery to let me know so that I can see if I can sort out an alternative.

Patient's Story

Retinal Detachment

Doctor's notes Eric Johnson, 61 years. PMH: Type 2 diabetes.

Medications: Metformin, Gliclazide, blood glucose testing strips.

How to act Very concerned.

PC *'My vision's gone blurred in my right eye.'*

History You are a 61-year-old businessman with diabetes that you struggle to manage well. Over the last couple of weeks, you have noticed slight reduction in VA in your right eye. You put this down to stress at work (financial viability of your company – selling tractors) or the diabetes being not well controlled, but last week you realised you couldn't see a car that was on your right-hand side when driving and had a near miss. This was very scary. You have always been short-sighted and wear quite thick lenses and contact lenses for sport. You try to keep fit by playing squash and were hit in the eye by a ball a few weeks ago. The eye was a bit sore for a few hours but then okay. You did not seek help at the time because you were busy and it is always hard to get an appointment at the doctors.

Social Married, with grown-up children. Businessman, working long hours. Important business meeting in the US next week – crucial you get to this as there is potential for a big order that could make or break the company.

ICE You are unsure what is causing it but wonder if it was the eye injury with the ball. You suspect your diabetes may be another possibility. You think the doctor will tell you off about your diabetes or tell you not to get so stressed (and this would annoy you). You are worried that either your vision is deteriorating or the doctor will say you can't fly.

Ask the doctor *'Am I going blind?'*

'Is it the diabetes?'

'Was it the squash ball injury?'

'If treated today, can I go to the US next week?'

Examination VA left eye – 6/9, right eye – 6/60.

Reduced visual field – lateral vision right eye.

Fundoscopy – difficult and retina not seen clearly.

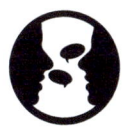

Eye Problems – 5

Learning Points   Retinal Detachment

Epidemiology	1 to 1.5/10,000 people per year.
	(One or two new cases per year in a medium-sized practice of 10,000 patients)
	Risk increases with increasing age: lifetime risk = 3% at 85 years
	Average age of occurrence = 60 years.
	Male = female.
Risk factors	Short-sightedness, FH, eye trauma, previous cataract surgery, diabetes (proliferative retinopathy), inflammatory eye problems, e.g. uveitis, scleritis, malignancy (secondary deposit or ocular melanoma primary), congenital eye disease (glaucoma, prematurity, cataract).
Symptoms	New onset of floaters (lines, haze, dots).
	New onset flashes of light.
	Sudden onset loss of vision – starts at edge of vision and progresses to centre. Often described as a 'curtain'.
	Reduced visual acuity– blurred vision.
	Contralateral eye affected in 10%.
Examination	Visual acuity – may be reduced to 'counting fingers'.
Management	Of new onset floaters/flashing lights:

1. Urgent (same-day ophthalmology) – if 'curtain', visual field loss, blurred vision, abnormal fundoscopy.
2. Less urgent (slit lamp within 24 hours) – if no reduction in VA, no field loss, fundoscopy normal.

Either case: PIL produced by RCO and RNIB – 'understanding retinal detachment'.

Hospital treatment

There are various ways of closing the hole and holding the retina against the eye wall. Surgeons often use a gas or oil bubble, then laser or cryotherapy to 'stick' it in place. The patient has to lie in a particular 'posture' to get the bubble in the right place. No air travel is permitted if gas has been used as the gas could expand and cause glaucoma and/or blindness.

When a patient has a chronic illness as well as the acute presentation (diabetes in this case), think about how the new problem will impact on their ability to manage their chronic illness. In this case, problems with sight could make it difficult to use and read a blood sugar monitor, with implications for diabetic control, ultimately risking further sight damage.

Extra Notes — The Red Eye

The primary care dilemma is to be able to confidently differentiate mild benign conditions (e.g. conjunctivitis) from those that need urgent referral.

What to ask: When did it start?

How did it start – quickly or gradually?

What eye symptoms (blurred vision, pain, photophobia, discharge)?

One eye or both eyes?

Contact lens wearer?

Any general symptoms (headache, nausea, fever, rash)?

Possible injury, foreign body or trauma?

PMH – eyes: Has it happened before?

Any eye operations?

Impact Work? Driving? Reading?

Examination VA, pupils, fundoscopy.

Eye Problems

Extra Notes

The Red Eye

Table adapted from http://patient.info/doctor/red-eye

	Age?	Pain	Symptoms	Signs	Urgent referral?
Conjunctivitis [Most are viral. Antibiotics do not significantly shorten bacterial conjunctivitis]	any	no	Itchy, gritty, discharge	Redness, watering Sticky discharge. VA normal	No, but refer if not settling/responding over 7–10 days or if suspect herpes. Swab for chlamydia in neonates
Subconjunctival haemorrhage	Older people	no	May start after coughing. Sometimes the eye aches	Deep redness. Usually unilateral. VA normal	No, but refer if lasts >1 week Check BP
Episcleritis	any	no	Mild discomfort	Defined wedge of redness. VA normal	No, but refer if >1 week
Trauma/FB	any	yes	Pain. Usually unilateral	Depends on trauma	Depends – immediate if ?penetration Slit lamp needed
Acute glaucoma	Older, usually >50	yes	Pain, haloes around lights, blurred vision, feels sick, ill, headache	Severe redness, ↓VA, pupil fixed, semidilated	Yes – immediate
Acute anterior uveitis	Usually 20–50 years	yes	Blurred vision, headache, light sensitive	Severe redness, ↓VA,	Yes – urgent same day
Corneal ulcer (ulcerative keratitis)	any	yes	Photophobia, watering, blurred vision	Stains with fluorescein	Yes – urgent same day
Scleritis	>50	yes	'Boring' eye pain + photophobia and ↓VA. Usually systemic disease, e.g. gout, herpes zoster, connective tissue disorder	Depends. Anterior = deep injection. Posterior = minimal signs	Yes – 24–48 hours
Endophthalmitis (inflammation of ocular cavities).	any	yes	Red eye, ↓VA, recent surgery, IVDU, trauma, immunocompromised	Hypopyon in anterior chamber, eyelid oedema	Yes – immediate. Rare condition but significant++

CHAPTER 19 OVERVIEW
Metabolic Problems

	Cases in this chapter	Within the RCGP curriculum: Care of People with Metabolic Problems RCGP Curriculum Online. March 2016[1]	Learning points in the chapter include:
1	Hyperparathyroidism	'Demonstrate a logical, incremental approach to investigation and diagnosis of metabolic problems'	Hypercalcaemia differential diagnosis Differential diagnosis of raised PTH
2	Diabetes Diagnosis	'Understand the need for early recognition and monitoring of complications in diabetes mellitus'	Diagnostic criteria Medication in diabetes
3	Type 2 Diabetes Review	'Recognise your central role as a primary care physician in managing diabetes mellitus' 'Understand the role of particular groups of medication in the management of diabetes, e.g. anti-platelet drugs, ACE inhibitors, angiotension-2 receptor antagonists, lipid-lowering therapies, GLP-1 agonists'	HbA1c targets Risk management Education and support
4	Tired All The Time	'Recognise that patients with metabolic problems are frequently asymptomatic or have non-specific symptoms and that diagnosis is often made by screening or recognising symptom complexes and arranging appropriate investigations'	Cushing's syndrome
5	Hyperthyroidism	'Manage appropriately primary contact with patients who have a metabolic problem'	Managing hyperthyroidism flow diagram
	Extra Notes		Antihyperglycaemics table

1. http://www.rcgp.org.uk/training-exams/gp-curriculum-overview/online-curriculum/applying-clinical-knowledge-section-2/3-17-metabolic-problems.aspx

CHAPTER 19 REFERENCES

Hyperparathyroidism
1. http://patient.info/doctor/hyperparathyroidism-pro
2. GP Update. Hypercalcaemia and primary hyperparathyroidism. Sep 2015. http://www.gp-update.co.uk/files/docs/Hypercalcaemia_and_primary_hyperparathyroidism.pdf
3. Taniegra E.D. Hyperparathyroidism. *Am Fam Physician*. 2004 Jan 15; 69(2): 333–9.

Diabetes Diagnosis
1. http://patient.info/doctor/glycated-haemoglobin-hba1c
2. Lilly M., Godwin M. Treating prediabetes with metformin. Systematic review and meta-analysis. *Can Fam Physician*. 2009 Apr; 55(4): 363–9.
3. NICE Guidelines. NG28. Type 2 diabetes in adults: management. Dec 2015.
4. NICE Guidelines. CG181. Cardiovascular disease: risk assessment and reduction, including lipid modification. Jul 2014.

Type 2 Diabetes Review
1. NICE Guidelines. NG28. Type 2 diabetes in adults: management. Dec 2015.
2. McCulloch D., et al. Treatment of type 2 diabetes mellitus in the older patient. May 2016. http://www.uptodate.com/contents/treatment-of-type-2-diabetes-mellitus-in-the-older-patient
3. Pierce M. Type 2 diabetes: prevention and cure? *Br J Gen Pract*. 2013 Feb; 63(607): 60–1.
4. http://www.dafne.uk.com/
5. http://www.desmond-project.org.uk/
6. https://www.nice.org.uk/guidance/ng28/resources/do-not-do
7. http://patient.info/doctor/antihyperglycaemic-agents-used-for-type-2-diabetes

Tired All The Time
1. http://patient.info/doctor/cushings-syndrome-pro

Hyperthyroidism
1. Wass J., Karavitaki N., Grossman A., et al. Joint management of thyrotoxicosis in primary and secondary care. Oxford University Hospitals NHS Foundation Trust. February 2012. http://occg.oxnet.nhs.uk/GeneralPractic.e/ClinicalGuidelines/Endocrinology/Thyroid/Guidelines%20for%20management%20of%20thyroid%20disorders%20%20FINAL%2016%2002%2012.pdf

Antihyperglycaemics
1. NICE. http://cks.nice.org.uk/diabetes-type-2. July 2016.
2. GP Update Summer 2012.
3. Hot Topics Spring 2014.
4. NICE Guidelines. NG28 Type 2 diabetes: management. Dec 2015.
   Algorithm for blood glucose lowering therapy in adults with type 2 diabetes.
5. NICE. https://www.nice.org.uk/guidance/ng28/resources/patient-decision-aid-2187281197 7. Dec 2015.
6. NICE Guidelines. NG28 Type 2 diabetes: management. Dec 2015.
7. https://www.gov.uk/drug-safety-update/sglt2-inhibitors-canagliflozin-dapagliflozin-empagliflozin-risk-of-diabetic-ketoacidosis. Contains public sector information licensed under the open Government Licence v 3.0.
8. http://patient.info/medicine/pioglitazone-tablets-for-diabetes-actos-diabiom-glidipion
9. http://patient.info/doctor/antihyperglycaemic-agents-used-for-type-2-diabetes

Doctor's Notes

Patient   Avani Virdee   57 years   F
PMH   No medical history
Medications No current medications
Allergies   No information
Consultations Bloods taken for routine health check
Investigations

3 weeks ago:
FBC	normal
U&E/LFT/TFT	normal
Lipids	normal
HbA1c	normal
eGFR	80 ml/min/1.73 m²
Corrected Ca	2.73 mmol/L (2.2–2.6 mmol/L)
Vitamin D	51 nmol/L (>50 nmol/L) = sufficient
	(30–50 nmol/L) = deficiency
	(<30 nmol/L) = severe deficiency

1 week ago:
PTH   7.9 pmol/L   (1.6–7.2 pmol/L)

Household   No household members registered

Example Consultation — Hyperparathyroidism

Open — Mrs Virdee, thank you for coming in. What led you to have these tests taken?

Sense — I can see you are worried and keen to know your result.

Impression — The blood test has shown that a little gland in your neck may be releasing too much hormone which increases the body's calcium level. This is called hyperparathyroidism. The hyper means too much and the parathyroid is a gland that sits in the neck. All your other blood tests are normal. This can be serious as high calcium levels can make you feel unwell. You are likely to have had it for many months but the good news is that we can often cure this problem.

Experience — Any questions so far? Calcium is good for you in moderation, like most things! Too much calcium can cause you to feel unwell but we don't usually advise calcium restriction in this condition.

History — To help me work out the best course of action, can I ask a little more about you? Have you felt unwell? Do you have any medical problems? Do you take any medicines?

Flags — Are you more thirsty recently? Passing more urine than normal? Any pain at all? Are your bowels okay? Have you ever had a kidney stone?

ICE — Before you came here today, did you have any thoughts about what may be wrong? Was there anything else you were hoping to talk about today?

Curious — You mentioned you were tired; what might be causing that do you think?

Summary — So to summarise, you were invited for a health check. We have detected a raised calcium level and raised parathyroid hormone level, which is likely to be due to a condition called hyperparathyroidism. Apart from feeling tired, which may be due to your work and family commitments, you feel well. You are keen to know what happens next. Have I got it right so far?

O/E — May I examine you; have a feel of your neck for lumps? All normal and reassuring.

Empathy — I appreciate that any new diagnosis causes worry and apprehension.

Options — This is a treatable problem. I think we need to send a referral to the hormone specialists called the endocrinologists. We should also do a few more blood tests, to recheck the calcium level as we haven't done this for 3 weeks. I usually also keep an eye on the kidneys to make sure you are not dehydrated. I would also suggest a bone scan, because some calcium will have come out of the bones which can weaken them.

Empower — You don't need to reduce the calcium in your diet, but it is important to avoid dehydration.

Future — I expect the endocrinologists will see you within the next month. At the hospital they will probably do further tests and may offer an operation to cure the problem by removing the gland. Sometimes no treatment is required, particularly if the calcium level stays below 3.

Safety net — If you ever start to feel thirsty, start passing more urine, have any pains or tummy upset, please come to see me as these may be symptoms of raised calcium. That is a lot of information; may I check I have been clear – what symptoms will lead you to contact the GP straight away? Thank you. Any other questions?

Metabolic Problems – 1

Patient's Story

Hyperparathyroidism

Doctor's notes Avani Virdee, 57 years. PMH: None. Medications: None.

Bloods taken for routine health check. Raised calcium and PTH.

Other bloods normal.

How to act Keen to know your results and what it means.

PC *'I was told to have a second blood test and then I've received another letter saying you wanted to see me about my tests … What's wrong?'*

History You have been a little tired but are otherwise very well.

You had a suspected kidney stone 4 months ago but the pain settled spontaneously so you didn't go for your USS. You have had no pain since.

Social You are married with 2 children.

You are a medical secretary. You are Sikh.

You are a new grandmother so are often on the road travelling to see the family.

ICE You thought you were tired because you are busy with work and the family.

You haven't slept well this week with fear over what the doctor may say.

You do not know what to expect.

You have never heard of hyperparathyroidism. You want to know all about it.

Ask the doctor *'I thought calcium was good for you.'*

'What has caused it?'

'Should I stop eating yoghurt and milk?'

Examination Examination of the neck is normal with no lymphadenopathy.

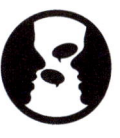

Metabolic Problems – 1

Learning Points — Hyperparathyroidism

PTH is released in response to low calcium.

Primary hyperparathyroidism
Causes include an adenoma on the parathyroid gland or familial endocrine disorders (e.g. multiple endocrine neoplasia).

Blood tests shows a raised calcium + raised PTH + reduced phosphate.

Symptoms[1]
- Asymptomatic — (often if calcium is below 3).
- 'Bones' — Fractures from reduced BMD, fatigue and myopathy.
- 'Stones' — Kidney stones.
- 'Groans' — Nausea, vomiting, constipation, gastritis and pancreatitis.
- 'Moans' — Malaise, confusion, depression or reduced GCS.
- Dehydration — Polydipsia, polyuria and dehydration.

Hypercalcaemia

Differential diagnosis	Investigations required/findings	
Myeloma	Normal PTH	Anaemia + renal impairment + monoclonal gammopathy
Bone metastases	Normal PTH	CT CAP if previous malignancy
Sarcoidosis	Normal PTH	CXR
Paget's	Normal PTH	Raised ALP
Addison's	Normal PTH	Low Na + raised K
Vitamin D toxicity	Normal PTH	Raised vitamin D
Thyrotoxicosis	Normal PTH	Raised T4

Differential diagnosis of raised PTH

Iatrogenic (e.g. lithium)

Vitamin D deficiency	Normal calcium
Secondary ↑PTH	Low/normal calcium drives the rise in PTH
Tertiary hyperparathyroidism	Similar picture to primary ↑PTH and occurs in CKD.[2]

Management of ↑PTH
Replace vitamin D deficiency.

Review medicines: anticonvulsants, steroids, thiazides and lithium.[2]

Refer to endocrinology. Same day if requires hydration or unwell.

Imaging: Biannual DEXA. USS/CT KUB if possible kidney stones.[2]

Parathyroidectomy.

Metabolic Problems – 1

Doctor's Notes

Patient	Dennis Peters	58 years	M
PMH	Hypertension		
Medications	Indapamide 2.5 mg		
	Atenolol 50 mg		
Allergies	No information		
Consultations	Bloods taken for annual medication review		
Investigations	BP 136/90		
	HbA1c 6.9% or 52 mmol/mol		
	eGFR 78 ml/min/1.73 m^2		
	Na$^+$ 142 mmol/L		
	K$^+$ 4.0 mmol/L		
	Total cholesterol 3.5 mmol/L		
Household	No household members registered		

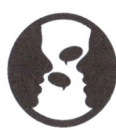

Example Consultation — Diabetes Diagnosis

Open — Mr Peters, I can see you are keen to know your result. Your blood sugar is high.

History — It would be helpful if I could understand your history to be able to decide what this means for you. I'm interested to know more about your health. And it's the first time we have met … do you have a family? I'm sorry to hear about your wife. How are you? Is there anyone else in your life? Do you work?

Flags — Do you: find you are thirsty often? Drink during the night? Frequently need to pass urine?

Risk — Do you smoke? Have you ever had any pain in the chest or legs when walking?

Curious — You asked straight away what treatment you may need. Are you worried about that? You mentioned your children will be very worried; what was going through your mind when you said that?

Impression — I think you have type 2 diabetes.

Sense — I can see this has come as a shock.

Experience — What do you know about diabetes?

ICE — Have you known anyone who has had diabetes? What is going through your mind?

Explanation — In diabetes, your blood sugar level is high but this is not because you have eaten too much sugar. The cause may either be that the muscles are not using the sugar in your blood or you are producing less insulin, a chemical which clears up excess sugar. Any questions so far?

Impact — How do you think this diagnosis might affect you day to day?

Empathy — I appreciate you are frightened especially after your uncle's experience.

Explanation — We need to keep the sugars low to keep the large vessels in the brain and heart healthy. If these vessels become damaged with fatty build-up, this can lead to angina or a stroke. The smaller vessels, for example in the eyes, feet and kidneys, can be affected. However, your other blood tests were excellent, including your kidneys and cholesterol. Any questions? It's a lot to take in and I'm happy to explain again.

Empower — Your blood sugar is not dangerous. We can control your blood sugars and pressure to protect your vessels in the future. There are things you can do to help too, watching your diet and exercising. I will ask the nurse to discuss foods with you. Do you feel these are steps you could take?

Options — We have a couple of options at this stage. We could see if your blood sugars reduce without tablets; we can try this if you feel there are changes you can make to your diet and exercise routine. However, if you don't feel there is much scope here, there is a tablet called metformin. What would you like to do? Okay, you start taking one tablet with your breakfast for a week, next week add a tablet with your evening meal and the week after that a tablet also with lunch so you are then taking three tablets a day. Side effects may include an upset stomach so if you feel unwell just let the GP know. Is that okay?

Future — Next time I'd like to tweak your blood pressure medications, as in diabetes there are better tablets for your blood pressure. So please make an appointment to see me next week. There is a lot to take in today; you may have further questions. Just write down questions you think of and we can go through them next week. Can you please make an appointment to see our diabetes nurse too? She will go through the lifestyle factors which can affect diabetes and explain more about monitoring and managing diabetes. She may also suggest that you attend a diabetes education course called DESMOND. Here is your prescription.

Metabolic Problems – 2

Patient's Story

Diabetes Diagnosis

Doctor's notes Dennis Peters, 58 years. PMH: Hypertension.

Medication: Indapamide 2.5 mg, Atenolol 50 mg. Blood tests for medication review BP 136/90, HbA1c 6.9% or 52 mmol/mol, eGFR 78 ml/min/1.73 m², Na 142 mmol/L, K 4.0 mmol/L, Total cholesterol 3.5 mmol/L

How to act Concerned and in disbelief

PC *'I've been asked to speak to you about my blood tests. What's wrong with them?'* After being told that the sugar is too high, ask *'What treatment will I need?'*

History You haven't noticed any polydipsia or polyuria until the doctor mentions it.

You do get up at night to go to the toilet and each time drink a glass of water.

You are always thirsty.

You have been in good health apart from your blood pressure.

Social Your wife died of breast cancer 3 years ago.

Since then you have not taken care of your diet but rarely drink alcohol.

No exercise. Never smoked.

You have three children and your two daughters *'will be very worried'*.

They took the news of their mother especially hard.

You see all your children often … they are always checking up on you.

If asked how you could change your lifestyle … you would like a dog to walk.

ICE You know diabetes happens when you have eaten too much sugar.

You are worried this will mean injecting yourself every day.

You did not expect this diagnosis.

Your uncle had diabetes and had to have his foot amputated.

You feel you could change your diet and exercise a little but when the doctor mentions a medicine you are keen to begin treatment.

Prescription Metformin before leaving the room.

Metabolic Problems – 2

Learning Points   Diabetes Diagnosis

When marking this case – did the doctor address this patient's incorrect health belief?
Watch out for type 1 diabetics: Osmotic symptoms, blurred vision, weight ↓ and generally unwell.
Type 2 symptoms: General itch, ED, infections, peripheral neuropathy.
Lactic acidosis: N&V, abdominal pain, LOC, thirst. Risk factors: nephrotoxic drugs or organ failure.
Blood ketones: If BM >12 test blood ketones, if >0.6 inform a doctor.

Diabetes diagnosis (not gestational): 2 of the following:

Symptomatic	Fasting blood glucose (FBG) >7 mmol/L
Random blood glucose >11.1 mmol/L	HbA1c >6.5% (48 mmol/mol)

HbA1c not accurate in[1]

<18 years	Gestational DM
Steroids	HIV
Renal failure	Iron deficiency
Pancreatic damage	Rapid onset symptoms
Haemoglobinopathy	Haemolytic anaemia
<2/12 postnatal	Antipsychotics in 1st 2/12 Rx

Pre-diabetes	HbA1c 6.1–6.4% (43–47 mmol/mol)
Impaired glucose tolerance	FBG <7.0 mmol/L and OGTT between 7.8 and 11 mmol/L
Pre-diabetes: Impaired fasting glucose	FBG 6.1–6.9 mmol/L

When to start medication depends on patient preference. Metformin can also be beneficial in pre-diabetes.[2]

Choosing the medication

Who is the patient?	Their lifestyle and wishes
What risk needs to be avoided?	Comorbidities and risk (live alone/work up ladders)
Do we need to treat more proactively?	Younger patient or signs of micro/macro disease
What is the aim of their HbA1c?	Tailored to them (hypo risk/comorbidities)

Adding in/changing diabetes medication
NICE have an 'Algorithm for blood glucose lowering therapy in adults with type 2 diabetes' – see guideline for useful flow diagram.[3]
Also see the Extra Notes at the end of this chapter for the table of antihyperglycaemics.

ACE inhibitor	Microalbuminuria (ACR >2.5 mg/mmol in men / >3.5 mg/mmol in women) or HTN
	Start ACEI with CCB or diuretic if treating HTN and Afro-Caribbean[3]
Atorvastatin 20 mg	Type 1 DM
	Type 2 DM and CV risk >10% or eGFR <60 ml/min/1.73 m^2 and/or albuminuria[3]
	Aim for total cholesterol <4 and LDL <2 mmol/L
Aspirin 75 mg	See antiplatelet therapy case.

Metabolic Problems – 2

Doctor's Notes

Patient	Margaret Timms	45 years	F
PMH	Type 2 diabetes		
Medications	Metformin 850 mg TDS		
	Gliclazide 160 mg BD		
Allergies	No information		
Consultations	Foot check normal		
Investigations	Creatinine 72 micromol/L		
	eGFR 68 ml/min/1.73 m^2		
	Na 140 mmol/L		
	K 4.0 mmol/L		
	HbA1c 8.5% (69 mmol/mol)		
	Total cholesterol 5.0 mmol/L		
	ACR 4.0 mg/mmol		
	BP 120/62		
	BMI 25		
Household	Charlotte Timms	12 years	F
	Philippa Timms	14 years	F

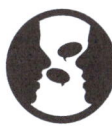

Example Consultation — Type 2 Diabetes Review

Open ☐	Thank you for coming in Mrs Timms. How do you feel things are going?
Curious ☐	You mentioned you have a busy schedule; tell me more about that.
Impact ☐	And how does your diabetes impact on your life?
Sense ☐	You seem frustrated by your sugars. I always like to check, are you okay or do you often feel low?
History ☐	It sounds like you are doing all the right things. Are you otherwise well?
Flags ☐	Do you ever have any hypos? Are your bowels okay? When was your last eye check?
Risk ☐	And your family – any history of heart disease at all. Do you smoke?
ICE ☐	Do you often worry about your diabetes? What goes through your mind? What did you think I might say today? What are your thoughts about where we go from here?
Impression ☐	Your blood pressure is reassuring. Regarding your blood tests, the HbA1c, which is an average blood sugar level over the past 8 weeks, is higher than we would like. It is 8.5% (69 mmol/mol).
Experience ☐	Do you know what we should be aiming for?
Explanation ☐	We should be aiming for 7% (53 mmol/mol) with you, as you are young and never have any hypos.
Summary ☐	To summarise, your blood sugars are often 7 pre-meals despite a healthy lifestyle. You are concerned that I may mention insulin and about your future health, but are keen to know your options.
Empathy ☐	You are very busy and any medication needs to work around your busy life. Have I understood your needs correctly? I appreciate you believe insulin is a 'slippery slope', I just want to explain that insulin doesn't put you at risk of needing higher doses, but the opposite; it is very helpful.
Options ☐	At this stage there are many options. Insulin isn't the only option; let's think about others. Firstly, insulin works the best – there are risk of hypos but it is otherwise safe, although you may gain some weight. Tablet options include saxagliptin, let's call this option 2, which should not affect your weight but there is an increased risk of hypos and there is also a risk of your pancreas becoming inflamed. Or trying an alternative tablet, dapagliflozin, option 3, which like gliclazide can give you hypos. You may lose some weight on this treatment, but it can cause water infections, and I would have to seek specialist approval before prescribing it. That is a lot of information. Shall I give you some information on all three options so you can take your time to compare them at home? Make a follow-up appointment when you're ready.
Future ☐	Now we did a few other tests too. The kidneys look good, a little protein is getting into the urine and this can be a sign that the vessels here could be starting to be affected by the sugar. Therefore, we may suggest a tablet called ramipril to help with this. We need to repeat the urine test with an early morning sample to double-check the result. I'll give you information on this too. Your cholesterol is 5 – let's discuss this next time as we should do a medical calculation to help us decide if we should consider treatment for this. There are a lot of additional suggestions but the aim is to keep a close eye on all aspects of your diabetes and vessels to protect you in the future. Any questions or thoughts?
Safety net ☐	Do you know what a hypo would feel like? If you do ever notice feeling shaky or unwell, check your blood sugar and have some Lucozade at the ready.

Patient's Story

Type 2 Diabetes Review

Doctor's notes Margaret Timms, 45 years. PMH: Type 2 diabetes.

Medications: Metformin 850 mg TDS, Gliclazide 160 mg BD. Recent results: Creatinine 72 micromol/L, eGFR 68 ml/min/1.73 m^2, Na 140 mmol/L, K 4.0 mmol/L, HbA1c 8.5% (69 mmol/mol), Total cholesterol 5.0 mmol/L, ACR 4.0 mg/mmol.

BP 120/62. BMI 25. Foot check normal.

How to act Happy to take any advice. You are here for your routine review.

PC *'Doctor, it's time for my annual check I believe.'*

History You are doing the best you can, you run twice a week even though you have a busy schedule and you eat very well, but your sugars are creeping up.

You did not tolerate 3 g/day metformin. You have not had any hypos.

You take pre-meal BMs and they are always around 7 at the moment.

You feel slightly frustrated and hope the doctor can help.

You are interested to know your results.

You have no family history of CVD. Your diabetes does not impact on your life.

Social You are a divorced legal adviser. You have two teenage children who are well.

You are busy because you are a single mum, work full time and are active.

Your mood is fine.

ICE You are concerned that your sugars are creeping up and fear your health is deteriorating. You have always been well and active.

You do not want to go on insulin, even if this is recommended.

You are happy to try any other medication but don't know what to try next.

You see insulin as a *'slippery slope'*. You expect the doctor will mention it.

You do not want any injections and would prefer a regime to be convenient.

You have forgotten what your HbA1c should be.

You have a low-GI diet.

Your foot check with the nurse was normal.

You had your eye check last week which was normal.

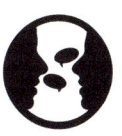

Metabolic Problems – 3

Learning Points — Type 2 Diabetes Review

Do not feel pressured into prescribing in the exam as you can always explain your thoughts, but signpost that you need to check carefully for interactions and cautions.

The elderly
If the HbA1c is suddenly 'better' consider anaemia or CKD.
Elderly/lives alone/risk of hypos consider 2nd line – gliptin but be aware of risks and cautions.
With renal impairment: Review/stop metformin. Reduce insulin and consider a glitazone.

Targets of HbA1c if an otherwise well patient without risk
However, these are a guide only; the aim should be adjusted to the individual (e.g. according to comorbidities, hypo risk and interactions). Use clinical judgement.

Pre-diabetes	<6%	(42 mmol/mol)
Diet or metformin alone	6.5%[1]	(48 mmol/mol)
1 Rx (not metformin) or ≥2 Rx	7%[1]	(53 mmol/mol)
Elderly and well	7.5%[2]	(58 mmol/mol)
Elderly + comorbidity	8%[2]	(64 mmol/mol)
End stage illness	8.5%[2]	(69 mmol/mol)

Hypoglycaemic prevention
Caution combining drugs with hypo risk.
Consider reducing the sulphonylurea to half dose.
Monitoring pre-meal BMs before titrating. Evening snacks if required.

Risk management
BP target 140/90 unless CKD or microalbuminuria or cerebrovascular disease 130/80.[1]
Weight: Aim 5–10% loss. If 15–20% loss and keep it off … a chance of cure.[3]
Low glycaemic index diet, high fibre, little saturated fat, oily fish, low salt.
Contraception counselling.
Pneumococcal and flu vaccine.
Review meds – e.g. thiazides and beta-blockers.

Diabetic education and support

Support	Diabetes UK, Diabetes 2gether, Diabetes 4ward.
Sick day rules	Discuss sick day rules including if becoming dehydrated stop metformin and ACEIs.
DAFNE	Education programme to adjust insulin doses according to diet.[4]
DESMOND	Education programme for T2DM. Identify health risks and set own goals.[5]
Monitoring	With glucose and ketone meters.

Monitoring: BM diary, mood, BP, bloods: cholesterol, HbA1c and eGFR/U&E and signs of small vessel disease – foot check, eye check and ACR.

When to offer BM testing kits: On insulin, history of hypoglycaemic episodes or taking medication which increase the hypoglycaemia risk or if pregnant, or planning pregnancy.[6]

Combinations to avoid unless advised by a specialist – seek advice
GLP-1 agonist and DPP4 – inhibitors
GLP-1 agonist and insulin.
Dapagliflozin and pioglitazone.[7]

Always refer to BNF and seek expert advice as not all combinations are licensed.

Metabolic Problems – 3

Doctor's Notes

Patient	Jayne Fitzpatrick	31 years	F

PMH Wrist fracture
Recurrent urinary tract infections – 3 in the past 6 months
Tonsillitis
Chlamydia
Termination of pregnancy
Stress at work

Medications No current medications

Allergies No information

Consultations Bloods taken for routine health check

Investigations No recent results

Household No household members registered

Example Consultation

Tired All The Time

Open ☐	Tell me more about how you feel. Any other changes? How are you sleeping?
Impact ☐	How is feeling so tired affecting you day to day? In any other ways?
Sense ☐	You seem puzzled as to what may be causing it.
History ☐	What medical problems have you had? How are you now? How is your mood now? Do you take any medicines from the pharmacy or supplements? Any stress in your life or worries? Is anyone at home with you? Do you have family? Are you in a relationship? Do you take any contraception? How did you break your wrist?
Flags ☐	Do you know if you snore or have any pauses in your breathing? Would you have a sleep if you were sitting down quietly in the afternoon, a passenger in a car or in a meeting? Is there any chance you could be pregnant? When was your last period? Was it a normal period? Are they regular? Or heavy? I see you had a urine infection in the past; do you have any symptoms of going more often or burning? Any weight loss or drenching night sweats? Have you felt flushed at times? Any headaches? Have your arms or legs felt different or floppy? Any visual changes? Any recent colds, ear or throat problems? Any problems with your breathing or in the chest? Stomach pain or change in bowels? Have you noticed any unusual dizziness or palpitations? Tell me more about the dizziness: room spinning or feeling lightheaded? What is your eating regime like? Do you avoid any food groups?
Risk ☐	Do you have any medical problems which run in the family? Have you travelled in the past couple of years? Or had any recent illnesses or rashes or bites?
ICE ☐	What do you think may be causing this? Is there anything you are particularly worried about or which has crossed your mind? Is there anything you were hoping we would decide today?
Examination ☐	I would like to measure your height, weight and blood pressure, look at your skin and hands, listen to your heart and lungs, feel your stomach, your neck and legs, look in your eyes and check your vision please. Can you provide a urine sample?
Impression ☐	I wonder if this may be a problem originating from the over- or under-production of a hormone, although there are many reasons why one may be tired.
Explanation ☐	The thyroid function, blood sugar level or red cell blood level can all cause tiredness.
Summary ☐	To summarise, you have been feeling exhausted for 4 months. It is unlike you to need time off work. You have also noticed a few symptoms: passing urine frequently, weight gain, light-headedness and absent periods. Your skin and hair are different. You believe you may be low and feel your thinking processes are perhaps slower. In the past 6 months you have broken your wrist and had urine infections.
Empathy ☐	It must be a real struggle when you feel so tired.
Options ☐	I would therefore like to arrange a blood test to check for anaemia, check your liver and kidneys, but also your hormones such as thyroid, the hormones that control your periods, and a blood test which shows the level of your steroid hormone. It would also be helpful if you could collect your urine for 24 hours, again to check for the amount of steroid in your body. I'll give you a container.
Empower ☐	I would avoid alcohol whilst you are feeling like this and try to go for walks even if you are feeling exhausted. You can take a multivitamin but this is unlikely to make a difference, especially as you are already eating a good diet.
Future ☐	Can we meet up again 2 days after you have handed in your urine and had your blood tests? Then I can explain further where the problem may lie. I may then ask a hormone specialist to see you. Depending on what the blood test shows you may need further blood tests or imaging.
Safety net ☐	If you do feel suddenly unwell with new symptoms, for example a headache or vomiting, please see a doctor straight away.

Metabolic Problems – 4

Patient's Story

Tired All The Time

Doctor's notes Jayne Fitzpatrick, 31 years. PMH: wrist fracture, recurrent UTIs – three in the last 6 months, chlamydia, tonsillitis, termination of pregnancy and stress at work. No current medications.

How to act Pleasant.

PC *'I just thought I'd see if there's a reason why I feel tired all the time.'*

History For the past 4 months you have felt increasingly tired. You sleep well and do not snore or have any pauses in your breathing. You have not fallen asleep during the daytime and even if you do try to rest you would not fall asleep. You already have 8 hours' sleep each night. Your periods are usually regular; however, you haven't had a period for 5 months. Your periods were not heavy. You did a pregnancy test 2 days ago, which was negative. You use condoms but you have not wanted to have sex recently. Being a veterinary nurse you know about some problems like diabetes and you have noticed a slight thirst and possible increased frequency. You have no symptoms of an infection. You have put on weight but don't know why. You have no night sweats or fevers. You have had no foreign travel other than Europe. You have had no recent rashes. You have had some spots on your face recently. Your bowels are normal. You do not have headaches and have no neurological or visual symptoms but your legs don't feel as strong, e.g. when walking up the stairs at work you have started to take the lift. You have noticed swelling around your ankles. If asked how this is affecting you – you had to take a day off work last week which you felt guilty about. You have been discussing with the vet how drained you feel. *'I've not needed a day off work since I fractured my wrist 6 months ago, even with urine infections I carry on.'*

You just tripped on the kerb when you fractured the wrist.

Your boss is worried about you; you are usually quite jovial. You feel your thinking is a little slower. You would like your hair to feel nice again. You did feel slightly lightheaded last week. Your ankles swell at the end of the day.

'The vet commented that I've lost my usual spirit.' He encouraged you to take another morning off work to see the doctor today. If asked about the conversations you have had with the vet: he suggested you need some blood tests and you are hoping the doctor will suggest this today. Straight after the conversation with the vet, you scribbled down a list of what the vet thought the doctor may do. You have this list for the doctor if he/she seems interested in your ideas. 'Anaemia, kidney, thyroid, diabetes, liver, hormones.' You feel saddened by what the vet said. You don't know why you have lost your spirit. Life should be good. You have not been crying and you don't think you are depressed but perhaps you are a little low.

Social You are a veterinary nurse. You are in a relationship of 2 years and you plan to move in together soon. Life is not stressful. You drink alcohol occasionally. You do not smoke. You do not currently exercise.

ICE You are just not sure what has caused it. You wondered if you should take a supplement.

Examination BMI 27, BP 150/92, Skin – some bruising, acne, abdominal striae.

No palpable thyroid or lymphadenopathy. No hepatosplenomegaly.

HS normal HR reg 70 bpm Apyrexial. Hands – no clubbing or nail changes.

Lungs clear. Urine dip negative. Fundi normal.

Metabolic Problems – 4

Learning Points   Tired All The Time

Complete CSA's motto   Common things are common ... but what mustn't I miss?

Have a look at the BMJ Easily Missed Series and have a think about how each of these conditions may present.

Cushing's syndrome[1]

Symptoms of Cushing's syndrome arise due to excess levels of glucocorticosteroids (e.g. cortisol).

There are 2 types of Cushing's syndrome based on the aetiology:

1. ACTH-dependent, e.g. excessive ACTH production by the pituitary (Cushing's disease), ectopic ACTH production, e.g. malignancy.
2. ACTH-independent, e.g. adrenal adenoma or carcinoma, excess glucocorticoid medication.

Symptoms and signs include: weight gain, buffalo hump, truncal obesity, moon facies, proximal muscle weakness, type 2 diabetes, hypertension, gonadal dysfunction, loss of libido, skin changes (e.g. striae), hypertension, oedema, headaches and visual disturbance if due to a pituitary adenoma.

Investigations: Dexamethasone suppression test. 1 mg oral dexamethasone at 11 pm and measure 9 am cortisol. More complex investigations are performed by secondary care.

'Tired All The Time'

This is a common presentation in general practice. In the majority of cases no medical cause can be found. Screen for obstructive sleep apnoea, mental health problems, perform a full systemic enquiry and take a detailed social history. If no cause is found, request routine blood tests and advise simple measures such as healthy eating, keeping hydrated, good sleep hygiene, avoiding caffeine and graded exercise can help.

Doctor's Notes

Patient   Fatima Sayed   47 years   F

PMH   Grave's disease – 1 year ago

Medications   Carbimazole 20 mg

                   Propranolol 40 mg TDS PRN (not issued for 6 months)

Allergies   No known drug allergies

Consultations 12 months ago – goitre palpable, confirmed on USS, no thyroid nodules. Diagnosis Grave's disease. Start carbimazole 30 mg.

                   10 months ago – T4 in the normal range. TSH remains low (expected). Decrease carbimazole to 20 mg. Repeat TSH/T4/T3 in 6 weeks. If TSH remains low or T4 increased again increase carbimazole.

                   8 months ago – TSH normal range. Asymptomatic. Decrease carbimazole to 10 mg.

Investigations

	1 month ago	1 year ago	
TSH	2.2 miu/L	<0.1 miu/L	(0.2–4.0 miu/L)
T4	8.0 pmol/L	32 pmol/L	(10–20 pmol/L)
T3	2.0 nmol/L	3.4 nmol/L	(0.9–2.5 nmol/L)

TSH receptor antibodies   positive

Household   Aaqil Sayed   49 years   M

Example Consultation — Hyperthyroidism

Open — Thank you for coming. How are you? How are you getting on with the treatment?

Experience — Would you mind taking me back to the start? I'm interested to know what it was like for you before you commenced treatment. What is your understanding of your condition? What is your understanding of the blood results?

History — Tell me more about yourself. Have you noticed any new or troublesome symptoms? What dose are you taking of the carbimazole? How often are you taking the tablet? Have you any other medical history? Any medical problems that are in the family? Do you take other medicines or supplements? Any stressors at work or home? Do you drink? Or smoke?

Flags — Is your weight stable? Did you ever have any problem with your eyes or vision?

Impact — And what impact has the Grave's disease had on your life?

ICE — Have you had previous conversations with a GP about when to stop treatment? Have you had anything on your mind that has been worrying you? You mentioned you would like to stop the treatment; is there anything else you were hoping for today?

Sense — I see you have not seen the GP for 8 months and I'm sensing there may be a reason why you have come to talk to me about the treatment at this time.

Curious — Tell me more about your thoughts about the treatment. I'm wondering why at this stage you feel it would be beneficial to see a specialist.

Examination — May I take your pulse, BP and examine your neck and eyes please?

Summary — To summarise, you feel well, all your symptoms of Grave's disease have gone. You started reading about when to discontinue the carbimazole and this led you to forums which discussed the risk of the drug which has alarmed you and led you to reassess the situation. You are wondering if the benefit of carbimazole no longer outweighs the risk and you would like to discuss stopping treatment with a specialist. Is that correct?

Impression — It does sound like you have had simple Grave's disease, meaning high thyroid levels without signs of eye disease.

Explanation — You are correct; there is a risk of agranulocytosis, 1 in 1000. With any treatment we are weighing up the benefit of the treatment versus the risk.

Empathy — I can appreciate that, when you hear about the frightening risks associated with a tablet and, particularly now that you are well again, it is natural to revisit the decision as to whether the benefits of the tablet continue to outweigh the risks.

Options — We usually treat Grave's disease for about 18 months. I see your recent thyroid levels were in the normal range, therefore I would usually suggest 5 mg carbimazole for the next 6 months then, if the blood tests remain normal, aim to stop it when you have completed 18 months of treatment. If you would like to stop it early that is your decision, but there is a risk of your symptoms returning and the disease not completely being treated. Looking at your blood tests and feeling your thyroid, a scan would not be helpful now. It was important to make the diagnosis at the beginning. I suggest decreasing the carbimazole to 5 mg for 6 weeks, then we can reassess in 6 weeks with a blood test after you have had a chance to think about it. Shall we do that?

Future — If at any stage the TSH drops below the normal range, we need to increase the carbimazole. Once we have stopped the carbimazole I would like to continue to check your TSH level initially after 6 weeks then every 3 months for a year.

Empower — If there were 100 people like you, at the end of the 18 months, 50 of them might need to continue carbimazole.[1] Smoking is a risk factor for this and if you are interested in stopping smoking I would like to help you.

Safety net — If you ever notice a sore throat, rash or infection then arrange a blood test straight away and withhold the medication until you know the blood test is normal.

Metabolic Problems – 5

Patient Story

Hyperthyroidism

Doctor's notes Fatima Sayed, 47 years. PMH: Hyperthyroidism – 1 year ago.

Medication: carbimazole 20 mg. Consultations: 1 year ago – goitre palpable, confirmed on USS, no thyroid nodules. Start carbimazole 30 mg.

	1 month ago	1 year ago	
TSH	2.2 miu/L	<0.1 miu/L	(0.2–4.0 miu/L)
T4	8.0 pmol/L	32 pmol/L	(10–20 pmol/L)
T3	2.0 nmol/L	3.4 nmol/L	(0.9–2.5 nmol/L)
TSH receptor antibodies		positive	

How to act Pleasant.

PC *'Good morning Doctor. I was hoping to discuss when I could stop my carbimazole please?'*

History Over a year ago you began to lose weight and feel just not yourself. You remember your bowels were loose and you felt quite jittery. Your doctor started Carbimazole for high thyroid levels.

Since the treatment you have felt much better. You have always been healthy, take no other medicines and have no FH.

You have read about Grave's disease and have a good understanding of the terms TSH, T3 and T4. You called a month ago and the receptionist said the blood tests were normal.

Social Barrister, married with 3 children who have now all left home.

You drink no alcohol but smoke 5 cigarettes a day.

You are active and attend art classes.

ICE *'I should come off it as soon as I can.'* A pragmatic suggestion you believe; however, if the doctor explores your thoughts behind this … You were reading about when to stop carbimazole and came across website forums which reminded you of the risk of the tablet. This led you down the path of reading frightening stories about agranulocytosis and you realised that now you feel well you should stop this tablet. You do not want this problem to happen to you. You wondered whether you should see the specialist again before you finished treatment so she could do a scan again to see if the treatment has to continue. You presume she would rescan and you would like this.

You follow the doctor's advice if he seems to know what he is doing. Otherwise you push to see a specialist.

Examination HR 70 bpm regular, BP 120/70, no palpable thyroid.

No sign of eye disease.

Metabolic Problems – 5

Learning Points

Hyperthyroidism

History: Heat intolerance, increased appetite, weight changes, increased bowel frequency, oligomenorrhoea and tiredness
Painful neck or 'sore throat', viral symptoms and fever. (De Quervain's thyroiditis)
Could it be secondary to amiodarone?

Examination: Cardiovascular: Raised heart rate and blood pressure. Possible AF or murmur
Thyroid: Palpable goitre or nodules. A thrill and bruit
Systemic: Weight ↓ and nails (onycholysis)
Hands (palmar erythema, telangiectasia and tremor)
Pre-tibial myxoedema
Brisk reflexes
Eye disease (exopthalmos, lid retraction, lid lag, chemosis, conjunctivitis, corneal ulceration, strabismus)

Next tests: Repeat TSH, T4, T3. FBC (anaemia)
Calcium and LFTs may be raised
Thyroid receptor antibodies (85% positive in Grave's). If positive no need to do a thyroid scintigraphy scan.
ESR (raised in Grave's or thyroiditis)
Thyroid scintigraphy scan if unsure on palpation of the thyroid. (GPs can request if antibody negative[1])

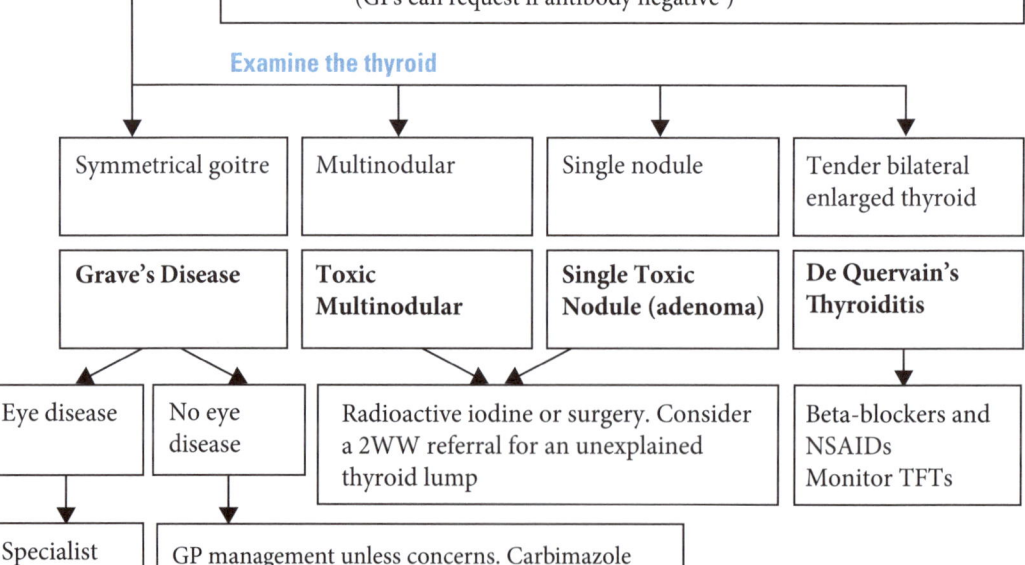

Examine the thyroid

Symmetrical goitre	Multinodular	Single nodule	Tender bilateral enlarged thyroid
Grave's Disease	**Toxic Multinodular**	**Single Toxic Nodule (adenoma)**	**De Quervain's Thyroiditis**

- Grave's Disease → Eye disease → Specialist referral
- Grave's Disease → No eye disease → GP management (see below)
- Toxic Multinodular / Single Toxic Nodule → Radioactive iodine or surgery. Consider a 2WW referral for an unexplained thyroid lump
- De Quervain's Thyroiditis → Beta-blockers and NSAIDs. Monitor TFTs

GP management unless concerns. Carbimazole 30 mg if fT4 <40 pmol/L. Carbimazole 45 mg if fT4 >40 pmol/L. 'Risk of agranulocytosis 0.1% and rash 4%'.[1] Initially TSH/T4/T3 4–6 weekly to guide the maintenance dose for 18/12. Propranolol TDS PRN. (50 mg Propylthiouracil = 5 mg carbimazole[1]).

Metabolic Problems – 5

Extra Notes — Antihyperglycaemics

Medication	Metformin	Sulfonylurea (S)	DPP-4 inhibitors
E.g.	Metformin	Glibenclamide, gliclazide, glipizide	Linagliptin, Saxagliptin, Sitagliptin
Advice – see BNF for the full list	Lactic acidosis risk. Warn the patient if D&V to stop metformin, ACEI, diuretics and inform the GP. Monitor B12	Review at 2 weeks. Titrate dose on pre-breakfast BMs	Stop if HbA1c not decreasing, e.g. by >0.5% or 5–6 mmol/mol at 6 months[9]
How given	Oral	Oral	Oral
How work	↓ glycogenesis ↓ intestinal absorption ↑ insulin sensitivity	↑ insulin secretion	DPP-4 blocks incretin production. Incretin ↑ insulin
Cautions and contraindications – see BNF for full list	Lactic acidosis risk. Recent cardiac respiratory, liver, renal disease. Caution: Creatinine >130 micromol/L or eGFR <45[6]. Stop if Cr>150 or eGFR <30[6]	Hypoglycaemic risk. Liver disease	Elderly. Hepatic or renal impairment. Pancreatic cancer. PMH pancreatitis
Hypoglycaemia risk	Low[5]	Yes[5]	Low[5] unless combined with another Rx with hypo risk
Weight	No change or lose[5]	May cause weight gain	Usually no change[5]
Risks and adverse events – see BNF for the full list	<1/10,000 Lactic acidosis[5]. D&V, ↓ appetite and abdominal pain[5]. Metallic/altered taste[5]. B12 deficiency	Hypoglycaemia. GI disturbance[5], photosensitivity, liver function changes and rarely haematological disorders	1–10/1000 – pancreatitis[5]. Headache, oedema, infections, GI disturbance[5]. Hypersensitivity reactions and rashes[9]

Always use the most up-to-date version of the BNF yourself before prescribing. Ensure you have checked all the cautions, contraindications, interactions and dose regimes.

Metabolic Problems

Extra Notes — Antihyperglycaemics

Medication	SGLT-2 inhibitors	Insulin	GLP-1 agonist	Glitazones
Example options	Dapagliflozin Canagliflozin		Lixisenatide Liraglutide Exenatide	Pioglitazone
Advice – see BNF	If sulfonylurea CI or risk of hypoglycaemia Seek specialist advice Monitor renal function[5]		Useful if BMI >35 Check U&E and eGFR before and 2 weeks later	May improve lipid profile Monitor LFT[5] Seek specialist advice Stop if HbA1c not decreasing, e.g. by >0.5% or 5–6 mmol/mol at 6 months[9]
How given	Oral	s/c	s/c	Oral
How work	'Pee out (urinate) sugar'	Replaces insulin	↑ insulin secretion	↑ Insulin sensitivity
Cautions and contraindications – see BNF for full list	Hypotension Elderly CVD Electrolyte disturbance Renal impairment Liver disturbance Prostate cancer Bladder cancer Ketoacidosis >75 years T1DM		Elderly AKI Caution if eGFR 30–50 and stop if eGFR <30 Caution with DPP4 Pancreatic cancer Thyroid cancer Gastroparesis MEN2 Consider stopping after 6/12 if HbA1c hasn't dropped >1% or 10–11 mmol/mol or weight dropped by >3%[9]	Risk of bladder cancer so avoid in smokers and those on chemotherapy Rx Oedema Heart failure Liver impairment DKA Osteopenia Bladder cancer Uninvestigated haematuria[6]
Hypoglycaemia risk	Low	High	Low/Medium	Low
Weight	Loss	Gain	Loss	Gain
Risks and adverse events – see BNF for the full list	UTIs, low BP Renal function Risk of DKA Thirst Thrush Constipation Dyslipidaemia[5,7]	Hypo	Pancreatitis Nausea and vomiting	Exacerbation of heart failure Bone #'s Liver function 1–10/1000 bladder cancer Visual disturbance[1,8]

Always use the most up-to-date version of the BNF yourself before prescribing. Ensure you have checked all the cautions, contraindications, interactions and dose regimes.

Metabolic Problems

CHAPTER 20 OVERVIEW
Neurological Problems

	Cases in this chapter	Within the RCGP curriculum: Care of People with Neurological Problems RCGP Curriculum Online March 2016[1]	Learning Points in the chapter include:
1	Peripheral Neuropathy	'Demonstrate empathy and compassion towards patients with disabling neurological conditions' 'Know the functional anatomy of the nervous system relevant to diagnosis'	Causes Blood tests Red flags
2	Normal Pressure Hydrocephalus	'Demonstrate a structured, logical approach to the diagnosis of "difficult" symptoms with multiple causes'	Symptom triad Cause Differential diagnosis
3	Migraine	'Understand principles of treatment for common conditions that are managed largely in primary care' 'Advise on the avoidance of triggers and prophylaxis for migraine'	Red flags Differential diagnosis Management options
4	TIA	'Understand the importance of continuity of care for patients with chronic neurological conditions' 'Demonstrate an understanding of the relevance to management and effective use of special investigations such as EEG, CT, MRI and nerve conduction studies' 'Know the indications for referral to a neurologist for chronic conditions that require ongoing specialist management and conditions that require early treatment to avoid permanent deficit'	$ABCD^2$ score High risk of stroke Low risk of stroke Secondary prevention
5	Multiple Sclerosis	'Know the epidemiology of common and/or important neurological conditions' 'Communicate prognosis, including any uncertainties, truthfully and sensitively to patients with disabling neurological conditions such as Parkinson's disease and multiple sclerosis'	Epidemiology Symptoms Diagnosis Differential diagnosis Blood tests

1. http://www.rcgp.org.uk/training-exams/gp-curriculum-overview/online-curriculum/applying-clinical-knowledge-section-2/3-18-neurological-problems.aspx

CHAPTER 20 REFERENCES

Migraine
1. http://patient.info/doctor/giant-cell-arteritis-pro
2. Dr Richard Wood. Migraine: Acute Therapy Guideline (Adult) and Prophylactic Therapy Guideline. OCCG, Version 11. Oxford University Hospitals NHS. Oxford CCG. (Sept 2015). Approved by APCO Sept 2015. Review date: Sept 2017. http://occg.oxnet.nhs.uk/GeneralPractice/ClinicalGuidelines/Neurology/Headache/Migraine%20Adult%20Prophylactic%20Therapy%20Guidelines%20-%20v10%20Sept%202015.pdf

TIA
1. NICE Guidelines. CG68. Stroke and transient ischaemic attack in over 16s: diagnosis and initial management. Jul 2008.
2. Scottish Intercollegiate Guidelines Network (SIGN). *Management of patients with stroke or TIA: assessment, investigation, immediate management and secondary prevention*. Edinburgh: SIGN 2008. 978 1 905813 40 7, Dec 2008. Available from http://www.sign.ac.uk/pdf/qrg108.pdf
3. NICE. http://cks.nice.org.uk/stroke-and-tia#!scenariorecommendation:3. Dec 2013.
4. Gent M., Beaumont D., Blanchard J., et al. A randomised, blinded, trial of clopidogrel versus aspirin in patients at risk of ischaemic events (CAPRIE). CAPRIE Steering Committee. *Lancet*. 1996 Nov 16; 348(9038): 1329–39.
5. Royal College of Physicians. *National Clinical Guideline for Stroke*. 4th edition. 2012.
6. Rothwell P.M., Algra A., Chen Z., et al. Effects of aspirin on risk and severity of early recurrent stroke after transient ischaemic attack and ischaemic stroke: time-course analysis of randomised trials. *Lancet*. 18 May 2016. http://dx.doi.org/10.1016/S0140-6736(16)30468-8

Multiple Sclerosis
1. http://patient.info/doctor/multiple-sclerosis-pro
2. http://bestpractice.bmj.com/best-practice/monograph/140.html

Doctor's Notes

Patient	Maggie Freestone 72 years F
PMH	Bereavement. Death of husband 2 years ago.
	2 × NVD
	Gastritis
	Miscarriage
Medications	No current medications
Allergies	No information
Consultations	No recent consultations
Investigations	No recent investigations
Household	No household members registered

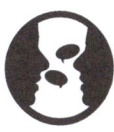

Example Consultation — Peripheral Neuropathy

Open ☐	Tell me about this problem from the beginning. Then what did you notice? Anything else that isn't right?
Curious ☐	When you say you don't trust your feet, what do you mean? Have you fallen?
History ☐	Any other symptoms? Are you otherwise well? Any other medical conditions yourself or which run in the family? I'm sorry that I am not aware, but what caused your husband's death? How are you getting on without him? Who else is in your life? Do you take any medicines? Did anyone in your family have a similar problem?
Risk ☐	Do you drink alcohol? Have you been unwell recently or had a cold or sore throat?
Flags ☐	Is it painful? What does it feel like? How are you on the stairs or rising from a chair? Any weight loss? Any change in your bowels or change in control of going to the toilet? Any episodes of sweating? Or weakness? Have you felt lightheaded on standing? Do you still feel hot and cold where the numbness is? Any dry mouth or problems with the skin or joints?
ICE ☐	What do you think has caused this? What has been on your mind? Is there anything you are worried about? What did you think or hope we may do today?
Sense ☐	I can see you a positive person but I'm worried how this is affecting you.
Impact ☐	Has this changed how you live or your behaviour? Or your mood?
O/E ☐	May I examine you; check the sensation and strength in your arms and legs, check your reflexes and watch you walk then check the spine for tenderness and movement please? I'd just like to look at the muscles in the legs now. Can I check your weight, pulse and blood pressure? Now I'd like to feel the pulses in the feet. May I feel your abdomen and the lymph glands in your neck, under the arms and groin? Lastly can I ask you to go to the toilet for a urine sample please?
Summary ☐	To summarise what you have told me, your feet have been gradually becoming more numb over the last year. This has stopped you cycling and you have fallen. You have been concerned about what may have caused this and so has your son. You weren't sure what I'd say today. You sometimes have pain in your feet too. Have I understood?
Empathy ☐	I can imagine it does knock your confidence when you can't trust your feet, especially after a fall.
Impression ☐	We call this peripheral neuropathy.
Experience ☐	Have you known anyone who has had a similar problem?
Explanation ☐	Peripheral means the parts of us furthest from the heart, and neuropathy means a problem with the nerve. Unfortunately, though, this is only a description of the problem rather than telling us the cause. There are several things that might cause it but no clues so far from what you have told me.
Options ☐	I'd like to start by doing a blood test for your routine health including for anaemia, your kidneys and liver, blood tests for inflammation, also check your cholesterol, your sugar level and vitamins called B12 and folate which, when low, can cause this. I would also like to check your urine for protein and sugar. We can try different pain relief – would you like to hear about the options?
Empower ☐	Have you any thoughts about what may give you more confidence on your feet? Perhaps something to give you some support when walking?
Future ☐	Can we meet up again after the blood tests? It is likely that I will, at that point, ask the neurologists – the nerve specialists – to see you. I expect they may talk to you about nerve conduction studies – a test which looks at the electricity flow in your nerves.
Safety net ☐	If ever you notice any weakness or new symptoms, or if you ever fall, please contact a doctor straight away as you would need to be examined again. I don't expect this to happen but if you ever notice a change in the control of your bladder or bowel or a new back pain or difficulty breathing, please let a doctor know straight away so we can make sure it is nothing serious.

Neurological Problems – 1

Patient's Story

Peripheral Neuropathy

Doctor's notes Maggie Freestone, 72 years. PMH: Bereavement. Death of husband 2 years ago. 2 × NVD. Miscarriage. Gastritis. Medication: Nil.

How to act Chirpy and chatty.

PC *'Hello Doctor. Well, it's the feet. Often I can't feel them. Very strange. What do you think it is then?'*

History You have always been very healthy. About a year ago you started to notice your left foot felt a bit odd at times and then the right started about 6 months ago. Now both feet don't really feel normal most of the time. You therefore watch your feet as you walk. You have no symptoms of diabetes. You drink no alcohol. You have never smoked. You take no medicines. Your memory is good. You have had no head injury. You have no back pain or bladder/bowel dysfunction. Your strength is good apart from when you can't feel what you are doing. You have no problems in the proximal muscles. You wouldn't describe it as pins and needles but *'peculiar ... like my feet have become sponge'*. You can still feel warm water.

You have no other symptoms. No FH.

Social You miss Des but you get on with life and love seeing people. Des died of prostate cancer which had spread to his bones and caused his kidneys to fail. You remain very active for the church, often raising money. You are very proud of how good you are for your age. You enjoyed riding your bike until last year when it became a problem.

'Now, I don't trust my feet.' Say this with laugh.

You live on your own.

ICE You try to laugh this off; however, you have been lying awake wondering what this is. But you like to stay positive and you shrug it off when your children mention it. Your son is worried since you fell and banged your shoulder. The shoulder recovered but it did knock your confidence. Only if the doctor specifically asks you, you mention the burning pain the problem causes but you do not want any medicine for this. Your son bought you a mobile phone just in case you ever fall.

Examination There is decreased sensation in both feet to just above the ankle. Arms are normal. The power in the legs is normal until L5/S1 which is 4/5 strength. Reflexes absent. Plantars downgoing. No muscle wasting. There is no spinal tenderness. BMI 25. BP 130/60. HR 62 reg. Normal ROM spine and straight leg raise. Sensory ataxic ('stomping') gait. Abdomen normal, no masses and no lymphadenopathy. Normal urine dipstick. Normal peripheral pulses.

Neurological Problems – 1

Learning Points   Peripheral Neuropathy

As well as sensory and motor symptoms, ask about features of autonomic dysfunction, which may include a change to the bowels, sweating, sphincter disturbance and postural hypotension.

Causes
- Alcohol
- B12/folate deficiency
- Diabetes or diabetic amyotrophy
- Lyme disease
- Sjogren's syndrome
- Amyloidosis
- Uraemia
- Guillain-Barré Syndrome/Chronic Inflammatory Demyelinating Polyneuropathy (CIDP)
- Porphyria
- Charcot-Marie-Tooth disease
- Malignancy or paraneoplastic syndrome
- Vasculitic neuropathy
- and more

Complete CSA's motto: **Common things are common … but what mustn't I miss?**

Ensure you are aware of how the rare conditions above may present.

Blood tests FBC, U&E, LFT, GGT, TFTs, CRP, ESR, ANA, B12, folate, serum and urine electrophoresis.
Urine dipstick for protein and glucose.
CXR – sarcoidosis, malignancy.
Consider – Lyme or HIV serology, urinary porphyrins and an autoimmune screen.

Red flags Always look out for cauda equina syndrome.

> **Gait**
> See the **Link Hub at CompleteCSA.co.uk** for a link to a helpful guide on the assessment of different gaits.

Doctor's Notes

Patient	Lionel Moore	84 years	M
PMH	TIA 3 years ago		
	Atrial fibrillation		
	Hypertension		
Medications	Warfarin		
	Atorvastatin 40 mg ON		
	Indapamide 2.5 mg OM		
	Ramipril 5 mg OM		
	Bisoprolol 5 mg OM		
Allergies	No information		
Consultations	No recent consultations		
Investigations	Blood pressure	130/70 one month ago	
Household	Sandra Moore	79 years	F

Example Consultation Normal Pressure Hydrocephalus

Open ☐	Tell me, when did either of you first notice something wasn't right? What symptoms followed? Has anything else changed with your health?
History ☐	I am interested to hear your story, Lionel. Sandra, feel free to add anything. Lionel, do you feel well? In what way 'not right'? Have you felt like this before? What happened when you had the TIA? Your tablets, please talk me through when you take each one. Let's now go through the different parts of the body. Any headaches? How did it start? Any nausea or vomiting? Any changes in the arms or legs? Any problems with your speech or swallowing? Eyesight problems? Any breathing difficulties or chest problems? Pain in the tummy? Have you had a temperature? Any back pain? Any increased frequency of urine? Or pain passing urine? Do you generally get up at night to pass urine?
Curious ☐	What do you mean by wobbly exactly?
Risk ☐	Has your INR been in the normal range? Have you fallen or banged your head?
Flags ☐	Have you lost weight over recent months? Have you had any change in behaviour?
Sense ☐	Lionel, you keep looking at Sandra, is that because you are struggling to tell me?
ICE ☐	Lionel, what did you think may be causing your symptoms? Is there anything you are particularly worried about? What did you think I may suggest today? How about you, Sandra – what have you been wondering? Is there anything that has been on your mind or troubling you? Did you hope I would do anything particular today?
Impact ☐	How has your memory affected you day to day, Lionel? Sandra, in what way have Lionel's memory troubles been difficult for you?
Summary ☐	To summarise, the unsteadiness came first 9 months ago and for 6 months your memory has been patchy. Sandra, you have been worried about what this may mean for the future; however with recent urinary incontinence you both wondered if you have a water infection and thought we needed to prescribe antibiotics for this.
O/E ☐	I would like to take a good look at you: listen to your heart, take your blood pressure, pulse, temperature, have a look at the nerves which supply the arms, legs and face and have a look at the back of your eyes. Now please stand up and walk across the room, turn around and return. Can you move your neck up and down? Now, lying down, I would like to lift your head and now raise your legs. May I check on the edge of the back passage to see if the nerve supply is normal? Could you provide a urine sample?
Impression ☐	I see why you worried about a urine infection and dementia but, with the additional symptom of feeling wobbly, I believe the diagnosis may be normal pressure hydrocephalus.
Experience ☐	Have you come across the term hydrocephalus?
Explanation ☐	Fluid surrounding the brain is continuously made then reabsorbed. If the reabsorption stops, this leads to less fluid being produced but overall the pressure increases. Usually three things happen: a change in mobility, followed by memory trouble then urine incontinence. The treatment involves redirecting the fluid so that it moves away from the brain to reduce the pressure. Sometimes there is no cause found, but a previous bleed in the brain is possible. Your age and drinking alcohol put you at risk of a bleed, but your headache symptoms are not typical.
Empathy ☐	I appreciate this must have come as a shock when you were expecting just antibiotics.
Options ☐	I think we need to ask the hospital doctors to look at you today. I expect they will want to scan the brain and may discuss a lumbar puncture, inserting a needle into the spine to measure the pressure of the fluid around the brain. I think this problem has been building for many months rather than a sudden change like a stroke. Sandra, do you feel comfortable driving Lionel to the hospital? I will call the specialist.
Future ☐	Lionel, when you are back home, please return to see me. We can reassess your memory to see if there are any ongoing concerns and check your general health.
Empower ☐	We could discuss the link between alcohol and risks to the brain.
Safety net ☐	I don't expect problems en route but if any problems arise, stop and call 999.

Neurological Problems – 2

Patient's Story

Normal Pressure Hydrocephalus

Doctor's notes — Lionel Moore, 84 years. PMH: TIA 3 years ago, atrial fibrillation and hypertension. Medication: Warfarin, Atorvastatin 40 mg ON, Indapamide 2.5 mg OM, Ramipril 5 mg OM and Bisoprolol 5 mg OM. Blood pressure: 130/70 one month ago.

You attend with your wife, Sandra, today.

How to act — You are quiet and often turn to Sandra to answer for you.

PC — Your wife Sandra is with you; she speaks first.

'Lionel has been incontinent the past few days.'

History

Sandra — You have found that he is damp and feel guilty that you shouted at him for wetting on the sofa. There has been no faecal incontinence. When the incontinence happened a third time you thought you had better see the doctor.

'Lionel's memory hasn't been too good.' For example, he can't remember if he has had dinner and repeatedly asks if the dog has been fed. He has not wandered and there have been no safety concerns.

'Over the last week he is not quite right.'

Lionel had a TIA. His INR levels have been good and were last checked 1 week ago.

There have been no further neurological signs unlike last time when, for 8 hours, his left side was weak. He has been *'a bit wobbly'*. You remember this started 9 months ago.

Lionel — You feel *'not myself.'* By this you mean you feel muddled. Your vision is normal.

No abdominal pain or dysuria. You can't remember any increased urinary frequency.

No prostate symptoms. You have no back pain. You have lost no weight.

You have no cardiac or respiratory symptoms. Your bowels are normal.

You have not fallen or had a head injury. You have a *'bit of a headache'* of gradual onset and no vomiting or nausea.

Social — Lionel enjoys two glasses of whisky every night. He stopped attending the pub quiz 6 months ago as it started to become embarrassing that Lionel's memory was fading. Lionel used to be a solicitor and has three children, grandchildren and now great-grandchildren. Lionel smoked until he was 38 years old.

ICE — Neither of you are worried that this may be another TIA as Lionel has had no weakness. You suspect a UTI. You expect antibiotics.

Sandra — Worried if he has the 'big D'. You have been very worried how this will progress.

Examination — BP 128/72. HR 68 bpm irregularly irregular. RR 14, Sats 97% 36.6°C.

Urine dipstick leucocytes only. HS normal. Abdomen soft, non-tender. Normal neurology apart from reflexes which are brisk bilaterally. CN normal examination. Unsteady gait. No other cerebellar signs. Fundi are normal. Brudzinski/Kernig's negative. No neck stiffness. Normal anal tone and sensation.

Neurological Problems – 2

Learning Points — Normal Pressure Hydrocephalus

Triad — Apraxia, progressive memory disturbance and sphincter disturbance/incontinence.

Cause — Idiopathic meningitis, subdural haematoma, head injury and radiotherapy.

Differential diagnosis in this case: all are possible and the scan will help differentiate.

Subdural haematoma — Secondary to age and alcohol.

TIA/cerebellar stroke — Secondary to risk factors but history and examination not typical.

Dementia, postural hypotension and UTI
All common. The symptoms and dipstick do not support a UTI.
With the above triad, NPH needs to be excluded.

Metastases — However, there was no reported weight loss or vomiting.

Cauda equina syndrome — However, no back pain or associated red flags.

Doctor's Notes

Patient   Yasmin Small   23 years   F
PMH   No medical history
Medications   No current medications
Allergies   No information
Consultations No recent consultations
Investigations No recent investigations
Household   No household members registered

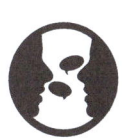

Example Consultation — Migraine

Open ☐	Tell me more about them from the beginning. Any other symptoms you've noticed? Is there a pattern?
History ☐	Is there one type of headache? How often does it occur? When does it occur? Where on the head? What does it feel like? Severity from 1 to 10? What makes it worse? Or better? Do you lie down or can you not keep still? Any visual disturbance? Do the arms or legs feel different or weak? Any medical problems? Sinus trouble? Do you take medicines? Four months ago what happened in your life? Are work and home okay? Any stress?
Risk ☐	Any FH? Contraception? Do you have much alcohol, caffeine, cheese or chocolate? Are you sleeping okay?
Flags ☐	Any weight loss? Nausea? Vomiting? What time of day do they start? Do they wake you? How long does it take to reach maximum severity? Are you ever confused or more sleepy? If you lean forward does this cause a headache? Has anyone said your behaviour has changed? Do you now struggle with anything you could easily do a few months ago? Any fevers? Does the light bother you? Any neck stiffness? Any injury to the head?
Sense ☐	I can see you touching your head; are you in pain now?
ICE ☐	What do you think may be causing them? Is there anything you are worried that it could be? Or have been wondering? What did you think I may suggest today?
Impact ☐	Since the headaches started how have they affected your life?
Curious ☐	What does your mum think? After 4 months why have you decided to see me today?
Summary ☐	Your headaches are impacting on your work and life. You believe it is likely to be migraine and would like to try sumatriptan. However, as the headaches are not resolving you have wondered about a brain tumour and seeking specialist advice.
O/E ☐	May I examine your BP, your eyes, arms and legs? Please walk across the room, now heel–toe like this.
Empathy ☐	I appreciate why you want to check that this frequent headache is nothing serious.
Impression ☐	I think you are right; these do sound like migraines.
Experience ☐	What do you know about migraines? Do you know anything that can trigger them?
Explanation ☐	A one-sided headache which takes you to bed is typical of a migraine.
Options ☐	It sounds like you thought seeing a specialist may be helpful for two reasons: to ensure there is no tumour and find the cause. Reassuringly, you have no symptoms of increased pressure in the brain. The headaches do not occur when the pressure is at its highest in the morning. You do not generally feel sick. You have not vomited. You also have no symptoms suggesting the nerve supply to your body is affected and your examination is normal. Regarding how frequently you have the headaches: both painkillers and foods can be triggers. Analgesia (which means painkiller) induced headaches are common and we advise going cold turkey for 6 weeks. In the meantime, you could try sumatriptan. I could write a letter to your employer if this would help?
Empower ☐	Could you try to avoid caffeine, chocolate and alcohol? Be prepared for rebound headaches initially. What are your thoughts so far if we tried this for 4 weeks? Does my explanation help to reassure you? Also general lifestyle measures – including regular healthy meals, a good sleep pattern and exercise – can all help.
Future ☐	Could we meet again in a month? If you still have migraines, we could discuss prevention tablets. I would be interested to see a headache diary. Would you like me to prescribe sumatriptan tablets, which is a treatment for migraine? Take one at the onset of your headache. Take a second after 2 hours if required. Side effects include tingling, blurred vision and feeling tired. Another tablet which may be helpful is called metoclopramide. This tablet helps with the nausea and helps the sumatriptan tablet to be absorbed. You can take one 10 mg metoclopramide tablet every 8 hours during migraines. There is a rare risk of it causing problem with movement. Would you like to try it?
Safety net ☐	If you start vomiting, feel unwell, have any new symptoms or the headaches wake you, see a GP.

Neurological Problems – 3

Patient's Story

Migraine

Doctor's notes	Yasmin Small, 23 years. PMH: Nil. Medications: Nil.
How to act	Currently in discomfort. Keep touching your head.
PC	*'I keep getting these headaches.'*
History	You started getting headaches 4 months ago. It is always the same headache.
	Left side or frontal. They originally occurred weekly but now twice weekly.
	Onset usually mid-afternoon. It develops over an hour and reaches 8/10 severity.
	Apart from nausea, only during the headache, you have no associated symptoms.
	You have not been under pressure; you are not stressed or depressed.
	You have a copper coil. The headaches are not related to your periods.
	You have no medical history and take no medicines. Your mum had migraines.
	You did have tennis elbow 6 months ago.
	You didn't see the GP as paracetamol and ibuprofen helped.
	When the headache comes on you lie down in a dark room after taking paracetamol and ibuprofen.
Social	You work in a clothes shop which you enjoy. You live with your boyfriend of 2 years.
	You drink a couple of glasses of wine weekly. You do not smoke.
	At work you take it in turns to buy each other a coffee and chocolate.
	You have had to have time off work.
ICE	You think you have migraines like your mother.
	You are worried that you will have to live with it.
	It has also crossed your mind it could be something worrying.
	'Well, I suppose you always worry you may have a brain tumour, don't you?'
	You saw a programme 3 nights ago about a girl who had a brain tumour.
	You are worried your boss will think you are 'pulling a sickie'.
	You spoke to your mum who told you to come and get some sumatriptan tablets.
	You would like to see a specialist, your reason being that the headaches keep coming back and you want to know what is wrong.
	You don't really know anything about migraines.
Examination	BP 110/60, Fundi normal. Visual acuity 6/6. Normal neurological examination.

Neurological Problems – 3

Learning Points Migraine

Please use your own judgement and refer to the full NICE guidance and BNF for further advice.

Red flags[2] Neurological or raised intracranial pressure symptoms or seizures.

Changes in behaviour, memory or skills.

Unilateral deafness or pulse synchronous tinnitus.

Drowsiness or loss of consciousness.

Ataxia.

Sudden visual loss.

Migraine with aura using OCP.

Differential diagnosis

Ear or dental infection	
Sub-arachnoid haemorrhage	'Thunder-clap headache' – severe, sudden onset.
Subdural haemorrhage	Risk factors include alcohol, being elderly and falls.
Temporal arteritis	>50 years + pain on chewing or combing your hair?
	Temporal artery 'absent pulse, beaded, tender or enlarged'.[1]
Acoustic neuroma	Pulse synchronous tinnitus or unilateral deafness.
	Sensorineural deafness or cranial nerve signs.
Obstructive sleep apnoea	Daytime somnolence.
Medication triggers	E.g. calcium blockers or analgesia induced.
Metastases/SOL	Previous cancer. Raised ICP symptoms and neurological signs.
Muscular, and many more	

Migraine management options to consider

Medication options	Ibuprofen.
	Aspirin.
	Metoclopramide or domperidone. Migraines cause gastric stasis so patients are likely to benefit from prokinetic treatment (with acute therapy) to assist absorption and decrease nausea. There is a risk of extrapyramidal side effects.
Triptans	Avoid if uncontrolled HTN and vascular disease.
	Check licencing: >60 years and children.[2]
Migraine prophylaxis	Propranolol. Amitriptyline or topiramate.[2]

See the **Link Hub at Completecsa.co.uk** for links to a very useful one page summary of:
Migraine – Acute Therapy Guideline
Migraine – Prophylactic Therapy Guideline

Neurological Problems – 3

Doctor's Notes

Patient	Ahmed Hidad 58 years M
PMH	Hypertension
	Hypercholesterolaemia
Medications	Indapamide 2.5 mg
	Atorvastatin 40 mg
Allergies	No information
Consultations	No recent consultations
Investigations	BP 3 months ago 132/80
	Blood tests 1 year ago HbA1c 5.8% (40 mmol/mol)
	Lipids – normal range
Household	No household members registered

Example Consultation — TIA

Open ☐	Tell me the story of what happened. How are you now? How is your health generally? Did you notice any other symptoms? How long did it last? What do the arm and leg feel like today? How do you feel today?
Flags ☐	Did the left side feel weak? Did you notice any changes in your vision or speech? Did you feel lightheaded, the heart racing or in pain at the time? Headache or vomiting? Has anything like this happened before?
History ☐	Talk me through when you take your medicines. Who is important to you in your life? Since your wife died, how are you doing on your own? Do you drink any alcohol?
Risk ☐	Has anyone in your family had a heart attack or stroke? Have you ever smoked? Do you have any pain in the chest or legs when walking? Have you had a fall or hit your head? Have you ever had a stomach ulcer?
Sense ☐	I see you are worried. It sounds like you were hesitant about calling for help.
Curious ☐	Why did you not call for help? What was going through your mind?
ICE ☐	What do you think the problem was? Is there anything else that you have been concerned about? What did you think I may suggest today?
Summary ☐	To summarise, you are usually well. You often forget the cholesterol tablet but take the morning BP tablet. You are worried that you have had a stroke as last night the left side felt weak, you lay in bed for hours uncertain whether to call for help but what stopped you is the fear that the ambulance crew would take you to hospital, which is a frightening thought.
Empathy ☐	You are a man who likes peace and quiet and the thought of going to hospital was what kept you from calling. It sounds as if you would have liked some support, but didn't feel there was a good option – your daughter was 2 hours away, is that correct?
O/E ☐	May I feel your pulse, listen to the heart and neck vessels, take your blood pressure, check the nerves in the face, arms and legs please. Please may I see you walk across the room?
Impression ☐	It sounds as if you had a mini-stroke called a TIA: transient ischaemic attack. Transient means short-lived and ischaemic means a lack of blood supply, in this case to the brain.
Experience ☐	Have you come across any of these terms before? Have you known anyone who has had a stroke? What happened to them?
Explanation ☐	Several factors increase the risk of having a stroke or mini-stroke. In your case it includes the high cholesterol and high blood pressure.
Options ☐	I would like to refer you to the rapid-access TIA clinic where you will be seen within 1 week. Please let me know if you have not received your appointment in 5 days. Are you happy to go to the hospital for a clinic appointment? I would also like to give you some aspirin to take until you have seen the specialist: 300 mg right away, then 75 mg once a day. It would be helpful to get a heart tracing done and some blood tests to help the specialist; could you book in for these at reception?
Empower ☐	There are things you can do meanwhile such as ensuring you remember to take all your medication regularly, including the aspirin.
Future ☐	At the hospital they will examine you and then discuss further tests such as a special brain scan (called an MRI) or a jelly scan of your neck arteries. When you have been seen by the hospital doctor, please return so we can discuss your general health and update your medicines.
Safety net ☐	There is risk this may happen again. I'm pleased that your symptoms went away which is why we call it a mini-stroke but a TIA can be a warning of a larger stroke and you could be left paralysed like your neighbour. This would have a huge impact on your life around the home and in the garden. Therefore, if this happens again, I would like you to call 999 straight away. The benefit of this is that they could give you treatment to help the blood supply to the brain and prevent some damage to the brain. Do you think you will call 999 if it happens again? Because of the risk of another episode like this, you are must not drive until you have been told it is safe to do so.

Neurological Problems – 4

Patient's Story

TIA

Doctor's notes	Ahmed Hidad, 58 years. PMH: Hypertension and hypercholesterolaemia. Medication: Indapamide 2.5 mg and Atorvastatin 40 mg.
How to act	Pleasant and respectful.
PC	*'Last night I couldn't use my arm and my leg felt weak.'*
History	You have always been well. You attend the doctors yearly for your blood pressure and cholesterol check. Last night you were sweeping the garage and your left arm dropped the brush. It felt as if it had gone limp and your left leg also felt strange and possibly weak. You went to sit down in the kitchen and weren't sure whether to call your daughter but it went away after 10 minutes. You lay awake for many hours unsure what to do but relieved it had gone away. Eventually you fell asleep. No symptoms this morning.
	You have never had anything like this before.
	You often forget to take your cholesterol medicine at night but you remember the blood pressure medicine with breakfast.
	Your vision was normal and you didn't speak to anyone. You didn't feel muddled in any way.
	You have not had a fall or head injury. You didn't call an ambulance as you thought they would send you to hospital and you have always preferred being alone and hate the thought of hospitals.
Social	You lost your wife to leukaemia 10 years ago.
	Your daughter lives 2 hours away so you didn't want to worry her.
	You used to be a gardener and still enjoy looking after your large garden for when the family is around. Your son lives abroad but tries to see you with his family every few months.
	You are independent with your ADL. You have never smoked and do not drink alcohol.
ICE	You are worried that you may have had a stroke.
	You expect the doctor may give you aspirin.
	Your neighbour had a stroke many years ago. He needed to be in a wheelchair afterwards.
	You follow all of the doctor's advice.
Examination	Normal examination of the arms, legs and cranial nerves. BP 132/88 HR 72 bpm regular. No carotid bruit. Normal gait.

Neurological Problems – 4

Learning Points

TIA

The ABCD² score:

'A — age: 60 years of age or more, 1 point.
B — blood pressure at presentation: 140/90 mm Hg or greater, 1 point.
C — clinical features: unilateral weakness, 2 points; speech disturbance without weakness, 1 point.
D — duration of symptoms: 60 minutes or longer, 2 points; 10–59 minutes, 1 point.
D — presence of diabetes: 1 point.'[1]

High risk of stroke ABCD² score ≥4 or 2 TIAs in 1 week or AF present or TIA already on anticoagulant.[1,2]
Aspirin 300 mg, 1 dose (or clopidogrel off label) unless taking an anticoagulant (± PPI).
'Do not delay treatment in people with uncontrolled BP.'[1]
Admit for specialist assessment within 24 hours of onset of symptoms.
Prescribe a statin.
Patients are likely to receive urgent brain imaging (preferably MRI) and carotid imaging within 1 week if a candidate for carotid endarterectomy.
Advise not to drive.

Low risk of stroke ABCD² score ≤3 or patients who present >1 week after their symptoms have resolved.[1,2]
Aspirin 300 mg, 1 dose (or clopidogrel off label) unless taking an anticoagulant (± PPI).
'Do not delay treatment in people with uncontrolled BP.'[1]
Continue aspirin or clopidogrel 75 mg OD until seen by specialist.[3]
Prescribe a statin.
Specialist assessment within 1 week of onset of event.
Are likely to be offered brain imaging (preferably MRI) and carotid imaging if a candidate for carotid endarterectomy.
Advise not to drive.

Secondary prevention Control of blood pressure.
Antiplatelet agents – see below.
Atorvastatin 80 mg.[2]
Diet and lifestyle advice.
Consider thiazides and ACE inhibitors regardless of BP unless CI[2].

After the CAPRIE trial[4] which recommends clopidogrel following atherosclerotic vascular disease, the 2012 Royal College of Physicians guidelines suggest 'For patients with ischaemic stroke or TIA in sinus rhythm, clopidogrel should be the standard antithrombotic treatment; clopidogrel should be used at a dose of 75 mg daily.'[5]

A study published in the *Lancet* (May 2016), 'Effects of aspirin on risk and severity of early recurrent stroke after transient ischaemic attack and ischaemic stroke: time-course analysis of randomised trials', suggests that the benefit of aspirin given as soon as possible after TIA has been underestimated in terms of preventing further stroke or severity of further stroke. Interestingly, it also mentions that benefits have been demonstrated for aspirin only, and not other antiplatelet agents yet![6]

TIA Booklet for patients
See the **Link Hub at CompleteCSA.co.uk** for a link to a SIGN's PIL following a TIA.[2]

Doctor's Notes

Patient	Lydia Cooper 25 years F
PMH	Tonsillitis – 3 years ago
Medications	No current medications
Allergies	No information
Consultations	No recent consultations
Investigations	No recent investigations
Household	No household members registered

Example Consultation — Multiple Sclerosis

Open ☐	Tell me what you've noticed from the beginning. Anything else that is unusual? How do you feel?
History ☐	Are you well usually? Have you had any recent illnesses or viral symptoms? Tell me more about you? Who are you close to? Do you work? What do you like to do – do you have hobbies?
Risk ☐	Has anyone in your family had similar symptoms in the past? Have you been abroad or noticed any insect bites? Have you ever had an infection through sex?
Flags ☐	Has your vision changed recently? What have you noticed? Has your speech changed? What about any weakness in the body where a leg or arm actually feels floppy? Have you noticed any difference in your control when going to the toilet? Have you lost weight? Any headaches or vomiting? Is your back painful? Have you had an injury?
Sense ☐	I can see you are upset and very worried.
ICE ☐	Have you had any thoughts about what may have caused this? What is going through your mind? Did you have any ideas about what I may say or suggest today?
Curious ☐	Tell me about your grandpa's experience.
Impact ☐	Have your symptoms stopped you from doing anything?
Summary ☐	To summarise, you have noticed unusual sensations now in both legs and your vision has been troubling you. You became very concerned when you realised you were wobbly on your feet. You have been passing urine more urgently. You fear it may be a similar problem to your grandpa's, but you are puzzled and worried by your symptoms. Is that correct?
O/E ☐	I would like to examine you please, take your pulse, blood pressure, breathing rate and temperature. Look at the nerves supplying the face, arms and legs and in the back of the eyes. Is that okay? May I check the nerve supply to the bottom? Because you mentioned urgency of urine, testing the sensation to the bottom is important. May I see you walk across the room … and can you produce a sample of urine please?
Empathy ☐	I appreciate it is frightening when you have symptoms which you cannot explain, especially when they come quickly together and it has made you wonder if this is similar to your grandpa's condition.
Impression ☐	I don't believe it is the same as what happened to your grandpa as the problem that elderly people have is usually very different from the cause of problems in young people and it sounds as if his symptoms were very different. However, I do think we need to ask the nerve doctors to have a look at you. I am questioning whether your nerves have become a little swollen, but the exact cause for why this has happened is not yet clear.
Explanation ☐	This can happen for several reasons: following an infection, low vitamin B, or where the nerve supply is irritated by something pushing against the nerve. The body can also attack itself by mistake and attack the nerves so they become weak and lose their protective layer. Instead of this protective layer, scar tissue forms and it blocks the normal signals from the nerves, which is why you may be feeling the strange sensations. I think the last reason may be the most likely but we need to do some tests to get the answer to why this has happened. Do you have any questions? You may find your symptoms go away and then come back again. Before we can give you the exact answer, we need to know what we are dealing with.
Options ☐	I would like to ask you to sit in the waiting room where a nurse will call you through for a blood test. Meanwhile I'm going to give the nerve doctors at the hospital a call to ask if they want to see you today or in their rapid-access clinic.
Future ☐	At the hospital I expect they will examine you like I have done today and, if they feel it is necessary, they may arrange an MRI scan. There may still be further tests you need before we have the answer.

Patient's Story

Multiple Sclerosis

Doctor's notes Lydia Cooper, 25 years. PMH: Tonsillitis – 3 years ago. Medications: None.

How to act Nervous and anxious.

Start to cry when you explain your symptoms.

PC *'I've got this strange feeling in my leg – it's the second time I've had it.'*

History Six weeks ago you noticed your right foot was tingling within the shoe. You thought it must have been your tight trainers but you noticed it again in bed last week but this time on the left foot and lower leg and today it has gone above your knee. You feel wobbly when you walk today. You feel like you are going to fall over.

A couple of months ago you realised that you needed glasses. Your right eye has been blurry this week.

No headache or weight loss.

You have noticed urgency of urine and nearly missed the toilet yesterday but no other urinary symptoms. Your bowels are normal.

No other symptoms on systemic enquiry.

Social You live with your boyfriend of 1 year. You are looking for work.

You left college aged 16 years. Since then you've found temporary work in offices.

You smoked in your teens. You do not drink alcohol.

ICE You don't know what may be causing it.

You hope you haven't had a stroke like your grandpa 2 years ago.

Your grandpa lost all movement on the right side and his speech was different.

You don't know what the doctor will say today.

Examination BP 120/60, HR 72 regular, apyrexial, RR 14.

No nystagmus, fundoscopy normal.

Visual acuity reduced right eye.

CN otherwise normal.

Reduced sensation from the left toes to L3.

Weakness L4/5/S1 – 3/5.

Knee/ankle jerk increase, clonus and extensor plantar response – left side.

Abnormal gait.

Reduced perianal sensation.

Urine dipstick normal.

Ask the doctor Will it get better?

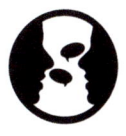

Neurological Problems – 5

Learning Points — Multiple Sclerosis

MS may take the course of relapsing-remitting, primary or secondary progressive.[1]

MS is usually a progressive disease.

Relapses may be triggered by infections.[1]

Epidemiology	Incidence F>M; common in young adults.
Symptoms[1]	Visual changes — E.g. acuity, colour vision, visual fields (optic neuritis). Reduced vision, loss of vision or double vision.
	Hearing loss.
	Facial weakness.
	Altered sensations.
	Limb weakness, gait problems.
	Bladder and bowel control may be affected.
	Altered temperature regulation, e.g. sweating.
	Altered sexual function/impotence.
	Lhermitte's phenomenon: the feeling of electricity down the spine on neck flexion.
	Cerebellar symptoms: ataxia, nystagmus, dysarthria and vertigo.
	Cognitive dysfunction (late symptoms).
Diagnosis	≥2 demyelinating lesions in the brain/spinal cord separated in time and space.[2]
	Investigations may include MRI, lumbar puncture and visual evoked potentials.
Differential diagnosis[1]	Sarcoidosis
	Spinal cord compression
	Vitamin B12 deficiency
	Neurosyphilis
	SLE
	Cerebrovascular disease
	SOL/tumours
	Lyme disease
Blood tests	FBC, U&E, LFT, calcium, glucose, TFTs, ESR, CRP, vitamin B12, ANA (antinuclear antibody), HIV (human immunodeficiency virus) ± syphilis.

CHAPTER 21 OVERVIEW
Respiratory Health

	Cases in this chapter	Within the RCGP curriculum: Respiratory Health RCGP Curriculum Online March 2016[1]	Learning Points in the chapter include:
1	Asthma Diagnosis	'Ensure that patients can use the inhaled medication they are prescribed, both routinely and in an emergency'	Asthma diagnosis – adult and child
2	Pneumonia	'Know the boundaries of primary care management and the role of specialist services in supporting the patient'	Management of pneumonia CRB65 score and AMTS
3	Acute Asthma	'Know the diagnostic and treatment guidelines for common respiratory diseases (asthma, COPD, lung cancer) in primary care'	Acute asthma management
4	COPD	'Understand the potential impact of the patient's family history, lifestyle and occupation on the subsequent development of respiratory disease' 'Explain, encourage and support self-management strategies for different respiratory diseases, according to the differing wishes and expectations of patients' 'Be able to explain to patients (and their carers) why they are breathless, the progression of their disease, benefits and limitations of treatments and how to recognise and treat exacerbations' 'Know how to interpret lung function measurements' 'Recognise the risk of co-morbid mental health problems in people with long-term respiratory problems, such as asthma and COPD, and the effect of these on morbidity and mortality'	Management of COPD Extra Notes: Spirometry
5	Cough	'Know the key points in your history-taking and examination with respect to specific respiratory diseases, e.g. in relation to occupation, smoking, "red flag" symptoms, family history, clubbing, lymphadenopathy'	Lung cancer
Extra notes	Spirometry	'Know how to interpret lung function measurements as performed in primary care, e.g. peak expiratory flow (PEF), spirometry, pulse oximetry, and know the expected impact of bronchodilators on such measurements' 'Be able to function as both diagnostician and respiratory team leader'	Spirometry Reversibility testing Restrictive lung disease

1. http://www.rcgp.org.uk/training-exams/gp-curriculum-overview/online-curriculum/applying-clinical-knowledge-section-1/3-19-respiratory-health.aspx

CHAPTER 21 REFERENCES

Asthma Diagnosis
1. Pellegrino R., Viegi G., Brusasco V., Crapo R.O., Burgos F., Casaburi R., et al. Interpretive strategies for lung function tests. *Eur Respir J.* 2005; 26(5): 948–68.
2. Scottish Intercollegiate Guidelines Network (SIGN). British Guideline on the Management of Asthma. May 2008. Revised Jun 2009. https://www.brit-thoracic.org.uk/document-library/clinical-information/asthma/btssign-asthma-guideline-2009/
3. Scottish Intercollegiate Guidelines Network (SIGN). Quick Reference Guide. British Guideline on the management of asthma. Oct 2014. https://www.brit-thoracic.org.uk/document-library/clinical-information/asthma/btssign-asthma-guideline-quick-reference-guide-2014/

Pneumonia
1. British Thoracic Society. Guidelines for the Management of Community Acquired Pneumonia in Adults Update 2009. A Quick Reference Guide. Nov 2009. https://www.brit-thoracic.org.uk/document-library/clinical-information/pneumonia/adult-pneumonia/a-quick-reference-guide-bts-guidelines-for-the-management-of-community-acquired-pneumonia-in-adults/
2. NICE Guidelines. CG191. Pneumonia in adults: diagnosis and management. Dec 2014.
3. Lim W.S., van der Eerden M.M., Laing R., et al. Defining community-acquired pneumonia severity on presentation to hospital: an international derivation and validation study. *Thorax.* 2003; 58: 377–82.
4. Hodkinson, H.M. (1972). Evaluation of a mental test score for assessment of mental impairment in the elderly. *Age and Ageing.* 1972; 1(4): 233–8. doi:10.1093/ageing/1.4.233. PMID 4669880

Acute Asthma and COPD
1. Scottish Intercollegiate Guidelines Network (SIGN). Quick Reference Guide. British Guideline on the management of asthma. Oct 2014. https://www.brit-thoracic.org.uk/document-library/clinical-information/asthma/btssign-asthma-guideline-quick-reference-guide-2014/
2. NICE Guidelines. CG101. Chronic obstructive pulmonary disease in over 16s: diagnosis and management. Jun 2010. https://www.nice.org.uk/guidance/cg101/chapter/1Guidance# management-of-exacerbations-of-copd
3. NICE. http://cks.nice.org.uk/chronic-obstructive-pulmonarydisease#! scenariorecommendation:17. Revised Sep 2015.
4. British Thoracic Society. Emergency Oxygen Guideline Group. Guideline for emergency oxygen use in adult patients. *Thorax.* Volume 63. Supplement VI. Oct 2008. https://www.brit-thoracic.org.uk/document-library/clinical-information/oxygen/emergency-oxygen-use-in-adult-patients-guideline/emergency-oxygen-use-in-adult-patients-guideline/

COPD
1. Fletcher C.M., Elmes P.C., Fairbairn M.B., et al. The significance of respiratory symptoms and the diagnosis of chronic bronchitis in a working population. *BMJ.* 1959; 2: 257–66.
2. British Thoracic Society. BTS Home Oxygen Guideline Group BTS Guideline for Home Oxygen Use in Adults. *Thorax.* Volume 70. Supplement 1. June 2015. https://www.brit-thoracic.org.uk/document-library/clinical-information/oxygen/home-oxygen-guideline-(adults)/bts-guidelines-for-home-oxygen-use-in-adults/
3. Iyer A.S., Dransfield M.T. Serum eosinophils as a COPD biomarker: ready for prime time? *Lancet.* 2016 May; 4(5): 341–3. http://www.thelancet.com/journals/lanres/article/PIIS2213-2600(16)30040-6/fulltext
4. NICE Guidelines CG101. Chronic obstructive pulmonary disease in over 16s: diagnosis and management. 2010.
5. https://www.gov.uk/drug-safety-update/tiotropium-delivered-via-respimat-compared-with-handihaler-no-significant-difference-in-mortality-in-tiospir-trial. Contains public sector information licensed under the open Government Licence v3.0.

Cough/Lung Cancer
1. NICE Guidelines. [NG12]. Suspected cancer: recognition and referral. Jun 2015.

Spirometry
1. The BTS COPD Consortium. Spriometry in Practice. A practical Guide to Using Spirometry in Primary Care. 2nd edition. 2005. https://www.brit-thoracic.org.uk/document-library/delivery-of-respiratory-care/spirometry/spirometry-in-practice/

Doctor's Notes

Patient	Peter Atkins	12 years	M
PMH	Eczema		
	Hay fever		
	Viral induced wheeze		
Medications	Current medication:	Oilatum cream PRN	
	Previous medication:	Salbutamol	
		Spacer	
		Loratadine	
Allergies	No information		
Consultations	3 months ago. Mild eczema – emollients encouraged.		
Investigations	No information		
Household	Rachel Atkins	40 years	F
	Alexander Atkins	40 years	M

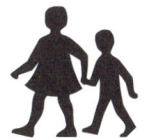

Example Consultation — Asthma Diagnosis

Open ☐	Why have you come to see the doctor today? Tell me more about this cough, Peter. Have you had any problems with your breathing? Are you well at the moment or are you poorly?
Flags ☐	Have you had a cold? Any phlegm? Does it hurt anywhere? Has Peter had a fever? When with your friends, do you run around like they do or do you need to stop more?
Risk ☐	I see Peter has hay fever and eczema. Has any family member had asthma at all?
History ☐	Any other medical history? Any complications when Peter was born? Or afterwards any other medical problems? And the medicines that he takes at the moment? Any allergies?
Curious ☐	Peter was previously given an inhaler; how often does he use it? When did he last?
ICE ☐	Why was Peter given the inhalers? Peter, why do you think you have a cough? You could be right Peter; why do you think that? Tell me more about your friend, Peter. Has John ever struggled with his breathing? Are you worried about your breathing too? And Mum, what do you think is causing this cough? Are you worried about anything in particular? And, today, what did you hope we would do at this stage?
Sense ☐	I can see you are both concerned.
O/E ☐	I would like to examine your chest, Peter, if you can lift up your shirt. Now check your pulse and oxygen level with this gadget. Have you seen this blowing tube (peak flow meter) before? I will demonstrate. Can you try?
Summary ☐	So, Peter, you have been coughing for months but otherwise feel fine. You are worried you could have asthma like John and would like an inhaler. Mum, you have had many doctors tell you this is viral wheeze not asthma and therefore thought his cough must be an infection as he has not been wheezy. Is that correct?
Impression ☐	Viral wheeze is very common as a young child but you are older now, Peter, and you feel your breathing isn't as good as your friends' so it sounds like this is asthma. Coughing can be the only symptom but, Peter, you think you have been wheezy at times too. Asthma is also more likely if you suffer with hay fever or eczema.
Experience ☐	Do you know what asthma is, Peter? What about you, Mum?
Explanation ☐	Asthma is where the air tubes in your lungs become narrow so there is less space for the air.
Empathy ☐	I appreciate this may worry you, Peter, after you have seen John go to hospital.
Options ☐	We can use inhalers to prevent this from happening. Firstly, to confirm the diagnosis, the nurse can do some special blowing tests. We should try a brown inhaler that is taken morning and night. The brown inhaler should prevent your cough or wheeze. But, if you are still coughing or wheezy, you can take the blue inhaler.
Empower ☐	So can I check I have been clear: when would you take the blue inhaler? And what about the brown inhaler? Peter, can you keep a diary of when you need your blue inhaler? Any questions so far?
Future ☐	The nurse can also check you are happy with your inhaler and give you an asthma plan which tells you what to do if your breathing gets worse. See the doctor again in 2 weeks, please, to see if the inhalers are working. If you need your blue inhaler more than twice a week, this may suggest you need a stronger brown inhaler so see the GP.
Safety net ☐	If you ever struggle with your breathing and need more than 10 puffs of your inhaler at once, then this is when an ambulance should be called but I don't expect that to happen as the brown inhaler should prevent this. So can you tell me, Peter, when you should ask for help? Yes, and if at any time your breathing gets worse, you should see a doctor. Any questions?

Respiratory Health – 1

Patient's Story

Asthma Diagnosis

Doctor's notes Peter Atkins, 12 years. PMH: Eczema, hay fever and viral induced wheeze.

Medications: Oilatum cream. Past medication: Salbutamol with spacer, loratadine.

How to act Peter is quiet and requires encouragement from the doctor to speak.

Mum speaks first if the question is not directed to Peter.

PC *'Doctor, Peter keeps coughing every night and it has been going on for months.'*

History **Mum** Peter has had a dry cough for months, especially at night and it keeps you awake.

He is not breathless and has no sputum or fever. He has not complained of pain.

He is well and you have not heard him wheeze.

Peter has had no other symptoms for months.

Peter has not used his (very) old inhaler for months, since winter.

He was born around his due date and was always well. Immunisations are up to date.

No FH. Eczema is mild and controlled with Oilatum.

History **Peter** You are *'fine'*. When you play football, you feel wheezy and out of breath.

Your friends can run around for longer. You have had no pain, no fever and no sputum.

You do not have an itchy nose at present. You recall that you used to use an inhaler.

Social No pets. Only child. Parents both smoke *'but not in the house'*.

ICE **Mum** You know that Peter has *'viral wheeze'* after multiple doctors have said so.

You are not worried but have brought him here today for antibiotics.

Peter has not told you about his friend John or his worries about asthma.

Peter If asked, you think the diagnosis is *'asthma'*.

Mention *'John has asthma too.'*

John is your friend and, if asked about John, tell the doctor that once John *'went to hospital because he couldn't play football'*. He was using his inhaler a lot that day and was sat on the football pitch with it.

You think you need the inhaler like John. You don't want to have to go to hospital too.

If asked what you understand about asthma, say. *'John uses his inhaler before he plays football.'*

Examination Height is 140 cm. Peak flow 270 l/min. Chest clear and no wheeze. HS normal.

Sats 98%. RR 17. HR 80 regular. Apyrexial.

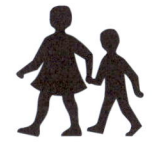

Respiratory Health – 1

Learning Points

Asthma Diagnosis

Symptoms Wheeze, cough, difficulty breathing and chest tightness. Especially at night or in the morning.

Triggers Exertion, weather, emotion, pets and hay fever.

Atopy PMH or FH of hay fever, eczema or asthma.

Medications Symptoms with aspirin, NSAID or beta-blockers.

Examination Widespread wheeze, reduced air entry, low saturations, FEV1 or PEF.

Investigations Usually no blood test required but may show eosinophilia. Spirometry.

Minus features which lower the probability: Only with a cold, no interval symptoms, moist cough, dizziness, light-headedness, no wheeze. Also in adults: smoking history, cardiac disease, voice change.

Management

High Probability	Intermediate Probability	Low Probability
↓	↓	↓
Start treatment	Spirometry if able	Further investigations or referral
	Diagnosis = FEV1/FVC <0.7 with reversibility*	
	If not able – trial of treatment	
	Continue treatment if effective	
	Investigate/refer if uncertain	

*__Reversibility__ 'A significant increase in FEV1 (>12% from baseline)[1] or PEF after bronchodilator indicates reversible airflow obstruction and supports the diagnosis of asthma.'[2]

'A >400 ml improvement in FEV1 to either β_2 agonist or corticosteroid treatment trials strongly suggests underlying asthma.'[2]

For treatment guidance see the BTS stepwise asthma management flow charts[3]

Trial of treatment and initiating treatment

Use clinical judgement to start treatment at the appropriate step according to symptom severity.

If <2 episodes wheeze a week, consider PRN salbutamol.

If >2 episodes wheeze a week, consider regular corticosteroid inhaler.

Respiratory Health – 1

Doctor's Notes

Patient	Lionel Morgan	82 years	M
PMH	Parkinson's disease		
Medications	Sinemet		
	Entacapone		
Allergies	No information		
Consultations	Medication review 3 months ago. No concerns.		
Investigations	No information		
Household	Betty Morgan	80 years	F

Wife Betty also present.

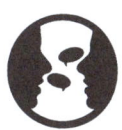

Example Consultation — Pneumonia

Open ☐	A chest infection? Anything else you have noticed? How do you feel about your health generally?
Flags ☐	Are you feeling SOB? Have you had a fever? Do you have any pain? What colour are you spitting out? Any blood? Any cold or sore throat at the moment?
Risk ☐	Are you managing to swallow food and tablets without coughing? Do you smoke? Have you suffered with lung trouble in the past? Have you been exposed to asbestos?
History ☐	I see you take Sinemet and Entacapone for your Parkinson's; is there any other medical history? Is it just the two of you at home?
ICE ☐	Any other concerns? Is there anything specific you were hoping I would do today?
Impact ☐	I'm interested to know how your Parkinson's is affecting you at the moment. Does it impact on your day? Since this cough, have either of you noticed any other changes?
Sense ☐	Lionel, you have turned to Betty a few times now. Are you feeling slightly muddled?
Curious ☐	Are you or your family worried about your memory?
O/E ☐	I'd like to examine you, check your heart rate and oxygen level, measure your blood pressure and listen to your lungs; if I can ask you to take your shirt off, is that okay? Can I test your memory by asking a few questions (AMTS). Would you normally be able to answer these questions more easily?
Summary ☐	So, for 4 days you have been struggling with your breathing and coughing up green phlegm, felt feverish and slightly more muddled than usual. You are both concerned this could be an infection.
Impression ☐	I think you do have pneumonia, Lionel.
Experience ☐	Pneumonia is an infection of the air sacs in the lungs which is usually significant enough to show up on a chest X-ray.
Explanation ☐	There is a pocket of infection in the left part of your lung that is making you feel very unwell.
Empathy ☐	I appreciate you said you are well cared for at home and prefer not to go to hospital but I think it may be necessary.
Options ☐	The other option is to give you antibiotics at home and keep a very close eye on you over the next couple of days but, due to your breathing, my recommendation would be to go to hospital for some oxygen and antibiotics into the blood to speed up your recovery.
Empower ☐	What do you both think? Lionel and Betty it sounds as if the two of you are looking after each other very well; however, should you need any help with carers then please let me know.
Future ☐	When you are feeling better, let's have another chat about your memory and Parkinson's in more detail: if you could please return to see me. Betty, it would be helpful to talk to you too about how you feel things are going.
Safety net ☐	How did you get here? Are you happy for your son to take you to the hospital? If, en route, you have pain or feel more short of breath or feel more poorly, stop the car and call for an ambulance. May I just check your son is comfortable with the decision to drive you there?

Patient's Story

Pneumonia

Doctor's notes Lionel Morgan, 82 years. PMH: Parkinson's disease. Medications: Sinemet and Entacapone. Wife Betty also present.

How to act Betty, your wife is with you. You turn to ask your wife Betty for answers.
Betty likes to answer for you.

PC *'Doctor, I think I've got a chest infection.'*

History

Betty Lionel is more muddled than usual. Your son is in the waiting room. He drove you here.

Lionel has been coughing green phlegm for 4 days,

He looks breathless but isn't wheezy. He is not choking on his food.

No blood seen. No other viral URTI symptoms. His fever was 102 degrees.

Lionel You have no pain. Your spit is green.

Social

Lionel You live with your wife, Betty, who does all your ADL and takes care of your medicines.

You are well looked after at home and your three children live close by.

You have never smoked. You drink no alcohol. No asbestos exposure.

ICE

Lionel You worry you have a chest infection.

'I would prefer you don't send me into hospital.'

However, you will do as the doctor suggests.

Betty You wonder if this is pneumonia.

'You will do as you are told, Lionel.'

Examination Bronchial breathing and crackles in the left base. Temperature 38.2°C. HR 90 bpm regular. Sats 95%, RR 24, BP 120/68.

AMTS score 6/10.

Betty states he would usually answer memory questions more easily.

Learning Points   Pneumonia

Pneumonia — An infection of the lung parenchyma (alveoli).

The BTS definition — 'Symptoms of an acute lower respiratory tract illness (cough and at least one other lower respiratory tract symptom).

New focal chest signs on examination.

At least one systemic feature (either a symptom complex of sweating, fevers, shivers, aches and pains and/or temperature of 38°C or more).

No other explanation for the illness.'[1]

CRB 65 score — This gentleman's CRB65 was 2.

1 point each for: Confusion (AMTS <8/10), RR>30/min, either BP <90/60 and age >65 years.

Mortality risk from CRB65 scores

0	'Low risk'[2]	<1% mortality risk[2,3]
1–2	'Intermediate risk'[2]	1–10% mortality risk[2,3]
3–4	'High risk'[2]	>10% mortality risk[2,3]

Sputum culture — 'Do not routinely offer microbiological tests to patients with low-severity community-acquired pneumonia.'[2]

CRP testing — Consider if clinically a diagnosis of pneumonia is not clear.[2]

<20 mg/litre — 'Do not routinely offer antibiotic therapy.'[2]

20 mg/litre–100 mg/litre — 'Consider a delayed antibiotic prescription.'[2]

>100 mg/litre — 'Offer antibiotic therapy.'[2]

NB: A fever is 100°F (= 37.8°C): a lot of older patients still use Fahrenheit.

AMTS[4]: to save time, ask the hard questions first, once they have got >2 wrong then move on.

Address to remember (42 West Street), age, time, year, where are we, 2 persons, DOB, queen, First World War, 20–1 backwards, ?recall address correct.

Treatment of pneumonia

Score= 0 — 5 days antibiotics + extend if no response after 3 days.[2] See your local guidance.

E.g. Amoxicillin (1st preference if possible[2]), erythromycin or doxycycline.

Score 1–2 — Consider either 7–10 days home Rx or hospital admission.

Consider dual therapy with a macrolide.[2]

Score = 3. — Usually admit where they may receive a 'dual antibiotic therapy with a beta-lactamase stable beta-lactam (e.g. co-amoxiclav) and a macrolide.'[2]

Safety net

See your GP if no response within 3 days and prior if worsening symptoms.

Asking about swallowing demonstrates you have considered the chronic comorbidities in this acute scenario and thought about aspiration pneumonia.

When a carer is present, acknowledge their role and if there is no time to discuss the impact of the disease in this first consultation, then signpost this suggestion. Practise holistically!

Respiratory Health – 2

Doctor's Notes

Patient	Daisy Fitton 24 years F
PMH	Asthma
Medications	Clenil 100 2 puffs BD
	Salbutamol PRN
Allergies	No information
Consultations	Last attended 9 months ago for asthma review with nurse. Peak Flow 450 l/min.
Investigations	No information
Household	No household members registered

Example Consultation — Acute Asthma

Open ☐	Oh dear, tell me more. What else have you noticed?
Flags ☐	How often have you been using your blue inhaler? With a spacer? How often do you usually use the blue one? What about the brown one?
Risk ☐	Have you ever been admitted with your asthma? Have you ever been in intensive care? Do you smoke? Has your asthma ever been as bad as this? Do you have a personalised asthma action plan?
History ☐	You are otherwise well, taking no medicines, is that correct? Is there anyone at home with you?
ICE ☐	What do you think has caused this? From your experience of your asthma, what do you believe is necessary?
Sense ☐	I can see you are struggling.
O/E ☐	May I examine you, listen to your chest, check your pulse and oxygen levels and your temperature and do the blowing peak flow test? Can I ask you to take off your top: is that okay?
Summary ☐	To summarise, you have had a cold and sore throat and now you are struggling with your asthma despite regular use of your blue inhaler.
Impression ☐	Your peak flow blowing test and your breathing and heart rate suggest this is a severe asthma attack. I think it has been caused by a viral infection.
Explanation ☐	There is no sign of a pocket of bacteria in the lung, you have not had a fever, you are not coughing green phlegm and your sore throat and cold are typical of a virus.
Empathy ☐	Normally, you have been able to manage the asthma at home so it is frightening when your asthma is so much worse than usual.
Options ☐	We need to give you a nebuliser and then see how you respond. I will also give you 40 mg of prednisolone, a steroid. I will ask the nurse to give you a nebuliser in the treatment room and I will see you again in 10 minutes. Let's see how your chest responds to that and make a decision then about whether you need to go to hospital. What are your thoughts about that? I would want you to be able to manage at least an hour without the inhaler, and then 4-hourly at home. I agree with you that you need steroids but as this attack is probably caused by a virus, antibiotics probably aren't going to be helpful.
Future ☐	When you are feeling better, let's meet up again to optimise your inhalers. In future if you are using your blue inhaler more than twice a week this suggests we need to increase the preventer, the brown inhaler. We can write all this down for you in your own asthma plan.
Safety net ☐	If you feel your breathing is deteriorating, tell us and we'll call an ambulance.

Patient's Story

Acute Asthma

Doctor's notes	Daisy Fitton, 24 years. PMH: Asthma. Medications: Clenil 100 2 puffs BD, Salbutamol PRN.
How to act	A little distracted by your breathing.
PC	*'My asthma isn't very good.'*
History	You've had a cold and sore throat and for the past 2 days you've become wheezy.
	You are not coughing any phlegm and have no pain but feel tight in the chest. No fever.
	Your chest always feels like this at this time of year.
	You were admitted once as a child but no ITU admissions.
	You use the clenil BD and usually your salbutamol 6 times a week, especially after hockey. You don't know your usual peak flow.
	You last took four puffs of salbutamol 1 hour ago.
Social	You are a solicitor. You live with your boyfriend. You have never smoked. All is well.
ICE	You believe the weather has caused this exacerbation. You are not too concerned.
	You expect the doctor will give you steroids and antibiotics.
	You will follow the doctor's advice regarding admission, stating: *'You are the doctor.'*
Examination	Peak flow 210 l/min, RR 24 Sats 95%, HR 104 bpm. Temperature 36.9°C
	Vesicular breaths and wheeze throughout. Good air entry, R=L, Expiration>Inspiration.

Respiratory Health – 3

Learning Points

Acute Asthma and COPD

Life-threatening asthma
Admit the patient **immediately**. Call 999. Features of life threatening asthma include:

Peak flow <33%, sats <92%, silent chest, cyanosis, poor respiratory effort, bradycardia, hypotension, confusion or exhaustion[1]

Acute severe asthma
Admit the patient and consider an ambulance. Features of severe asthma include:

Peak flow 33–50%, RR≥25, HR ≥110 and not able to complete sentences.[1]

Moderate asthma
Start treatment and if they remain well following treatment then advise the patient they must have a further assessment if they require further treatment within 4 hours. Features include:

Peak flow 50–75% and no signs of acute severe/life-threatening asthma.[1]

Management of acute asthma – adults
Oxygen to keep the saturations between 94 and 98%.[1]

Prednisolone 40–50 mg stat then daily to complete 5 days in all cases of acute asthma.[1]

For life-threatening asthma give salbutamol 5 mg nebuliser and repeat continuously if required whilst waiting for the ambulance. A patient with features of severe asthma may respond to salbutamol via inhaler and large volume spacer, but may require nebulisers.

Ipratropium bromide 500 mcg × 1 if features of severe or life-threatening asthma or poor response to salbutamol whilst waiting for an ambulance.[1]

If the actor is really struggling to answer your questions, advise a nebuliser +/− phone ambulance early in the consultation. It is kinder to the patient to ask them more questions after their breathing feels better. You can always indicate to the examiner that you know you require more information by stating that you will need to ask some more questions once their breathing has improved.

Safety netting
On discharge. If requiring more than 10 puffs of salbutamol though a spacer within 4 hours, they will then need to see a doctor again or go to hospital.

Acute COPD
There is a useful chart of signs to guide the decision regarding home or hospital care.[2,3]

For the patient at risk of hypercapnic respiratory failure:

The target saturation is 88–92%[4]

Provide oxygen through a venturi mask at 24% and increase to 28% if saturations remain <88%.

Doctor's Notes

Patient   Chao Lin   82 years   M

PMH   COPD
                 Current smoker

Medications Salbutamol
                Tiotropium

Allergies   No known drug allergies

Consultations COPD review 1 year ago with the nurse – no changes made. Using Salbutamol on hills. Tiotropium daily. Saturations 96%. MRC dyspnoea scale – 2. Weight 72 kg.

Spirometry 1 year ago.

FEV1 = 48%, FVC = 80%, FEV1/FVC = 0.6. FEV1 following salbutamol 52%.

Letter to patient

'Dear Mr Lin. Please make an appointment to see me at the surgery. I would like to discuss your breathing and inhalers to see if any adjustments are required and take this opportunity to discuss your general health and if there is anything that you may need. Best wishes. Dr Blount.'

Investigations No information

Household   No known household contacts

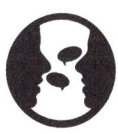

Example Consultation — COPD

Open □ — Thank you for coming in Mr Lin. How are you? This is the first time we have met so please tell me about your health. What is most difficult? What has changed?

ICE □ — Is there anything you wanted to talk to me about? Or other aspect of your health? Has anything been on your mind or worrying you? What is your biggest fear? And did you have any thoughts about what we may talk about or decide today?

Sense □ — I noticed that when you came in your breathing was harder – it seems to have eased.

History □ — Apart from your breathing, have you had any other medical conditions in the past? Or other parts of your body which don't work as they used to? Tell me more about your breathing. When do you take your inhalers? Every day? Can you show me how you use your inhaler please? Do you have any allergies? Who else is important to you in your life? I'm sorry, that must still be very painful. How are you managing on your own? How often do you see your son? What did you do for a living?

Risk □ — Are you still smoking? Where were you born? Growing up, were you exposed to much pollution or smoke? Did your family in China have any health problems?

Flags □ — Do you feel breathless or wheezy around the home? Do you cough up any phlegm or blood? Do you ever have any chest pain? When did you last have a chest infection? Do you feel breathless at night? How many pillows do you use? Do your legs swell up? Have you lost or put on any weight? You seem concerned about infections.

Curious □ — Why might that be? How is your mood? Do you feel isolated? Or depressed? Do you ever want to not wake up? Do you have a faith? With your faith is there anything important to you that I should know about now or in the future?

Impact □ — What are you not able to do? How long can you walk for? Do you have stairs in your home? Do you do your meals and shopping? Are you able to keep the home clean?

O/E □ — I'd like to listen to your heart and lungs, check your BP and a breathing test and have a look at your neck, hands and legs – if I may ask you to remove your top please.

Summary □ — Mr Lin, you have noticed that, for the past 6 months, you struggle to walk as far as before without having a rest. You worry about getting a chest infection and also how your breathing may change over time and fear dying and struggling to breathe.

Impression □ — Mr Lin, I'm afraid your airway disease does seem to have progressed.

Experience □ — What do you know about the term COPD? Or chronic airways disease?

Explanation □ — It is a long-term condition of the airways which have been damaged over time.

Empathy □ — I can imagine it is frightening to notice that your breathing does not allow you to do what you used to, and fear that soon you will not be able to reach the shops.

Options □ — I would like to help your lungs be as good as they can be. There are things we can do to make things better for you. You can take a course of prednisolone 30 mg daily (steroid) if your breathing gets worse, with amoxicillin (antibiotic) if you get more phlegm or it changes colour. Would it be reassuring to have these medications at home?

Empower □ — Are you interested in our stop smoking service? It can really help to slow the disease progression. I would advise the flu and pneumococcal vaccine. May I also refer you to our rehabilitation service aiming to optimise your lungs as much as possible? I would like to swap your capsule inhaler for a stronger one. We have two options here and usually I recommend an inhaler called Fostair which contains a steroid to calm the airways, but you must be aware that there is an increased risk of infection with a steroid inhaler. I can see you are not keen, another option would be an inhaler called Duaklir which you take one puff morning and night. I will ask the pharmacist to show you how to use it. Does this sound okay? This is to replace your capsule inhaler.

Future □ — Can we meet again in 1 month to talk about what might happen to your breathing over time? We can create a care plan where we talk through different scenarios and what you might like doctors to do. I'd also like to talk more about how you are generally.

Safety net □ — If you are more breathless, in pain or unsure please speak to a doctor straight away.

Patient's Story

COPD

Doctor's notes Chao Lin, 82 years. PMH: COPD. Medications: Salbutamol and tiotropium. Smoker. Consultations: 1 year ago, COPD review with PN. Sats 96%. MRC 2. Letter to patient: COPD review now due.

How to act Breathing initially fast when enters but this settles after being seated.

PC *'Hello, Doctor. I had a letter asking me to attend for my check-up.'*

History You don't like to bother the doctor. Apart from your breathing you are well and you have no significant PMH. You are compliant with your tiotropium and use the salbutamol twice daily. You have no allergies. You remember your grandparents were heavy breathers. You never knew your father and your mother died when you were small. You believe you are 82 years old but don't know exactly. Your breathing hasn't been very good for the past 6 months. You started to wheeze about 3 years ago. You wheeze when walking to the shop but you are okay in your home but occasionally wheeze after a shower. You have no orthopnoea and sleep on two thin pillows. You have no fluid collecting in the legs. You have no cardiac symptoms. Where you grew up, your grandparents used to light fires throughout the day to keep you warm. You had no siblings. You had three infections last winter and once you were in hospital overnight. This was a frightening experience as you had never been in hospital.

Social You moved to the UK when you were 36 years old and worked in the shipyards. You live alone and find life tiring. You walk to the local shop a couple of hundred yards away and stop for a rest midway. You use a shopping trolley to wheel your food back to the house but this is getting harder. You do not drive. Your son owns the local garage in the next village and he always offers to help you and you see him twice a week. He takes you wherever you need to go. You lost your wife to bowel cancer 3 years ago. You feel quite lonely but feel you should not complain. Your mood is a little low but you have no thoughts of not wanting to be alive and generally you feel grateful for life. Your faith (Buddhism) is important to you. You continue to smoke and would like to stop. The surgery is on the next door street to your home so walking to the appointment is okay. You have no problems within your bungalow.

ICE You worry about an infection or whether you will one day struggle with your breathing. Is it likely you will die of not being able to breathe? You have no expectations from the consultation and would follow any advice that the doctor gives. However, a preference would be to avoid any risk of infection if possible.

Examination Chest – air entry and wheeze throughout. No accessory muscle use. Saturations 94%. Heart sounds normal, HR regular 72 bpm. No leg oedema or raised JVP. Weight 72 kg. BP 130/70. Peak flow 200 l/min. No supraclavicular lymphadenopathy. No clubbing.

Respiratory Health – 4

Learning Points   COPD

MRC dyspnoea scale[1]	Determine the exercise tolerance.
Pulmonary rehab	Offer if MRC ≥ 3 or recent hospitalisation.
Pneumonia risk	Discuss if offering an ICS inhaler.
Home oxygen	'Patients with a resting stable oxygen saturation (SpO2) of ≤92% should be referred for a blood gas assessment in order to assess eligibility for LTOT.'[2]
Health promotion	Smoking cessation. Flu and pneumococcal vaccine.
Carer support	Involve the carer in the management plan.
Self-management plan	For exacerbations – when to step up inhalers and take rescue medications.

The treatment of COPD

Exclude asthma/reversibility – see *Reversibility in the Learning Points of Asthma Diagnosis.

  Why? – It is dangerous to prescribe a LABA without a steroid in asthma.

Use steroids with lower strength in COPD (e.g. beclomethasone = Fostair).

  Why? – Because of the risk of pneumonia in COPD.

  So avoid high potency steroid (fluticasone = Seretide 500, Relvar or AirFluSal Forspiro) if possible.

Raised serum eosinophils may be an indication for the use of steroid treatment.[3]

Always review the patient for step-up as well as step-down treatment.

The patient should receive an explanation of how to use their inhaler. Following this, prescribe the same brand.

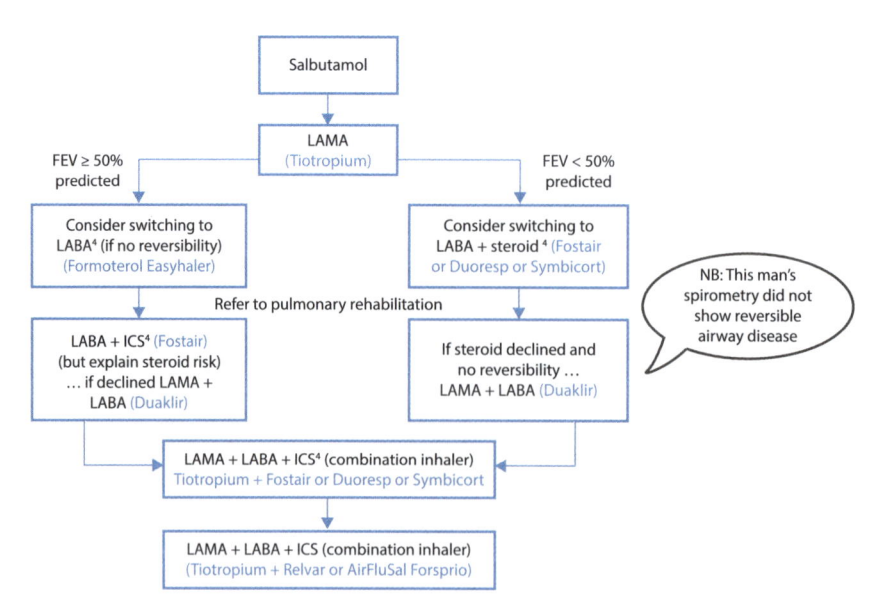

```
                        Salbutamol
                            ↓
                          LAMA
                       (Tiotropium)
       FEV ≥ 50%          ↓            FEV < 50%
       predicted                       predicted
           ↓                               ↓
   Consider switching to          Consider switching to
   LABA[4] (if no reversibility)  LABA + steroid[4] (Fostair
   (Formoterol Easyhaler)         or Duoresp or Symbicort)
                                                           NB: This man's
          Refer to pulmonary rehabilitation                spirometry did not
           ↓                               ↓               show reversible
   LABA + ICS[4] (Fostair)        If steroid declined and  airway disease
   (but explain steroid risk)     no reversibility ...
   ... if declined LAMA +         LAMA + LABA (Duaklir)
   LABA (Duaklir)
                 ↓               ↓
           LAMA + LABA + ICS[4] (combination inhaler)
           Tiotropium + Fostair or Duoresp or Symbicort
                            ↓
           LAMA + LABA + ICS (combination inhaler)
           (Tiotropium + Relvar or AirFluSal Forsprio)
```

If a patient who requires tiotropium is not able to use the device and they also have a cardiovascular history – be aware of the advice in reference[5].

Respiratory Health – 4

Doctor's Notes

Patient	Betty Diggens 68 years F
PMH	Lower respiratory tract infection 1 year ago
	Smokes 20 cigarettes/day
Medications	No current medications
Allergies	No information
Consultations	LRTI 1 year ago.
	Health check 2 months ago – BP 120/60
Investigations	Health check bloods 2 months ago:
	FBC, U&E, LFT, HbA1c, lipid profile – all normal.
Household	Percy Diggens 70 years M

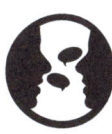

Example Consultation   Cough

Open ☐ — Oh dear, what symptoms have you noticed? Anything else? Tell me about your breathing.

History ☐ — What medical problems have you had in the past? Do you take any medicines? Do you bring up any phlegm with this cough? And how is your breathing? Do you ever make a whistling sound called a wheeze? Have you had any pain in the chest? Sometimes a cough can be from irritation of the gullet; have you had any acid taste or indigestion? When the cough started, did you have a cold?

Impact ☐ — Have you had to stop any activities recently? Does the cough keep you awake?

Flags ☐ — Have you coughed up any blood? How is your appetite? Have you lost any weight? Are you feeling generally tired lately?

Risk ☐ — On my records I see that you smoke approximately 20 cigarettes a day; is that correct?

ICE ☐ — What are your thoughts about this cough? What worries have gone through your mind? Anything else that you've been wondering? What do you feel we should do?

Curious ☐ — You mentioned your chest infection last year. Did you have similar symptoms then?

Sense ☐ — It sounds like you enjoy life but at the moment you are irritated by this cough.

O/E ☐ — I'd like to listen to your lungs, if you could please take off your jumper: I'd also like to feel your pulse, check your breathing rate, oxygen level and temperature. Is that okay? May I look at your hands and fingers and feel for lymph nodes above the collar bone?

Summary ☐ — To summarise, you have waited for a month but the cough remains. Therefore, at this stage you wondered about antibiotics as you fear another chest infection developing as happened last year. This time you feel well and have no phlegm, your breathing is fine, it's just the cough. Is this correct?

Impression ☐ — I'm not sure this sounds like a chest infection. You have no signs of infection; you are not bringing up any phlegm, you have no temperature, your breathing is fine and you feel very well. But I am pleased you have come today as you are right, if a cough persists for a month we need to know what may have caused this. You may have picked up a virus, which can cause an ongoing cough but unfortunately viruses do not respond to antibiotics at all. I want to make sure this is nothing more serious. My feeling is at this stage we should get a chest X-ray. If it does show infection that I can't hear then we can treat this, but the reason for the chest X-ray is to make sure there is no sign of a lung cancer.

Explanation ☐ — At present the only symptom you have is a cough and you have no other worrying symptoms, for example you have not coughed up any blood or lost any weight. However, as smoking increases your risk of a cancer and with a cough that has lasted for longer than a month, I feel we should rule it out.

Experience ☐ — Have you ever known anyone with a lung problem or a lung cancer?

Empathy ☐ — I appreciate this is not what you thought I was going to say; has it come as a shock?

Options ☐ — As you say, there is always a chance antibiotics can help, but from what you've told me, I think that chance is low. We prefer not to use antibiotics when they are unlikely to help because this can prevent the antibiotics working when we need them to. For example, if you were in hospital with pneumonia we would need antibiotics to work for you at that time. Also antibiotics may irritate your bowels. Are you happy to wait and see what the X-ray shows?

Future ☐ — If the X-ray is negative, we could keep a close eye on you but, if you continue to cough for another couple of weeks, I would want to refer you to the lung doctors who may do further investigations. Can you make an appointment to see the doctor again in a few days to discuss what to do, based on the X-ray results? If in the meantime the X-ray is reported as an infection, a doctor will give you a ring.

Safety net ☐ — If in the meantime you start to become breathless, cough up phlegm or blood or have a temperature, please inform the doctor.

Respiratory Health – 5

Patient's Story   Cough

Doctor's notes	Betty Diggens. 68 years. PMH: Lower respiratory tract infection 1 year ago. Medication: None. Smoker 20/day.
How to act	Pleasant.
	You have not considered a lung cancer and act shocked if this is mentioned.
PC	*'Doctor, it's my chest again. I can't quite get rid of this cough.'*
History	You have now had a cough for 3 weeks. No viral symptoms.
	You are not short of breath. You do not wheeze. You have no pain. No fevers.
	You have not got any sputum and no haemoptysis. You are not tired.
	You continue to eat well. You feel well in yourself.
	You have never had chest problems before last year. You have no reflux symptoms.
	Last year you had green sputum and felt dreadful. You feel well this time but don't want that to happen again and would prefer to treat with antibiotics before this happens.
	You don't know anyone who has had a problem with their lungs or cancer.
Social	You live with your husband and are enjoying your retirement from teaching.
	You volunteer in the hospital twice a week.
	You have always smoked approximately 20 cigarettes a day. You drink no alcohol.
	You continue to have great fitness, enjoying hill walking and gardening.
ICE	You believe you need some antibiotics as last time, when you had a chest infection, antibiotics cleared up your cough and you have been well since.
	You have lost no weight.
	You try to push for antibiotics if the doctor says no, *'just in case it helps'*.
Examination	HS normal, chest clear, HR 60 bpm regular. Saturations 96% RR 14 and apyrexial.

Respiratory Health – 5

Learning Points

Cough/Lung Cancer

Lung cancer and mesothelioma[1]

Type of referral	Indication
2WW Lung cancer referral	'Have chest X-ray findings that suggest lung cancer'[1]
	'Are aged 40 and over with **unexplained** haemoptysis.'[1]
2WW Mesothelioma	'Have chest X-ray findings that suggest mesothelioma'[1]
Chest X-ray within 2 weeks	If ≥40 years and at least two of the following unexplained symptoms (or one symptom if patient has ever smoked or had asbestos exposure):

    cough
    SOB
    chest pain
    fatigue
    weight loss
    appetite loss.

Consider if ≥40 years with any of the following:

    persistent or recurrent chest infection
    finger clubbing
    supraclavicular lymphadenopathy or persistent cervical lymphadenopathy
    chest signs **consistent with** lung cancer or pleural disease
    thrombocytosis.

Extra Notes   Spirometry

	Normal	Obstruction	Restrictive
FEV1/FVC (FEV1%) and	>0.7	<0.7	>0.7
FEV1 and	>80% predicted normal	<80%	<80%
FVC	>80% predicted normal	normal/low	<80%

If overweight the spirometry may suggest they have a restrictive airway disease.

If VC > FVC the spirometry may not have taken this into account.

Reliability: 3 consistent readings (within 5% or 150 ml).

Restrictive
E.g. Fibrotic lung disease: Extrinsic allergic alveolitis (farmer's lung), sarcoidosis, silicosis, pneumoconiosis and cryptogenic fibrosing alveolitis.

Obstructive
Obstruction which is non reversible confirms COPD. The severity of COPD is determined by the FEV1 result.

Mild = FEV1 50–80%. Moderate = FEV1 30–49%. Severe = FEV1 <30%

Reversibility testing
Reversibility testing can be performed before and 20 minutes after 2–4 puffs salbutamol.

Or before and after a steroid trial (prednisolone 30 mg) for 14 days.

Always interpret the results of reversibility testing with the clinical history.

See *Reversibility in the Learning Points of Asthma Diagnosis.

	COPD	Asthma
Smoker or ex-smoker	Nearly all	Possibly
Symptoms under age 35 years	Rare	Often
Chronic productive cough	Common	Uncommon
Breathlessness	Persistent and progressive	Variable
Night time waking sob/wheeze	Uncommon	Common
Variability	Uncommon	Common

See the Link Hub at CompleteCSA.co.uk for useful links to
Flow Volume and Time Volume Curves
A guide to how to use and interpret spirometry in the GP practice
A flow chart – interpreting spirometry

Respiratory Health

CHAPTER 22 OVERVIEW
Musculoskeletal Problems

	Cases in this chapter	Within the RCGP curriculum: Care of People with Musculoskeletal Problems RCGP Curriculum Online March 2016[1]	Learning points in the chapter include:
1	Low Back Pain	'Identify "red flags"' 'Be aware of the concept of "yellow flags"'	Causes Flags Guidelines Imaging – MRI
2	Knee Pain	'Refer those conditions which may benefit from early referral to an orthopaedic surgeon'	ACL injuries Investigating knee pain NICE Guidance. CG 177 Osteoarthritis: care and management. Feb 2014
3	Osteoporosis	'Identify those patients at risk of bone disorders, such as osteoporosis, and understand the principles of primary and secondary prevention of fragility fractures'	NICE Guidance. CG146. Osteoporosis: assessing the risk of fragility fracture. Aug 2012
4	Plantar Fasciitis	'Use simple techniques and consistent advice to promote activity in the presence of pain'	Gout Differential diagnosis of foot pain.
5	Shoulder Pain	'Diagnose common, regional soft-tissue problems that can be managed in primary care'	Anatomy Rotator cuff tendonitis Adhesive capsulitis Osteoarthritis Referred pain to the shoulder

1. http://www.rcgp.org.uk/training-exams/gp-curriculum-overview/online-curriculum/applying-clinical-knowledge-section-2/3-20-musculoskeletal-problems.aspx

CHAPTER 22 REFERENCES

Low Back Pain
1. Chronic low back pain. *BMJ*. 2003; 326 http://dx.doi.org/10.1136/bmj.326.7388.535. 8 Mar 2003.
2. http://patient.info/doctor/low-back-pain-and-sciatica
3. Collison K., Russ R. Oxfordshire CCG. MRI Referral Guidelines for cervical, thoracic and lumbar spine for adults. June 2014.

Knee Pain
1. NICE Guidelines. CG177. Osteoarthritis: care and management. Feb 2014.
2. Kobayashi H., Kanamura T., et al. Mechanisms of the anterior cruciate ligament injury in sports activities: a twenty-year clinical research of 1,700 athletes. *J Sports Sci Med*. 2010 Dec; 9(4): 669–75.

Osteoporosis
1. NICE Guidelines. CG146. Osteoporosis: assessing the risk of fragility fracture. Aug 2012.
2. http://www.shef.ac.uk/FRAX/tool.aspx?country=1
3. http://www.qfracture.org/
4. http://www.shef.ac.uk/NOGG/
5. Michaëlsson K., Melhus H., Warensjö E., Lemming E. Long term calcium intake and rates of all cause and cardiovascular mortality: community based prospective longitudinal cohort study. *BMJ*. 2013; 346: f228. http://www.bmj.com/content/346/bmj.f228
6. NICE. http://cks.nice.org.uk/osteoporosis-prevention-of-fragility-fractures#!scenario:1. Mar 2016.
7. http://cks.nice.org.uk/osteoporosis-prevention-of-fragility-fractures#!prescribinginfosub:9. Mar 2016.
8. NICE Guidelines. TA 160. Alendronate, etidronate, risedronate, raloxifene and strontium ranelate for the primary prevention of osteoporotic fragility fractures in postmenopausal women. Oct 2008. Updated Jan 2011.
9. http://patient.info/medicine/alendronic-acid-for-osteoporosis-fosamax
10. http://www.cgem.ed.ac.uk/research/rheumatological/calcium-calculator

Plantar Fasciitis/Differential Diagnosis – Foot Pain
1. Cooper A., Blythe J., Wise E. BMJ Masterclass for GPs. Musculoskeletal Medicine. Course Materials Apr 2013.
2. http://www.mdcalc.com/ottawa-ankle-rule/
3. NICE. http://cks.nice.org.uk/gout#!scenario. Apr 2015.

Shoulder Pain
1. http://www.physio-pedia.com/Supraspinatus_tendonitis
2. http://patient.info/leaflets/painful_arc_syndrome.htm
3. http://patient.info/health/frozen-shoulder-leaflet

Doctor's Notes

Patient	Rachel West	43 years	F
PMH	Irritable bowel syndrome		
Medications	No current medications		
Allergies	No information		
Consultations	No recent consultations		
Investigations	No recent investigations		
Household	Arthur West	45 years	M
	Jennifer West	6 years	F
	Timothy West	4 years	M

Example Consultation — Low Back Pain

Open □ — Rachel, it is a pleasure to meet you and I'm sorry you are in this much pain. What has happened? Tell me more about the pain. Are you having any other symptoms?

History □ — Back pain can sometimes be due to kidney problems: any problems passing urine? Is your tummy okay? When was your last period? Tell me more about you. Do you have family? Are you otherwise well? Is everything okay at home?

Flags □ — I just need to ask a few questions to check that both the spine and you are healthy. Any weight loss? Any fever? Does the pain wake you at night? Have you ever injured your back? Any weakness or numbness in your legs? Any problems controlling your bladder or bowels? Any numbness around your bottom?

Curious □ — What do you think is keeping you awake all night – the pain or something else?

Sense □ — I see how much pain you are in. You said this is the 'last straw'. What do you mean?

Risk □ — Work sounds tough. Have you been feeling low even before this happened?

ICE □ — What do you think has caused this? What did you feel we should do today? Is there anything that you are especially worried about? What pain relief have you tried?

Empathy □ — I appreciate this amount of back pain is going to be very difficult, especially with your work and small children. We can do a work-note but your back needs to keep moving or you will stiffen up.

Impact □ — Tell me which important areas of your life are affected by the back pain.

O/E □ — May I examine your back with you standing and then check your legs on the couch?

Summary □ — So, to summarise, your back suddenly became worse after you bent forward yesterday and you have been in agony since. You have been finding work life difficult, with your boss, and feel this is the last straw; you need time away from work. You fear it will impact on picking up and playing with your children. You believe this is a slipped disc and you need a scan. Have I understood you correctly?

Impression □ — It sounds like you have sciatica.

Experience □ — Have you known anyone with this problem? What do you know about it?

Explanation □ — In sciatica, the sciatic nerve becomes irritated or squashed which causes pain all the way down your leg. As there are no worrying features – you have not lost weight or had an injury – I do not believe there is anything nasty happening in your spine so a scan would not help. This is probably due to a 'prolapsed disc'. In this situation, the whole disc doesn't usually move, it's just the soft jelly centre.

Future □ — Back exercises can help this problem and are important but improvement can take weeks. We need to manage your pain. You can self-certify for a week whilst the pain is severe but let's meet again in a week to see how you are. If the pain is not controlled, let us know.

Options □ — Naproxen, taken every 12 hours, decreases any swelling and codeine, every 6 hours, is a good painkiller. Side effects can include nausea, constipation or drowsiness. If this isn't helping and your back continues to feel in spasm, there is a tablet called diazepam. I can give you a 3-day supply of this which you can take three times a day but, together with the codeine, you may feel drowsy or nauseated so don't drive or use machines. It is not a drug we can continue to use due to its risks. What would you like me to prescribe? I would expect that over the next few days the intensity of the problem should decrease. If you are not getting back to normal after 4–6 weeks of exercises, please see a doctor, or sooner, if you have worsening symptoms. I will also refer you to physiotherapy.

Empower □ — This PIL has some exercises, e.g. lying on the floor, knees up and swing them side to side. Avoid lifting the children in the meantime.

Safety net □ — If your legs feel different, you need to inform the doctor. Also – I don't expect this to happen – but I tell everyone that, if you lose control of going to the toilet or develop weakness in your legs, you must let a doctor know immediately.

Musculoskeletal Problems – 1

Patient's Story

Low Back Pain

Doctor's notes — Rachel West, 43 years. PMH: IBS. Medications: None.

How to act — You are in a lot of pain.

PC — *'It's my back. I'm in agony.'*

History — You have often had lower back pain in your life.

It has increased over the past few months.

Then last night *'I was picking up toys and I felt my back go.'*

'This is the last straw!' If asked, you mean regarding your work – you need time off.

The pain goes down your left leg. It doesn't wake you but *'I am awake all night'*.

You have not had any numbness or weakness. Full control of bladder and bowels.

There are no abdominal, urinary or gynaecological symptoms. LMP 1 week ago.

You have IBS but are otherwise well. No weight loss or fever. No injury.

You have no other symptoms systemically. Paracetamol hasn't helped the pain.

You have been feeling low but no features of depression.

You haven't known anyone with this back pain. You don't know what sciatica means.

Social — You work in IT. Your work has been very difficult. Your marriage is good.

You have two children. Your husband is a director of a building supplier company and busy.

There are problems with your manager and you do not get on.

You hope you can find alternative work.

Work has been very stressful. You think about it through the night.

ICE — You feel you need a scan. You think you have *'slipped a disc'*.

You expect the doctor will tell you to rest and take time off work.

You fear it may take months to heal. You would like some strong pain relief.

You worry about playing with the children with this pain.

Your mother is coming to help.

Examination — No spinal tenderness, tender L para-spinal muscles. Slightly reduced ROM.

Reduced straight leg raise left leg – 50 degrees.

Normal neurological examination.

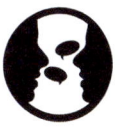

Musculoskeletal Problems – 1

Learning Points   Low Back Pain

Causes   Mechanical low back pain, malignancy – primary or secondary, infection (e.g. spinal TB), ankylosing spondylitis, pyelonephritis or kidney stone or referred pain, e.g. AAA.

Flags[1,2]
Red flags (* refers to criteria within Oxford guidance – see below)
- Unexplained weight loss*
- Previous or suspected malignancy*
- Drug abuse, HIV, immunosuppression or corticosteroid use
- Abnormal bloods (ESR >50[4])* or fever
- Thoracic or night pain
- Trauma*
- <20 or >55 years (worsening/new onset)
- Disturbed gait or progressive neurological deficit
- Comorbidity or unwell patient
- Abnormal function/control of bladder or bowel or saddle anaesthesia
- Known osteoporosis and suspected crush fracture[3]*
- Severe morning stiffness
- Consider cauda equina syndrome if on examination there is gait disturbance, urinary retention, abnormal perianal sensation or anal tone with lower limb weakness

Yellow flags: (psychosocial factors)
- 'A negative attitude that back pain is harmful or potentially severely disabling'[1]
- 'Fear, avoidance behaviour and reduced activity levels'[1]
- 'An expectation that passive, rather than active, treatment will be beneficial'[1]
- History of depression, low mood and social withdrawal[1]
- 'Social or financial problems'[1]

<20 years   Consider HLAB27 testing for AS if morning stiffness and pain awakens the patient.

>55 years   Consider an ESR, electrophoresis (myeloma screen), urine dipstick, palpating for AAA, PSA in men and CA 125 in women.

So should all >55 years with new onset back pain have an urgent MRI if they have no other red flags and bloods are normal? This is where 'clinical judgement' comes in and follow your local guidance.

Oxford CCG guidance[3]

Cauda equina Widespread neurological deficit or infection	Refer as an emergency to the spinal team.
Red flag symptoms* (no mention of age)	Direct referral for urgent limited MRI.
Suspected osteoporotic crush fracture only	Lateral X-ray then routine MRI.
No red flags and persistent pain >6 weeks	Review diagnosis, conservative Rx and refer to the MSK assessment team.
Progressive deformity (kyphosis) Intractable pain Deteriorating neurology	Review diagnosis and refer to spinal team if patient will consider surgery and is a surgical candidate

Occasionally an MRI will report that it cannot exclude malignancy in which case consider a bone scan.

For simple back pain offer analgesia and exercises. Give a realistic prognosis.

Musculoskeletal Problems – 1

Doctor's Notes

Patient	Robert Hayes 27 years M
PMH	No known medical history
Medications	No current medications
Allergies	No information
Consultations	No recent consultations
Investigations	No recent investigations
Household	No household members registered

Example Consultation — Knee Pain

Open ☐ — What happened? Talk me through the injury in slow motion if you can please. Then what did you notice?

Flags ☐ — Did the knee swell straight away? Could you walk on it? Does the knee lock into a certain position stopping you from straightening or bending it? Has it given way?

Risk ☐ — Have you injured your knee before? Any other injury?

History ☐ — Are you otherwise well? Tell me more about you. Do you work? What sports do you enjoy?

ICE ☐ — What do you think may have happened inside the knee? Has anything else gone through your mind? Anything else you fear about this injury? Is there anything you thought I might say we should arrange? Is there anything else you were hoping we could do? Are there any other thoughts you had about what may be helpful?

Impact ☐ — And the past couple of days, has it stopped you from doing anything? How would a knee injury impact on your work, hobbies or home life?

Curious ☐ — Is there a reason why you would prefer to avoid the orthopaedic doctors?

O/E ☐ — I would like to examine your knee. That would involve taking off your trousers, having a look at the knee, then doing some movements to work out what may have caused the swelling. If you feel any pain during the examination, it would be helpful if you could tell me where exactly. Is that okay?

Summary ☐ — So Robert, you were playing football 2 days ago when your foot seemed to stick in the mud causing your knee to twist. Since then the left knee has been swollen and painful to walk on. You believe you may have torn a ligament and fear needing an operation after your experience with your right ankle. You are hoping that I will organise an MRI scan to guide physiotherapy but would like to get better quickly because you don't want to be sat out for the rest of the season. Is that correct?

Impression ☐ — I think you may be right. The examination shows it is likely that you have torn a ligament, called the anterior cruciate ligament. This can be very painful, as you have described.

Sense ☐ — I can see you are very disappointed about this injury.

Experience ☐ — Have you heard of this injury?

Explanation ☐ — This ligament in the knee prevents your knee from overstretching, but unfortunately if you have had an injury which causes the leg to overstretch, it can tear.

Empathy ☐ — It sounds like you have been lonely since the end of your relationship so I appreciate that not being able to play football with friends is a huge disappointment.

Options ☐ — I think to get an answer and to get you on the mend as soon as possible we should refer you to the trauma clinic today. I will give the trauma registrar a call.

Future ☐ — You mentioned you were keen for physio; I think that sounds a good idea but wonder if we should get the orthopaedic opinion first. If surgery is needed, keyhole surgery may be an option. I can also prescribe some codeine for you for additional pain relief if you need it. Does this sound okay?

Empower ☐ — In the meantime, please keep it elevated with some ice on it to reduce the swelling. Whilst waiting to see the trauma team, I'd recommend paracetamol and an anti-inflammatory like ibuprofen but can prescribe something a little stronger if you need it.

Patient's Story

Knee Pain

Doctor's notes	Robert Hayes, 27 years. PMH: None. Medications: None.
How to act	Pleasant but concerned.
PC	*'I've injured my knee playing football.'*
History	Two days ago you were playing football. You felt something pop as you were changing direction – your studs seemed to stick in the mud. There was no contact with another player at the time. It was extremely painful and you could not continue the game.
	You applied ice to your swollen knee and the swelling is still present. The knee doesn't lock but has given way. You have had no previous knee injury.
	You have not been able to drive since the injury despite taking paracetamol and ibuprofen. You also find it painful walking and weight-bearing.
Social	You work as a project manager.
	You enjoy running, badminton and football. You live with a flatmate.
	If the doctor asks you about what impact this may have, you have recently broken up with your long-term girlfriend and it wasn't until the football season started that you began to spend more time with your friends.
ICE	You believe you may have torn a ligament.
	You are worried that you will be *'out for the season'*.
	You also fear you may need an operation. You fractured your ankle falling out of a tree as a child and remember a lot of pain after the operation. You would rather see a physio than be referred to orthopaedics for this reason; however, you will follow the doctor's advice. You would like an MRI of your knee – if asked why, you think this would help a physiotherapist.
	If the doctor asks you about your understanding of the diagnosis, you remember that Michael Owen couldn't play in the 2006 World Cup due to a cruciate ligament injury. The doctor is giving you terrible news as you fear you will now be isolated from your friends this season.
Examination	The left knee is swollen with an effusion. The knee is not hot or red.
	There is tenderness along the medial side.
	The anterior drawer test is positive. The rest of the examination is normal.

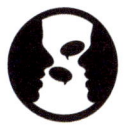

Learning Points   Knee Pain

Osteoarthritis

Diagnosis
'Diagnose osteoarthritis clinically without investigations if a person:
- is 45 or over and
- has activity-related joint pain and
- has either no morning joint-related stiffness or morning stiffness that lasts no longer than 30 minutes. [new 2014]'[1]

Atypical features include 'history of trauma, prolonged morning joint-related stiffness, rapid worsening of symptoms or the presence of a hot swollen joint'.[1]

Differential diagnosis includes gout, septic arthritis, inflammatory arthritis, malignancy[1] and injury from trauma.

NICE advises a holistic assessment of a person with OA: social situation and impact, health beliefs, mood, quality of sleep, support network, other MSK pain, attitudes to exercise, influence of comorbidity and a full pain assessment. See guidance for more detail in a helpful diagram.[1]

GP management options include: NSAIDs, muscle strengthening exercises, advice about aerobic fitness and footwear, physiotherapy, steroids injection. Consider the additional need for TENS or aids.

When to consider surgery[1]
- Mechanical locking or loose bodies on X-ray for arthroscopic lavage and debridement.
- After at least three core (non-surgical) treatment options.
- Symptoms causing a significant impact on life or ongoing functional limitation.

ACL injury

Mechanism	Most commonly associated with a non-contact mechanism – 'knee in and toe out'[2]
	The risk is greater in females.[2]
Injury triad	Anterior cruciate ligament + medial collateral ligament + medial meniscus.

Acute injuries
Refer acute injuries to orthopaedics for assessment, imaging and management options. NB: Immediate effusions following trauma/injury are often due to haemarthrosis which is associated with more significant joint injuries. Have a low threshold for referral of such cases (possibly same day or urgently to trauma/fracture clinic). If presenting as a chronic injury, you may be able to refer for direct access MRI to guide diagnosis and management – check local protocols.

Doctor's Notes

Patient   Shirley Warner   72 years   F
PMH   Wrist fracture
Medications Codeine phosphate 30 mg
Allergies   No information
Consultations 2 months ago: telephone consultation – codeine prescribed following wrist fracture
Investigations DEXA   Score –2.7
                  Corrected calcium   2.36 mmol/L
                  Vitamin D   40 ng/mL
Household   Tina Wright   76 years   F

Example Consultation — Osteoporosis

Open ☐	Thank you for returning. What led to you having this test?
Impact ☐	How is the arm? How has the broken arm affected you day to day?
Flags ☐	How did you fall? I see: when a break occurs after a low-impact injury, we must check the bones.
History ☐	Before I explain, may I learn more about you to help me interpret the result and what we may need to do? Are you well? Any medical problems? Any medicines? How do you spend your time? Who is at home? Any family history of medical problems?
ICE ☐	Have you had thoughts yourself about what the scan may show? Do you have any fears about what I may say today? And what did you think I might suggest today?
Risk ☐	A few questions, now, about factors that may affect the bones. What age was your menopause? Have you ever taken any steroid treatment? Do you smoke? How much alcohol do you drink? Have you had any other broken bones?
Curious ☐	When you fell, had you been drinking any alcohol?
Sense ☐	You've mentioned your mum a few times. Her experience is important to you; what happened?
Empathy ☐	I understand your fear of another fracture especially after your mother's experience.
O/E ☐	May I just check your weight and height?
Summary ☐	To summarise, a low-impact fall caused a fracture which led to the scan. You suspect this is due to low calcium which will need replacing and fear another fall, having watched your mother suffer. Is this right?
Impression ☐	The scan has confirmed that you have osteoporosis.
Experience ☐	Do you know anything about osteoporosis?
Explanation ☐	Osteoporosis means the bones are not as strong as they should be. Sometimes calcium tablets are taken but actually your calcium levels are already good. Osteoporosis is a lack of bone strength but not necessarily a lack of the nutrients such as calcium. Many things lead to osteoporosis. In your case, I suspect it is a mixture of things such as being a postmenopausal woman, an ex-smoker, drinking more than 14 units of alcohol a week and having a family history of osteoporosis.
Options ☐	Thankfully there is treatment available which should reduce your risk of more broken bones in the future. Alendronate is a tablet that prevents bone breakdown. It is taken once weekly. Like all tablets there are potential side effects – for this tablet that includes diarrhoea or headaches. There are also risks: it can damage the jaw bone. Although this is rare, we recommend seeing your dentist prior to starting treatment. To prevent acid reflux we advise taking the tablet 30 minutes before your breakfast and any medication, with a full glass of water and remain upright (either sitting or standing) for 30 minutes. I will give you an information sheet which explains again how to take the tablet. Are you happy to start this medication?
Empower ☐	We also need to consider your calcium and vitamin D. Your calcium blood test was normal but your vitamin D was a bit low. To decide if you need extra calcium, we need to assess your dietary intake of calcium. If it is low, we will give you a tablet with both calcium and vitamin D. If it is adequate you will only need vitamin D. This is because recent research suggests that too much calcium can be harmful. Could I give you a questionnaire to fill out about your diet? There are other things you can do to protect your bones such as reducing your alcohol intake and doing weight-bearing exercises. I will send you a sheet of these exercises.
Future ☐	Can we meet again in a couple of weeks to go through your questionnaire? I suggest every 5–10 years you give your body a rest from the alendronate for 3 years. We will need to repeat your scan in 2–3 years' time.
Safety net ☐	With alendronate if you notice black stools, reflux or heart burn, jaw pain or a loose tooth, inform a GP.

Musculoskeletal Problems – 3

Patient's Story

Osteoporosis

Doctor's notes	Shirley Warner, 72 years.
	DEXA Score −2.7. Corrected calcium 2.36 mmol/L. Vitamin D 40 ng/mL (low).
	PMH: Wrist fracture 2 months ago. Medications: Codeine phosphate 30 mg.
How to act	Friendly.
PC	*'Doctor, I've come for my scan result.'*
History	You were referred for a DEXA scan by the hospital doctor.
	2 months ago you fractured your wrist when you tripped on a kerb.
	Your mother broke her hip when she was in her 80s.
	'Mum was low in calcium and took calcium tablets.'
	You have no other medical history. You have taken no other medicines.
	The arm is improving.
	Your menopause was aged 52 years.
Social	You are a retired seamstress. You live with your partner, Tina.
	You drink 16 units of alcohol a week.
	You *'tripped after the golf party'* (3 glasses of wine).
	You are an ex-smoker.
	You enjoy yoghurt, full fat milk and eat very well.
	You are happy to keep a food diary to calculate your calcium intake.
ICE	You understand that you have weak bones lacking in calcium.
	You are worried you will get a hip fracture like your mother.
	Your mum was in hospital a long time and then had to start warfarin for a DVT.
	You expect the doctor will start calcium tablets.
Examination	Your BMI is 24.

Musculoskeletal Problems – 3

Learning Points   NICE Guidance.[1] Osteoporosis

+ Risk factors:	♀, BMI <18.5, smoking, alcohol (units >14/week ♀ or >21/week ♂). Previous fracture or history of falls, immobility, FH osteoporosis or hip #. Medical comorbidity
++ Risk factors:	Corticosteroids, premature menopause, previous osteoporotic fracture.
+++ Risk factors:	>7.5 mg prednisolone daily for >3 months (current or recent). Previous major osteoporotic fracture. Multiple fragility fractures.
Who do we screen:	♀ >65 years or <65 years with any risk factor. ♂ >75 years or <75 years with any risk factor. Anyone <50 years with a ++ or +++ risk factor OR <40 years with a +++ risk factor.
How do we screen?	1. History – is the patient at risk? 2. Calculate the FRAX score[2] if aged 40–90 years or Q fracture[3] if aged 30–84 years 3. Once the data is inserted into the tool, use the link to NOGG[3] to guide management – lifestyle advice (low risk) – DEXA scan (intermediate risk) → recalculate risk with BMD – start treatment (high risk).

'Above the upper age limits defined by the tools, consider people to be at high risk.'[1]

>80 years 'predicted 10-year fracture risk may underestimate their short-term fracture risk.'[1]

Assessment tools underestimate risk in: multiple #'s or vertebral #, alcohol abuse, steroid Rx or comorbidities[1]

T score   T score between –1 and –2.5 = osteopenia.

T score <–2.5 = osteoporosis.

For reversible causes consider testing: TSH, PTH, Ca^{2+}, vitamin D, testosterone, LH and FSH to investigate for hyperthyroidism, hyperparathyroidism, osteomalacia and hypogonadism respectively.

Who should have calcium and vitamin D replacement?

Due to new studies[5] demonstrating the risks of calcium treatment, consider vitamin D replacement alone if dietary calcium intake is >700 mg/day.[6] 'If calcium intake is inadequate: Prescribe 10 micrograms (400 international units) of vitamin D with at least 1000 mg of calcium daily. Prescribe 20 micrograms (800 international units) of vitamin D with at least 1000 mg of calcium daily for elderly people who are housebound or living in a nursing home.'[6]

Who should have bisphosphonates?

NOGG guidance has indicated Rx is required or following a confirmed osteoporosis diagnosis.

'Only alendronate (OD tablets) and risedronate (once-weekly tablets) are licensed for use in men.'[6]

The following is recommended reading: counselling prior to bisphosphonate use – see reference.[7]

Also for information regarding Rx in postmenopausal women – see reference.[8]

Patient.co.uk has a useful patient leaflet on how to take alendronic acid.[9]

Management of osteopenia

Lifestyle: smoking, exercise and weight-bearing exercises.

Test bone profile, albumin, U&E, LFT, FBC, ESR and TSH. Rescan 2–3 years.

There are several calcium calculators available online. It is a good idea to save one to your desktop at work to allow calcium intake calculation in consultations. An example is given in the references[10].

Musculoskeletal Problems – 3

Doctor's Notes

Patient	Selina Richards	31 years	F
PMH	No known medical history		
Medications	No current medications		
Allergies	No information		
Consultations	No recent consultations		
Investigations	No recent investigations		
Household	Craig Richards	38 years	M
	Alexander Richards	8 years	M
	Maria Richards	6 years	F
	Amelia Richards	5 years	F

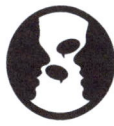

Example Consultation — Plantar Fasciitis

Open ☐	Please tell me the story of the pain from when you first noticed it. Anything else you have noticed? When does the pain come and go?
Flags ☐	Have you noticed any swelling? Can you move the ankle and foot normally?
Risk ☐	Have you ever had any injury in the past?
History ☐	Any medical problems? Have you tried any pain relief yet? I'm interested to know more about you …
ICE ☐	Have you had any thoughts as to what may be causing it? What worries have gone through your mind? Is there anything else you hoped we would arrange today?
Impact ☐	And since this problem started, what has the pain stopped you from doing?
Sense ☐	So this has come at a very difficult time for you?
Curious ☐	What did your friend suggest?
O/E ☐	I would like to examine your foot and ankle; if I may please ask you to remove your socks and shoes?
Summary ☐	To summarise, you have told me that the pain in the right foot has been building over a month but, especially in this past week, it has stopped you from walking the dog, something that you enjoy, but have also had to do more since you have separated from your husband. You wondered if it was gout.
Impression ☐	I think what is causing your pain is a plantar fasciitis. Have you come across this before?
Explanation ☐	The plantar fascia is a sheet of tissue which supports the bones of your foot. Sometimes it can become painful and inflamed. It may be triggered by an increase in physical activity. There is no sign of a broken bone. I don't think you have gout as your foot is not red, hot or swollen and the site you point to is typical of plantar fasciitis. X-rays do not show this inflammation so are unlikely to be helpful.
Empathy ☐	This is an additional stress, especially as the dog is whining and you have three children to care for. I also hear that you are very fond of the dog. I appreciate why you feel you need to fix this problem straight away. The problem can unfortunately take many months to settle completely. However, for this common condition I have some suggestions.
Empower ☐	The ibuprofen could be changed for a tablet which is slightly stronger and lasts 12 hours, called naproxen. You take one tablet twice a day but, like ibuprofen, it can irritate your stomach lining so stop it if this becomes a problem. There is a useful exercise for PF too. The exercise aims to stretch the tissue to help the repairing process. It uses a frozen litre drinks bottle. Put the bottle under the arch of your foot and roll the bottle forwards and backwards. The movement helps stretch the tissue and the ice helps reduce pain and swelling. The more you do, the sooner it will improve but, like any exercise, time is needed. Padded footwear can also help.
Options ☐	There is a PIL which explains this. It also mentions steroid injections into the feet, which is an option but some do not find it effective and there are risks to injecting in the foot, such as infection or injury to the tendons there. We therefore don't recommend the injections as first line. What are your thoughts about what I have said?
Future ☐	How do you feel about trying this option for the next 6 weeks? If you have seen no improvement after a month, come back and we can think about either physiotherapy or the injections.
Safety net ☐	I don't expect this to happen but, if you do notice any swelling or heat in the foot, please see the GP earlier.

Patient's Story

Plantar Fasciitis

Doctor's notes Selina Richards, 31 years. PMH: None. Medications: None.

How to act Slightly pushy for the doctor to fix this problem.

PC *'It's a pain in my foot – it's a nightmare.'*

Point to the tendon insertion at the calcaneus.

History You walk your dog every morning and recently have pain in the right foot whilst walking. You have had no injury or swelling.

You started to notice this a month ago and over the past week you have had enough of this discomfort. You have always been well. Ibuprofen only helps slightly. You drink minimal alcohol and don't smoke.

Social You do not work. You have three children and a dog.

Your children are all in primary school.

Your husband has just left the marriage and he used to walk the dog in a morning.

You spend your days meeting your friends, doing housework, dog-sitting and food shopping for your mother. Financially you have always been very lucky and have never worked since you were married. You would like to have a job but don't know how or where. You are going to volunteer at the school with cooking classes.

ICE Your friend told you that the problem may be gout as she had the same thing and you have not had an injury. Therefore, you expect the doctor will give you colchicine, the tablet your friend was given. You would also like a blood test and an X-ray.

You plan to pay for a dog walker, but will miss the time out of the house with the dog.

Impact The dog has been whining as you couldn't walk him and you need to get this sorted straight away. Apart from walking the dog, the pain has not stopped you from doing anything else. You are coping well without your husband; he was always away on business anyway. The divorce proceedings, however, are stressful. You also want to keep the dog and fear your husband will want him if he is not being walked.

You have never come across plantar fasciitis.

Examination No swelling or abnormality of the foot, ankle or Achilles tendon.

Tender at the plantar surface of the calcaneus.

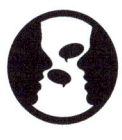

Musculoskeletal Problems – 4

Learning Points   Differential Diagnosis – Foot Pain

Soft tissue	Chronic heel pad inflammation	'Warm dull throbbing pain over weight-bearing area of the heel ... worse when first getting up'[1]
	Acute synovitis	Throbbing pain made worse by movement.[1]
		Rule out systemic causes.
	Acute inflammation of anterior metatarsal heads	
		Common in women wearing slip-on/heeled shoe.
		Burning and throbbing on walking.[1]
	Plantar metatarsal bursitis	'Throbbing pain under the metatarsal head ... persists at rest and exacerbated when the area if first loaded.'[1]
Bone	Fracture	Has there been impact? Use the Ottawa rules.[2]
	Stress fracture (March fracture)	Palpable tender lump.
	Osteoarthritis	Common at 1st MTPJ, tarsus joints and midfoot.[1]
	Rheumatoid arthritis	Swelling and deformity, may describe walking on pebbles due to swelling/subluxation.[1]
	Sever's disease	E.g. boys 8–13 years and exacerbated by jumping.[1]
	Hallux valgus	Great toe moves towards/overlies the 2nd toe.[1]
	Bunion	Inflamed and painful metatarsal head.[1]
Red hot	Gout	
	Septic arthritis	Requires urgent aspiration/culture/Rx
Nerve	Morton's neuroma	Burning and numbness ... often the 3rd/4th toe.[1]
	Peripheral neuropathy	E.g. tarsal tunnel or 2° to ↓B12, alcohol or DM.
Arterial	Ischaemia	Absent pulses, signs of PVD and check ABPIs

Gout

Risk factors Thiazides, ACEI, alcohol, obesity.

Do not start allopurinol during an acute attack.

'Do not stop allopurinol or febuxostat during an acute attack'[3] if treatment is already established.

Acute medication[3] 1st line NSAID (diclofenac, indometacin or naproxen)

2nd line colchicine

3rd line if NSAIDs contraindicated – consider systemic corticosteroids

When initiating allopurinol, consider a course of NSAID or colchicine. If in 2/12 you need to ↑ the allopurinol give another overlap of colchicine to prevent an acute attack as the urate levels ↓ again.

Uric acid levels Measure 4–6 weeks after an acute attack.

Aim for normal levels of uric acid if the decision has been made to start allopurinol.

Self-management[3] Rest, avoid trauma, keep the joint cool. Lifestyle: reduce alcohol, weight loss and dietary changes and avoid dehydration.

Doctor's Notes

Patient   David Meadows   47 years   M
PMH   Cruciate ligament injury
Medications   No current medications
Allergies   No information
Consultations   No recent consultations
Investigations   No recent investigations
Household   No household members registered

Example Consultation   Shoulder Pain

Open ☐	Mr Meadows, how can I help? Shall we start from when you first noticed the problem?
Flags ☐	Have you had an injury? Any pain elsewhere –chest, neck or arm? What are you doing when the pain comes on? Which movements specifically? Does other activity cause pain? Does it wake you?
Risk ☐	Have you ever damaged the shoulder?
History ☐	I see you have injured your knee. Any other medical problems? And tell me more about you.
ICE ☐	What do you think has caused this? Is there anything else you have been wondering? Is there anything else you are worried about? What did you think I might say we should do today? Is there anything specific you would like to be done today?
Curious ☐	Has someone you know had a shoulder pain that was from their heart?
Impact ☐	Are you having to do anything differently? Is it stopping you do anything else?
Sense ☐	You seem very disappointed about having to stop golf.
O/E ☐	Please can you remove your top so that I may feel your shoulder, neck and arm and check their movements?
Summary ☐	So, 2 weeks of shoulder pain is now affecting you daily. You wonder whether this may be caused by golf or from arthritis. You wanted to clarify that this is not coming from your heart. You fear it will prevent you from playing in the golf competition. You wondered whether imaging would be helpful.
Impression ☐	I believe you have painful arc syndrome. This pain is not coming from your heart. I can reassure you of this because it is painful moving the shoulder joint but not when exercising.
Experience ☐	Other names for it are tendonitis or impingement. Have you come across painful arc?
Explanation ☐	The problem lies within the shoulder at the tendons. Tendons attach the shoulder muscles to the arm. There is a narrow tunnel in the shoulder for these tendons to pass through. Repeated use or an injury can cause swelling of the tendon or wear and tear of the bones that form the tunnel. Both make the narrow tunnel smaller. Lifting the arm makes this space smaller again. This causes friction and is why you get pain with that movement.
Empathy ☐	I appreciate the need to fix the shoulder quickly. I will try but I fear 6 weeks is optimistic.
Options ☐	Firstly, we need to reduce the inflammation with anti-inflammatory tablets. If this doesn't help a steroid injection may be beneficial. Secondly, you need to rest your shoulder from heavy exercise but perform some physio exercises. I will demonstrate a good exercise. Hold a weight, like a can of beans, in the right hand directly below the shoulder, leaning to that side and then make circle movements. This helps to increase that gap. I suggest a 2-week trial of exercises and anti-inflammatories.
Future ☐	If it is not on the mend, consider the steroid injection guided by an USS and physiotherapy. What are your thoughts? I will send you a PIL with this and other exercises. Any questions?
Empower ☐	With the exercises, the more you do, the sooner you will notice a difference.
Safety net ☐	I will prescribe some naproxen, an anti-inflammatory which is stronger than ibuprofen and lasts longer, so is taken every 12 hours with food. Like any tablet it has its risks including tummy ulcers so let me know if it is causing tummy pain. Inform me if you develop shoulder swelling.

Musculoskeletal Problems – 5

Patient's Story

Shoulder Pain

Doctor's notes	David Meadows, 47 years. PMH: Cruciate ligament injury. Medications: None.
How to act	Relaxed and pleasant.
PC	*'I've done something to my shoulder doctor.'*
History	Right shoulder pain (no radiation) began slowly 2 weeks ago. No specific injury.
	It is painful inside the shoulder especially when raising the arm: 5/10 severity of pain.
	You have still managed to cycle on your cycling machine to keep fit without discomfort.
	No neurological symptoms in the arm and no problem at the neck or elbow.
	You once injured your knee playing football.
	You have otherwise been well.
	You are very active and never have any chest pains.
	There are no contraindications to starting an NSAID.
Impact	It has stopped you from playing golf. You are right-handed. You fear having to pull out of a competition in 6 weeks which you have been looking forward to.
	It is not painful at night.
	You are struggling to wash your hair so you are leaning forward and using your left hand.
Social	Work for local council – the practice is near your office.
	Wife and 2 children at home. Occasional alcohol. Never smoked.
ICE	You wonder if this could be arthritis or maybe you have injured it playing golf.
	At the back of your mind you hope it isn't your heart.
	You have heard heart pain can be in the shoulder or arm.
	You have heard this from an old boss whilst he was telling you about his heart attack.
	You expect the doctor will send you for an X-ray and give you some pain relief.
Examination	Allow the doctor to examine.
	No swelling or deformity.
	The shoulder is not hot. Painful arc at 30 degrees.
	Pain on lifting the arm against resisted movement and reaching to the back.
	The neck and elbow are normal.

Musculoskeletal Problems – 5

Learning Points

Shoulder Pain

The three joints of the shoulder   Sternoclavicular, acromioclavicular and glenohumeral joint.

The four rotator cuff muscles: Supraspinatus (initiation of abduction)

Infraspinatus (external rotation)

Teres minor (also external rotation)

Subscapularis (internal rotation)

These join together to form the rotator cuff tendon which travels through the sub-acromial space.

Rotator cuff tendonitis[1-2] is where inflammation which causes **impingement** (where the tendon becomes trapped) reduces the range of movement, hence a **painful arc**. For example, if there is a supraspinatus tendonitis there is compression of the supraspinatus tendon between the humeral head and acromion.

Causes: Tendonitis secondary to an injury or repetitive strain or calcium deposits.

Sub-acromial space narrowing: bony spurs from wear and tear or enlargement of the bursa.

An USS may be helpful to diagnose and guide a steroid injection. It may also diagnose tears in the rotator cuff tendons, some of which require surgical repair. Most tendonitis settles with rest, physio and NSAIDs/steroid injection. Occasionally (e.g. if chronic/bony spurs) arthroscopic decompression is necessary.

Frozen shoulder (adhesive capsulitis)[3] is generalised inflammation within the capsule, which causes pain and limits any ROM of the glenohumeral joint. It usually affects the non-dominant shoulder. Frozen shoulder may occur after rotator cuff injury or spontaneously and the cause is unknown. There are typically three phases:

1. 'Painful freezing' stage – most painful stage with gradual loss of movement, may last up to 9 months
2. 'Frozen/Adhesive stage' – reduced movement but less painful, lasts up to 1 year.
3. 'Thawing/Recovery phase' – gradual return to normal function which may take 1–3 years.

Tell patients that symptoms may last between 18 months and 3 years, although the vast majority of patients have recovered by 2 years. The treatment is physiotherapy. A steroid injection may be helpful within the first 8 weeks. Patients with diabetes or thyroid conditions have an increased risk of a bilateral frozen shoulder.

Osteoarthritis: In an older patient it may be helpful to see if there is OA present.

Dislocations usually occur after an impact injury.

Consider **referred pain** from the diaphragm (ruptured ectopic pregnancy) or heart (MI).

If you are ever giving a PIL then describe what is on it!

If unable to abduct the shoulder the first 10 degrees, consider a complete tear of the supraspinatus and speak to a specialist about arranging a clinic appointment.

Musculoskeletal Problems – 5

CHAPTER 23 OVERVIEW
Skin Problems

	Cases in this chapter	Within the RCGP curriculum: People with Skin Problems RCGP Curriculum Online March 2016[1]	Learning points in the chapter include:
1	Skin Lesion	'Be able to advise regarding risk of long-term exposure to ultraviolet and sunburn' 'Be able to distinguish benign from malignant skin conditions and make appropriate referrals' 'Understand the "alarm symptoms and signs" for skin cancers that necessitate fast-track referral'	Skin Lesions – advice from the Primary Care Dermatology Society Solar keratosis
2	Acne	'Empower patients to adopt self-treatment and coping strategies, where possible, in such conditions as mild eczema and mild acne'	When to refer Treatment
3	Melasma	'Recognise the spectrum of patterns and distributions of rashes of different skin disorders'	Triggers When to investigate Management
4	Eczema	'Appreciate the quantities of cream/ointment/lotion that should be prescribed to enable patients to treat their skin condition appropriately, and when to use each vehicle' 'Appreciate the importance of the social and psychological impact of skin problems on the patients' quality of life'	Cause Management Red flags Fingertip units
5	Psoriasis	'Know the association between psoriasis and arteriosclerosis'	Triggers Associations Limb/trunk treatment Scalp psoriasis treatment

1. http://www.rcgp.org.uk/training-exams/gp-curriculum-overview/online-curriculum/applying-clinical-knowledge-section-2/3-21-skin-problems.aspx

CHAPTER 23 REFERENCES

Skin Lesion
1. http://www.dermnetnz.org/lesions/lichenoid-keratosis.html
2. www.pcds.org.uk
3. http://www.pcds.org.uk/ee/images/uploads/general/skin-cancer-detection-patient-advice-07-2012.pdf
4. http://www.dermnetnz.org/lesions/solar-keratoses.html

Acne
1. http://www.pcds.org.uk/ee/images/uploads/general/Acne_Treatment_2015-web.pdf
2. http://patient.info/health/acne-leaflet

Melasma
1. http://www.dermnetnz.org/colour/melasma.html
2. http://www.britishskinfoundation.org.uk/SkinInformation/AtoZofSkindisease/Melasma.aspx
3. http://melasmatherapy.com/melasma-area-and-severity-index-masi/

Eczema
1. http://www.pcds.org.uk/clinical-guidance/atopic-eczema

Psoriasis
1. http://www.pcds.org.uk/clinical-guidance/psoriasis-an-overview
2. NICE guidelines. CG153. Psoriasis: assessment and management. Oct 2012.

Doctor's Notes

Patient	Paul Robson	65 years	M
PMH	No medical history known		
Medications	No current medications		
Allergies	No information		
Consultations	No recent consultations		
Investigations	No investigations		
Household	No household members registered		

Example Consultation   Skin Lesion

Open ☐	Tell me about the skin changes from the beginning please. Anything else that you noticed?
Impact ☐	Has this been worrying you?
ICE ☐	What do you think it is? An SCC – tell me what you understand by this. You mentioned your daughter. What does she think? Is there anything else you hoped we would discuss today?
Sense ☐	I can see you have written everything down for me which is helpful. Would you like to go through what you have written?
Curious ☐	Is your daughter medical? Did you have any other ideas between you?
History ☐	Tell me about you. Your general health? Any other problems to report whilst we have the opportunity today? Do you work? Have you ever smoked? How much alcohol do you drink? Is anyone else at home? Tell me about your lifestyle or hobbies.
Risk ☐	Have you had much sun exposure? Sunburn?
Flags ☐	Has the lesion changed? Over what time period? Have you noticed changes in size, colour, shape, thickness? Has it bled?
O/E ☐	May I take a closer look at this lesion as well as the skin on the head? May I check other areas of skin now? Please could you first take off your shirt so I can look at your chest and back, then put it back on and we'll check the legs. Is that okay?
Summary ☐	To summarise, you have noticed for a few years that the skin on parts of your scalp and face is discoloured but then, over the past month, the patch on your right temple became darker and thicker. Then your daughter, who is a GP, believes it changed again over a week and she thinks it may be an SCC because it has changed quickly. You would like to be referred promptly for a biopsy and hope that I can give you my opinion as well as explain what is likely to happen at the hospital appointment. Is that correct?
Impression ☐	I agree there is sun damage to the face and scalp, which we call solar keratosis. We try to keep this under control with creams as it has the potential to become cancerous and change to the SCC which your daughter talked about. But I agree it is not typical, because of the pigment. Therefore, we also need to rule out a melanoma.
Explanation ☐	Sometimes we can only be sure what we are dealing with by taking a biopsy of the skin and looking at it under a microscope. This is certainly necessary if a lesion changes quickly.
Options ☐	At the hospital, it is likely that they will first have a look at your skin and may or may not do a biopsy on the same day. They may also talk to you about creams for the sun-damaged skin. They will write to me with their findings and advice if any treatment is required.
Empathy ☐	I appreciate it is a worry when anyone points out something which is potentially a cancer. You said you were on holiday at the time – I hope you still managed to have a good time!
Empower ☐	You have come promptly – well done – and I hope this can be dealt with quickly. Do wear a hat and factor 50 sun cream when outside. Now you're someone we don't see very often, so I was wondering if we could arrange some general health checks? Regarding your blood pressure, sugar and cholesterol – how do you feel about seeing the nurse next week to check all of this?
Future ☐	I would like to refer you on the suspected cancer pathway, which means you should be seen within 2 weeks. If this doesn't happen, I need to know straight away please.
Safety net ☐	If you ever notice any other skin changes or you are not sure, see your GP straight away.

Skin Problems – 1

Patient's Story

Skin Lesion

Doctor's notes	Paul Robson, 65 years. No medical history or medications.
How to act	Pleasant. You have written down what you need and hope to be an efficient patient. You show the doctor the examination description with your opening statement.
PC	*'I am concerned about the sun damage on my face.'*
History	You have had this skin damage on your right temple for about 3 years and there are other parts of the head which look similar but are not as dark and not as noticeable.
	If asked about a change, over the past month it has become darker and possibly thicker. It has not changed in size.
	You have no other medical problems. You are very well in yourself.
Social	You are a retired physics lecturer. You have never smoked.
	You drink a glass of wine most nights.
	You live with your wife and keep very active playing golf.
	You have had lots of sun exposure and have been burnt several times, you enjoy spending time outside both in the garden and playing golf and try to go on a couple of sunny holidays a year. You don't always wear sun cream in the UK.
ICE	You think it is fine. You are not worried and wish to be pragmatic.
	'Well, my daughter noticed it whilst we were on a family holiday.'
	If asked, your daughter is a GP.
	If asked what she thinks, explain: *'My daughter thinks it may be the beginning of an SCC because it's scaly and she thinks it has changed from the week before, but she says she isn't sure because it is pigmented.'*
	If asked what your daughter thinks: *'She said I should have a biopsy.'*
	You hope the GP will give you his/her opinion, refer you to a dermatologist and tell you what is likely to happen at the hospital.
	However, you are aware how busy GPs are and are satisfied with a referral.
	If the GP does not refer you, follow his/her advice.
	You are not interested in a general health check at the moment. You will, however, talk to your daughter about it.
Examination	Description of the lesion for the doctor: On the patient's right temple there is a 1 cm pigmented lesion with a scale and irregular outline. The base is thickened. There is no ulceration or induration. Central hyperpigmentation which is raised and surrounded by flat irregular slightly pigmented areas. There is no rolled edge or central telangiectasia. Pigmented areas over the scalp. There are no other lesions of concern on the body.

Skin Problems – 1

Learning Points

Skin Lesion

The biopsy returned as a lichenoid keratosis. DermNet NZ provides an excellent educational resource[1] including pictures and descriptions of common and not so common lesions.

Skin Lesions – Advice from the Primary Care Dermatology Society

> **Primary Care Dermatology Society (PCDS)** website is recommended reading.
> See the **Link Hub at CompleteCSA.co.uk** for a useful patient advice leaflet for skin lesions and useful diagnostic tables from PCDS.[2]

PCDS encourages looking at the body (not the individual lesion alone) for 'pattern comparison'[2] and spot 'the ugly duckling'.[2]

A change in a lesion or the following features (A–G) should raise concern.[3]

Asymmetry	In shape or colour
Border	Uneven, notched or irregular
Colour	Either several colours within 1 lesion, or a different colour to other moles.
Dimensions	Change and size
Elevated	
Firm	
Growth	

Solar (actinic) keratosis

Features	Sun-exposed sites
	May be flat or thickened, with scale or a wart/horn surface, tender or asymptomatic and the colour can vary from skin coloured, red or pigmented.[4]
At risk of	Developing into a cancer (e.g. SCC and BCC) or cutaneous horn or actinic cheilitis.[4]
Treatment	Aimed at removing the affected cells so the epidermis can regenerate.[4]
Minor surgery	Options include cryotherapy with liquid nitrogen; shave, curettage and electrocautery of hypertrophic tissue or horns, or excision.[4]
Field Rx's	'Creams are used to treat areas of sun damage and flat actinic keratosis.'[4]
	'Pre-treatment with keratolytics (such as urea cream, salicylic acid ointment or topical retinoid), and thorough skin cleansing improves response rates.'[4]
	E.g. Diclofenac gel, 5-Fluorouracil, Imiquimod, Photodynamic therapy and Ingenol mebutate gel[4] – see DermNet NZ for further advice.
	'Tender, thickened, ulcerated or enlarging actinic keratoses should be treated aggressively. Asymptomatic flat keratoses may not require active treatment but should be kept under observation.'

Doctor's Notes

Patient   Adelaide Bukoski   23 years   F
PMH   No medical history known
Medications   No current medications
Allergies   No information
Consultations No recent consultations
Investigations No investigations
Household   No household members registered

Example Consultation — Acne

Open ☐	Please tell me more about your skin. Anything else that you have noticed?
History ☐	Have you had any medical problems? Or in the family? What have you tried for your skin? Do you take any medicines? Do you smoke? What is your facial washing regime?
Risk ☐	A few questions about hormones now: do you use hormonal contraception such as the Pill, implant or a hormonal coil?
Flags ☐	Have you noticed any hair on your face? Is your weight stable? Are your periods regular? Have you noticed that the spots increase around your period?
Impact ☐	How does your skin affect you and your self-esteem?
ICE ☐	What do you believe is causing the spots? What do you hope a hormone specialist will do? Is there another reason why you think there is a problem with your hormones? What concerns you most about your skin? Were you hoping I would start treatment today?
O/E ☐	May I take a closer look at the skin on your face and back and check your weight?
Impression ☐	You have acne, which affects 12% of women over 25.
Experience ☐	What do you know about acne? Do you know why it happens?
Explanation ☐	Pores, tiny holes in the skin, become blocked due to the skin thickening at the surface or dead skin cells blocking the pore. Oils usually come out of the pores to keep the skin soft. Some people generate more oil than others. When the oil collects behind these blocked pores, bacteria start to collect and the skin can become painful and swollen. Sometimes hormonal imbalances can be a cause of excess oils, e.g. PCOS or excess male hormone. Every woman has male hormone but some women have more. You have no other symptoms of these hormone problems but we can do blood tests to check. The progesterone and oestrogen levels fluctuate throughout the period cycle but the LH, FSH and testosterone levels will help us rule out hormonal causes for your acne.
Options ☐	As cream alone hasn't worked, and the back is hard to reach, we could try a combination of a cream called Epiduo with an antibiotic tablet, called lymecycline, taken every day. The Epiduo contains two treatments which kill the germs, unblock the pores and reduce the inflammation. It is especially helpful for the white and blackheads you have, but is used in all severities of acne. Lymecycline is an antibiotic which kills the skin bacteria and will help treat the pustules. Like all tablets, side effects are possible; the cream can irritate the skin and the tablets can cause nausea or headaches, but usually people feel fine. Even if you did have PCOS or a raised male hormone, which we will find out from the blood test, treatment options are similar including a hormone pill used for acne. There is another treatment, called isotretinoin, which is only prescribed by skin specialists because it has risks, e.g. to the liver. It is an option for you and, if you were interested in this treatment, we could refer you to the skin specialists should your skin not improve with the treatment I have suggested. I can give you information on all these treatments to read.
Sense ☐	Is your priority finding out if there is a hormone problem? I can see you are unhappy.
Curious ☐	What would your GP in Poland do? What do you believe the GP's role is for you?
Empathy ☐	I can imagine it is frustrating that my suggestions are different from your other doctor's.
Options ☐	Because acne is so common, GPs know a lot about it and we don't need to refer everyone to a skin specialist. The specialists are there for anyone thinking about isotretinoin or who doesn't respond to treatments from the GP. We can start treatment today. Would you like me to prescribe you something appropriate?
Empower ☐	At first, you may want to use the cream every other day, as irritation is more common in the beginning. There is no evidence that different foods make acne worse. Wear clothes like cotton, which can breathe, to avoid your back from getting sweaty. Clean your face and back twice a day. Cleaning too much may cause excess oil to be produced.
Future ☐	Shall we meet again in 3 months? The treatment prevents new spots forming so it may be 8 weeks before you notice a big improvement. If you notice scarring or increased inflammation, please return earlier. You must stop this treatment before falling pregnant.

Skin Problems – 2

Patient's Story

Acne

Doctor's notes	Adelaide Bukoski, 23 years. New patient.
How to act	Demanding.
PC	*'I would like to see an endocrinologist for my spots.'*
History	You moved to the UK from Poland 6 months ago.
	In Poland you were given a cream for your spots but this was not effective.
	You do not know what the cream was called.
	You are otherwise well. You have never taken any regular medication.
	You had a copper coil inserted 2 weeks ago.
	You have regular periods and no symptoms of PCOS.
	The acne is on your face and back. You have tried eating a healthy diet.
	You wash your face four times a day and have spent lots of money on cleansing products.
Social	You work in a café. You drink minimal alcohol and have never smoked. You have a new partner.
ICE	You believe there is a problem with your hormones.
	You would like to see a specialist as you want to know why you have spots at your age.
	You presume the GP is not able to solve the problem and demand to see an expert.
	Before you left, your GP in Poland wrote down a list of blood tests which you could have. *'LH, FSH, oestrogen, progesterone, testosterone.'* You would like these checking.
	If the doctor does not refer, you become angry as you want to find the cause.
	You have just started a new relationship. The spots on your back are especially bad and you feel embarrassed and self-conscious about this.
Examination	A few open and closed comedones on the face and back and some papules. No scarring, pustules, nodules or cysts. No hirsutism.
	BMI 22.

You leave dissatisfied unless you are referred to an endocrinologist. You accept the suggested treatment but walk out looking unhappy with the doctor.

Skin Problems – 2

Learning Points — Acne

This was a challenging case with an unhappy and demanding patient, with high expectations. You may have a patient in the exam who looks disgruntled when you explain why their request is not appropriate, no matter how hard you try to provide suitable alternative suggestions. If this is the case, question what you may be missing – ICE, impact, experience – and be curious. Verbalise that you have sensed their dissatisfaction and explain why you feel their request is inappropriate. Negotiate and take time to educate the patient, which may also demonstrate that you do know what you are talking about!

If a patient leaves the room looking unhappy, you may have done everything appropriately and it may be that the nub of the case is to see how you manage the challenging consultation. So don't dwell on it!

It is difficult to justify using NHS resources inappropriately simply because a patient has high expectations. E.g. a referral to an endocrinologist for acne without abnormal blood tests!

Acne can affect 12% of woman and 3% of men over the age of 25 years.[1]

'Red flags – Refer immediately if
- Severe psychological distress
- Uncontrolled acne developing scarring
- Nodulo-cystic acne (Rx can be initiated, but refer)
- Diagnostic uncertainty
- Patients failing to respond to multiple therapeutic interventions.'[1]

Refer for oral isotretinoin, if the patient wishes, for moderate/severe or Rx resistant acne or scarring.

On examination Comedones, papules, pustules and nodules/cysts.

Treatment

See reference[1] for an excellent table advising which treatment works best for each grade of acne.

E.g. benzoyl peroxide (BPO), topical antibiotics, Duac, OCP or oral antibiotics.

PCDS[1] advise:
- Adapalene should be used in all acne.[1]
- Do not combine a topical and oral antibiotic.[1]
- Do not use lymecycline alone due to resistance – combine with BPO or/and a topical retinoid.[1]
- Azelaic acid is helpful in darker skin at risk of hyperpigmentation.[1]

Possible regimes
- Azelaic acid 20% – Skinoren.
- Either BPO or Adapalene alone but they work well in combination (Epiduo).
- Topical Retinoid/Antibiotic Combination Treclin (resistance may limit duration of use).[1]
- Epiduo at night + Duac in the morning.
- Lymecycline + Epiduo.
- Combined oral contraceptives containing co-cyprindiol, e.g. Dianette and any of the above.

Avoid pregnancy With oral tetracyclines, topical retinoids and isotretinoin.

Rarer causes of acne Exposure to halogenated hydrocarbons in the workplace.[1]

Skin Problems – 2

Doctor's Notes

Patient	Francesca Reece	32 years	F
PMH	NVD 1 year ago		
	Migraines		
Medications	No current medications		
Allergies	No information		
Consultations	GP consultation 1 month ago – advised sun protection for melasma		
Investigations	No investigations		
Household	Oliver Reece	34 years	M
	Jennifer Reece	13 months	F

Example Consultation — Melasma

Open ☐	Tell me about this problem from the beginning. What thoughts have you had about it?
Impact ☐	How has this affected you? Has this changed how you live, your behaviour, or mood?
Curious ☐	I see that you saw another GP a month ago. How did that go?
History ☐	Before this, any problems with your skin at all? Have you any other symptoms which cause you trouble? Are you otherwise well? Tell me more about your migraines. Any other medical conditions or skin problems which run in the family? Do you take any medicines? How is Jennifer? Do you have a partner? What does he think? How is your relationship? Have you spoken to anyone else about this? Are you working as well as being a mum?
Risk ☐	Do you spend much time in the sun? Is there stress in your life? How often are you taking ibuprofen for your migraines?
ICE ☐	What do you think has caused this? Is there anything you are worried about? What would be most helpful to you before you walk out of the door today?
Empathy ☐	This problem is causing you to change your lifestyle and lowering your self-esteem.
Sense ☐	I can see how important this is to you. You look saddened by the change to your skin.
O/E ☐	May I have a closer look at your skin? May I also check the skin on your hands?
Summary ☐	To summarise, since your pregnancy you feel upset and embarrassed by the uneven pigment on your face. You want to enjoy the outdoors with Jennifer. You feel out of shape, through not running, and therefore your skin is having an impact on your life. You also feel embarrassed and upset that your partner agreed with your comment. You hope a dermatologist can suggest a treatment or a prescription today. Have I got it?
Impression ☐	This is called melasma. Unfortunately, pregnancy can sometimes cause this.
Experience ☐	May I explain about melasma or do you already know about it?
Explanation ☐	Melasma is increased pigment in the skin. The exact cause is unknown but contributing factors are thought to be hormones, stress and sun exposure. There may be a family history. Some perfumed cosmetic products can make it worse.
Options ☐	I appreciate you hoped to be seen by a dermatologist; however, I know about treatments for this condition and can recommend something. You were worried this would not go away. Hopefully we can improve things but it's important to be realistic. Melasma is difficult to treat and may persist but, gradually, treatments should help to control it. You should avoid all things that can make it worse. Ibuprofen can cause a pigment reaction. I would stop taking ibuprofen and perhaps we can discuss alternative treatments for your migraine next week? I agree with the previous GP's advice to wear factor 50 sun cream 2-hourly throughout the year. All hormones can make this worse. Most of the hormone in the Mirena stays in your womb, but some may be in your bloodstream. This could be changed to a copper coil. Have a think about the risks of using non-hormonal methods, such as a copper coil or condoms, vs the benefit of being hormone free. Changing the Mirena may, however, make no difference. Could you talk to your partner about this? You can use an unperfumed cleanser, moisturiser and make-up. There are lots of creams for melasma. To start with, we could try azelaic acid 15% in the morning and adapalene at night. All creams can cause irritation, so give the skin a break for 1–2 days if this occurs. Perhaps start by using them on alternate days for a week. The risks of creams are that irritation can cause inflammation and make the pigmentation worse. If this doesn't help we could try a different combination of creams. These suggestions may start to make a gradual improvement. As you are otherwise well I don't think blood tests will help. I believe this is melasma but we can do a biopsy to check for other diagnoses if you wish? How do you feel about the suggestions?
Empower ☐	How could you help your fitness? Wear a cap, use sun cream and enjoy running again.
Future ☐	Can we meet again next week to discuss your migraines, then for your skin in 3 months? If you are feeling frustrated, see me sooner but, remember, change will take time.
Safety net ☐	If you ever notice any new skin lesions, see a GP straight away.

Skin Problems – 3

Patient's Story

Melasma

Doctor's notes Francesca Reece, 32 years. PMH: NVD 1 year ago. Migraines. Medications: None.

GP consultation 1 month ago – advised sun protection for melasma.

How to act Quiet but make it clear that you would be grateful for the doctor's help.

PC *'My skin around my face still looks brown.'*

History Since your pregnancy with Jennifer you have had a discolouration around your face.

You have not been on holiday.

You saw another GP before you moved to the area and felt they did not help at all. He just suggested sun cream which you used, but this did not help so you now prefer to stay indoors, which is a shame as you would like to spend time outside with Jennifer.

You have occasional migraines; you have had a few recently so take ibuprofen several times a week for this. You want to talk about the melasma today. If the doctor asks questions about your migraine, they are a unilateral headache which takes you to bed, with no raised ICP symptoms. They have been with you since teenage years and have not changed.

You have no features of depression but the problem does get you down.

You have no other symptoms on systemic enquiry.

You have no FH of this condition.

Social You enjoy meeting up with your friends.

You work in an office selling online sports equipment.

You do not smoke or drink alcohol.

Your partner once agreed when you said, 'It doesn't look nice, does it?' You know he didn't mean to hurt your feelings but knowing he doesn't like the look of it has made you feel more down. You are already feeling out of shape after the baby and haven't managed to lose much weight.

You have a good relationship with your partner who is supportive.

He hasn't said anything else that is negative. You have a good group of friends but it has not happened to them so they don't understand.

You used to be very active and go running. You don't want to pay for gym membership as you will hardly have the chance to go with the baby and work.

ICE You are worried this will never go away.

You don't know what the doctor may be able to do but hope you can see a dermatologist.

You believe it is your hormones as it started in pregnancy. Do you need a blood test?

You wonder if going back on the Pill might help.

You have the Mirena coil fitted and have had no complications with this.

If the doctor mentions changing the Mirena, you will consider this.

You would like, if possible, to be given a prescription to start treatment today.

Decline a biopsy if offered – you don't like the sound of that.

Examination Melasma around the forehead and upper lip only.

Skin Problems – 3

Learning Points   Melasma

Ask	? Family history (1/3 report a family history[1])
	Sun exposure
	Contraception
	Impact on life and self-esteem
	Medications can trigger a hyperpigmentation reaction, e.g. NSAID or minocycline.[1]
Blood tests	Thyroid levels if symptomatic.
	U&E if suspect Addison's disease.
Advice	Sun protection – hat and factor 50 sun cream, applied 2-hourly – throughout the year.[1]
	Avoid perfumed cosmetics, deodorants or soaps.[1,2]
	All hormonal contraceptives can contribute, so discuss the risk/benefit of trying non-hormonal methods.
	Use a mild cleanser and moisturiser if required.[1]
	The response to the advice and treatments can be slow.[1]
	Use make-up to disguise and camouflage the pigment.
Pregnancy	Usually melasma will start to fade a few months after pregnancy.[1,2]
Differential diagnosis	Post-inflammatory pigmentation[1]
	Solar lentigines/lentigo[1]
	Drug-induced pigmentation[1]
	Lichen planus[1]
	Naevus of Ota and naevus of Hori[1]
	Guttate hypomelanosis[1]
	Addison's disease
Severity	Melasma Area and Severity Index (MASI).[3]
Refer	For biopsy to confirm the diagnosis if uncertain.
	Consider dermatology email advice.
Treatment	'The most successful formulation has been a combination of hydroquinone, tretinoin, and moderate potency topical steroid.'[1] This is available in combination as a private prescription called Pigmanorm.
	See reference[1] (DermNet NZ) for the full list of treatments.
Risks of treatment	Irritation – see BNF for individual treatment.
	Contact dermatitis, further post-inflammatory hyperpigmentation.[1]

Doctor's Notes

Patient	Arthur Miller	12 years	M
PMH	Eczema		
Medications	Eumovate		
	Oilatum		
Allergies	No information		
Consultations	No recent consultations		
Investigations	No investigations		
Household	Gary Miller	49 years	M
	Anita Miller	45 years	F
	Sophie Miller	8 years	F

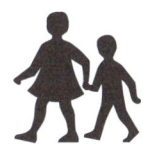

Example Consultation

Eczema

Open ☐	Thank you for coming in. Arthur, how is your eczema? Mum, what are your thoughts? We can certainly make sure Arthur has a prescription back on repeat.
History ☐	Are you otherwise well? How often do you need to use the Eumovate cream, Arthur? Is that once a day? And in between times how is the skin? Is it completely back to normal? How often do you use the Oilatum? Do you like the Oilatum? Does anyone else in the family have eczema? Are there any other conditions which run in the family? What is the worst your skin has been like? Tell me more about that.
Risk ☐	Do you have any allergies? Pets? Is anything making you unhappy? At school?
Sense ☐	I can see it is very important that you never run out of creams.
ICE ☐	I'm just wondering if we can improve things further. What do you think, Arthur? Are you happy with your skin? Why not? What would you like to change? What did you think we may say today? Is there anything else you would like? Mum, what are your thoughts? Is there anything else you thought would be helpful today?
Curious ☐	What do you use for soap, Arthur? And to wash your hair? Is your head itchy?
Impact ☐	How does your skin impact on your life, Arthur? How about using your medication? How would you feel about using the Oilatum four times a day? What would stop you?
O/E ☐	May I have a look at your skin now? Please show me wherever it is a problem.
Summary ☐	Arthur, your skin is always itchy but it becomes red every 2 weeks when you need to use the Eumovate, usually twice a day for a couple of days, then it settles down.
Impression ☐	I agree with you both. The eczema is slightly flared up and it is important to make sure it doesn't get worse. It sounds as if the eczema is rarely completely absent and therefore I'd like to help with that, to prevent you needing to use the Eumovate every 2 weeks.
Experience ☐	Arthur what have you been told about how to use the Oilatum cream? What about the Eumovate? Do you know why we don't suggest using the Eumovate every day?
Explanation ☐	Oilatum is a strong moisturiser. If you use this cream four times a day, it stops the dryness which causes the itching and leads to flare-ups of the eczema. Eumovate is quite a strong steroid cream. The moisturiser won't cause any harm so we can use lots of it, but the steroid creams can cause problems; for example, the skin can get thinner and bruise or it can cause problems inside the body such as weak bones or diabetes. You haven't been using a large amount of steroid, so I am not concerned that you will develop these problems. You are welcome to use the steroid when it flares up, as you have been doing, but I would like to help you to have healthier skin that is less itchy and not so prone to cracks and infection. How does that sound?
Options ☐	I'm wondering what we need to do to help you feel happy with your moisturising creams: change the cream or make it stronger so you need to use it less? Or both? Great – let's do that. Another cream, Doublebase Dayleave, lasts longer. Can we try it every morning?
Empathy ☐	Do you think you could tell your friends about your eczema so they know why you need the cream? Okay, can we be sneaky then and wash out your current shower gel container and fill it with Oilatum? Then your friends won't notice. Showering can wash off the morning moisturiser but using Oilatum as a soap will help.
Empower ☐	Your current shower gel and shampoo strip away all your good work with the moisturiser. There's a better shampoo for eczema – shall we try it? If you can put another layer of moisturiser on after a shower where no one can see, e.g. in the toilet, then do so. Shall I give you a small tube to keep in your bag? If you need the Eumovate, just use this once a day. Mum, what do you think?
Future ☐	Shall we meet again in a month and see if that's made a difference? You may find that you no longer need the Eumovate. I will add the creams to your repeat prescriptions. If you also book an appointment for your daughter, we can check how she is getting on.
Safety net ☐	If your skin does ever look red or oozing, see the GP as this may be a sign of infection.

Skin Problems – 4

Patient's Story

Eczema

Doctor's notes	Arthur Miller, 12 years. PMH: Eczema. Medications: Eumovate and Oilatum.	
How to act	**Mum**	Demanding. Intelligent.
	Arthur	Articulate.
PC		*'We need more steroid cream for Arthur but apparently Arthur needs a medication review.'*
History	**Mum**	Arthur always responds well to the Eumovate, which he's been using for years.
		Arthur was born by NVD at term and had no antenatal or postnatal problems. He has had all his immunisations. There is no family history.
	Arthur	You have no other medical problems. You currently use the Oilatum cream twice a day when the eczema is bad and you don't use it the rest of the time. You have to use the Eumovate every 2 weeks for a couple of days for your arms, wrists and legs. You use it twice a day. In between times it can be itchy, even on the head, but it doesn't always look red. You use Lynx shower gel and Head and Shoulders shampoo. You don't like using the emollient as it makes you feel sticky. You never take it to school with you and you never apply it after showering after sport. You think your friends would laugh at you putting moisturiser on but it does help.
		In the past your skin has been cracked and painful and you needed an antibiotic.
		You have no other medical conditions. You have a younger sister who also has eczema and you have been using her hydrocortisone cream when you ran out of Eumovate.
Social	**Arthur**	You play sport every day. You are happy at school.
		You live with your parents and sister. You have no pets.
ICE	**Mum**	You would like a prescription for the Eumovate to be on repeat so you don't have to keep coming back. You will tell the doctor if there is a problem. You have no concerns.
	Arthur	You think the cream works well. You think your skin is itchy at times and this bothers you but otherwise have nothing to say.
Examination	Mild-moderate eczema on the arms and behind the knees.	

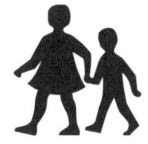

Skin Problems – 4

Learning Points   Atopic Eczema

Ask
- Atopy
- Family history
- Impact
- Compliance and regime with emollients and use of other soaps
- Stress

Cause
- Genetic and environmental
- Mutation in the filaggrin gene in atopic eczema causing a defect in the skin barrier layer ... 'immunological changes are probably secondary to enhanced antigen penetration through a deficient epidermal barrier. The relevance of this finding is that it reinforces the importance of the regular use of emollients to help manage eczema.'[1]

Flags
- Sign of infection.
- Overuse of steroids and underuse of emollients.
- Admit if painful vesicular or ulcerated lesions which may be eczema herpeticum.

Management
- Moisturiser '20 minutes before applying the topical steroid'.[1]
- Take the time to find out why compliance may be an issue and consider how to adapt the management plan for the individual to increase their emollient use.
- 'In both children and adults it is more effective and safer to "hit hard" using more potent treatments for a few days than it is to use less potent treatments for longer periods of time.'[1]

Other Rx's
- Antihistamines for itch.
- Bath and shower emollients.
- Scalp preparations and shampoos.
- Bandages and dressings.
- Antibiotics – topical or oral.
- Topical immunomodulators – tacrolimus and pimecrolimus.[1]
- Coal tar and ichthammol.
- Salicylic acid.
- Potassium permanganate.

See the **Link Hub at CompleteCSA.co.uk** for helpful links to Patient information for eczema

The Primary Care Dermatology Society Website is very helpful. See reference[1] http://www.pcds.org.uk/clinical-guidance/atopic-eczema for further information.

Doctor's Notes

Patient	Maureen Staples	70 years	F
PMH	Psoriasis		
	Pre-diabetes		
	2 × normal vaginal deliveries		
	Hypertension		
Medications	Dermovate		
	Cetraben		
	Ketoconazole scalp shampoo		
	Amlodipine 5 mg		
Allergies	No information		
Consultations	No recent consultations		
Investigations	18 months ago	HbA1c 44 mmol/mol	
		BP 130/70	
Household	Brian Staples	72 years	M

Example Consultation   Psoriasis

Open ☐	Thank you for coming in to see me. Any problems at all? Tell me about you. Tell me about your medical history please.
Impact ☐	What aspect of the psoriasis troubles you the most? In what way is it a nuisance?
History ☐	I'd be interested to know more about your psoriasis from the beginning please. Where is it a problem at present? How bad is it at the moment? And what treatments have you used? How often do you apply the Cetraben? What do you wash with? What shampoo do you use the rest of the time? What do you think about this cream? How often do you apply the Dermovate? Does it make a difference? Every day? How many days within the month would you not apply it? When was the last time you had more than a week's break from it? The scalp shampoo: does this work? How often do you use this? Tell me about a time when your psoriasis was particularly a problem. Do you have any other symptoms elsewhere in the body? Are your eyes and joints okay? How is your general health? Do you have a family history of any medical problems?
Sense ☐	You seem very relaxed about your health. We do like you to see us at least once a year and more often if there are any issues.
Curious ☐	What would you change or try to improve if you could?
ICE ☐	Is there anything you have been worried about or would like to talk about, as we certainly have time? Is there anything you thought or hoped we may decide today?
O/E ☐	May I have a look at your skin, wherever it is a problem? May I also take your blood pressure. Thank you. May I feel your pulse and listen to your heart? Please step onto the scales, I'd like to check your height and weight.
Summary ☐	To summarise, you feel well but the psoriasis has always been a nuisance, rubbing on and damaging clothes and, if you could improve this, it would be helpful. You like the Cetraben which you use twice a day and also use this in the shower.
Impression ☐	Your psoriasis is moderate in severity. Your high blood pressure is currently under control. I'm wondering how your blood sugars are now and also, because you are a postmenopausal woman, we should have a think about your bones.
Experience ☐	What do you know about psoriasis? Has anyone explained to you the risks of too much steroid cream?
Explanation ☐	Psoriasis is caused by increased cell turnover. The Dermovate is a very strong steroid. You can use this daily for 8 weeks but then you should have a 4-week break as there are risks of too much steroid being absorbed into the body. For example, it can lead to changes in your hormones, a rise in blood pressure, diabetes and thinning of the bones.
Options ☐	I wonder if we can take this opportunity to look at your general health to aim for improvements as well as changing your treatment for psoriasis. I notice that last year's blood test showed that your blood sugar was in the range of pre-diabetes. Was this explained to you? That is correct. I will also put your numbers into a calculator to determine risk of frail bones so we can discuss this next time. How does this sound?
Empathy ☐	You've lived with a troublesome condition all your life – it must have been wearing.
Empower ☐	Continue the Cetraben at least 4 times daily and please now stop the steroid cream for at least 4 weeks and use instead a cream which contains vitamin D for the next 4 weeks. It is called Dovonex and you put it on twice a day. For the scalp I would suggest trying Cocois ointment at night and wash it off in the morning with Capasal shampoo. If these don't work, we could try coal tar for the body and a steroid mousse for the scalp.
Future ☐	It would be helpful if you could please arrange a fasting blood test with the nurse where we can check your cholesterol, kidney function and sugar, then a further appointment to discuss your results and response to the skin treatments please. Perhaps in 1 month? If we are not winning we can ask the dermatologist to see you, you may be suitable for UV treatment. What are your thoughts about this?
Safety net ☐	If ever the skin looks red and is weeping, it may be an infection, so see a doctor.

Skin Problems – 5

Patient's Story   Psoriasis

Doctor's notes	Maureen Staples, 70 years.
	PMH: Psoriasis, pre-diabetes, 2 × NVD and hypertension.
	Medication: Dermovate, Cetraben, Ketoconazole shampoo and Amlodipine.
	Investigations: 18 months ago, HbA1c 44 mmol/mol, BP 130/70.
How to act	Polite and playing down symptoms.
PC	*'I have come for my annual review please.'*
History	You do not like to bother the doctor.
	The pharmacist told you that you are due for your medication review.
	The psoriasis has been present all your life. You do not think about the impact it has on your life as you are used to it. But it does bother you: *'It is a nuisance.'* By this you mean it itches, rubs against clothes and the dry skin ruins your clothes.
	You use the Dermovate most days so you are unsure if it makes a difference. Your last steroid break was 4 months ago. You apply this to your elbows and knees.
	You like the Cetraben and use this in the shower and morning and night.
	Your head irritates you the most. It is itchy. You use the shampoo twice a week and OTC anti-dandruff shampoo the rest of the week.
	You have taken your blood pressure in the waiting room it is 120/60.
	No family history.
Social	You have never worked since you were married. Your husband is well.
	You are a proud grandmother of seven grandchildren.
	You enjoy a whisky with your husband every night. You have never smoked.
ICE	Your psoriasis has been with you ever since you can remember. You remember the doctor saying last year that pre-diabetes means nearly diabetes. Since then you cut out sugar and swim most days.
	You were very interested in the psoriasis in your 20s and read all about it – but you have forgotten most of it now. You have no concerns.
	You expect the doctor will just give you the same creams.
	You are interested in any suggestions the doctor has.
Examination	The psoriasis plaques are moderate in severity. There is psoriasis on the scalp. HS normal. HR regular 70bpm. BMI 20. BP 120/60.

Skin Problems – 5

Learning Points   Psoriasis in Adults

Psoriasis in the RCGP online curriculum includes:
'Know the association between psoriasis and arteriosclerosis.'
'Be aware of inheritance of common skin diseases, such as eczema or psoriasis.'

Ask/Triggers	Trauma, infection, pregnancy, sunlight, drugs, stress, alcohol, smoking and HIV.[1]
Associations	Autoimmune conditions
	Psoriatic arthropathy 'In 30% … early intervention can reduce joint damage.'[1]
	Cardiovascular disease
	Venous thromboembolism
	Depression
Examine	Joints and nails, BP, BMI.
Investigate	CVD: BP, lipids and HbA1c.
NICE suggest	Explain the risks of steroid Rx. Stop steroids when the skin is nearly clear. Prescribe a maximum of 8 weeks of topical potent or very potent steroids, followed by a 4 week break. Encourage emollients. Offer referral with second and third line treatments if required.[2]

For limb/trunk psoriasis[2]

1st	4 weeks of a potent steroid am and vitamin D/or analogue (e.g. Dovonex) pm.
2nd	Continue the steroid for a maximum of 8 weeks.
3rd	Continue vitamin D (or analogue) twice daily until 8–12 weeks.
4th	Either a potent corticosteroid BD for 4 weeks or coal tar (e.g. Exorex) BD or combined steroid/vitamin D (Dovobet) daily for 4 weeks.

Very potent corticosteroids only if:
'In specialist settings under careful supervision when other topical treatment strategies have failed for a maximum period of 4 weeks.'[2]
'Do not use very potent corticosteroids in children and young people.'[2]

Scalp psoriasis
NICE suggest:[2]

1st	Commencing with a potent corticosteroid daily for up to 4 weeks.
2nd @ 4 weeks	Change preparation or add ointments to remove scale. Apply before the steroid.
3rd @ 8 weeks	Combined calcipotriol + steroid or if mild/don't tolerate, a vitamin D product alone.
4th @ 16 weeks	A very potent steroid for 2 weeks or coal tar or seek advice.

If mild – an example regime as advised by a dermatologist

Start with	Ointment at night and wash off with a shampoo in the morning.
Ointment	Sebco scalp ointment (coal tar, salicylic acid, sulphur) or Cocois.
Shampoo	Capasal shampoo (coal tar 1%, coconut oil 1%, salicylic acid 0.5%), T gel or Polytar.
No improvement	Above plus steroid and vitamin D preparation.
Steroid	Betamethasone valerate 0.1% (potent).
Vitamin D	Calcipotriol scalp solution.
When improved	Stop the Sebco and continue shampoo and the Bettamousse.
When controlled	Stop the steroid (Bettamousse) and continue antipsoriasis shampoo PRN.

Skin Problems – 5

CHAPTER 24 EXAMINATION CHECKLISTS

Examinations   Informed Consent

To gain **informed consent** explain what you would like to do and why it would be helpful.

'I would like to examine your chest by bringing you to the examination couch. It would be helpful if you could please remove your top (keeping your bra on) and then I'd like to take your temperature, feel your pulse and have a listen to your chest to see if there are any signs of infection. Would that be okay?'

If an intimate examination is required then either **state** you need a chaperone or, if you feel comfortable without, **offer** a chaperone. (In real consultations always document this discussion.)

You need to inform the patient of everything you would like to examine just in case you do not have the opportunity to carry out the examination. Do not turn to look at the examiner to ask if you should examine! Presume you are proceeding with the examination (even if an intimate examination) and **move** after gaining consent to either a chair or couch as appropriate. You may be stopped and given information (by card, on the iPad or verbally) at this point.

Be aware that there may be a second page on the iPad with further information and this may be signposted at the bottom of the iPad.

Candidates often ask:
1. Should I examine in the chair or on the couch?
   The chair is acceptable if you can obtain all the information you require without cutting corners.
2. Should I complete a thorough and formal examination of a system?
   The extent to which you examine should be appropriate and guided by the history. E.g. if a patient presents with angina, we suggest a formal/full approach to the cardiovascular examination.

When examining, always use the phrase a '**good look**' not a 'quick look'.

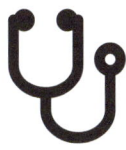

Examinations

Cardiovascular

Example description
'I'd like to **thoroughly** examine your chest and heart by asking you to come over to the couch and take off your top, please. I will then feel your pulse, take your blood pressure and listen to your heart. This will help me to check the heart and blood vessels. Is that okay?'

Checklist
- 'I'd like to start by measuring your blood pressure and checking your pulse.'
- 'Now may I feel both pulses together?'
- 'May I see your hands?'
- 'And now just the one pulse and I will lift your arm.' (Collapsing pulse.)
- 'Look up to the ceiling for me ... and stick out your tongue.' (Anaemia.)
- 'Now please turn your neck to the side.' (JVP – if appropriate from history.)
- 'May I feel your heart?' (Apex, thrills and heaves.)
- 'Now I'll listen.' (Apex with bell for mitral stenosis.)
- 'And now please roll slightly to your left.' (Mitral regurgitation.)
- 'Please roll back.' Switch to diaphragm to check the other valves.
- 'I will now listen to the arteries in your neck.' (Carotid bruit.)
- 'Now please sit forward.' (Listen for aortic regurgitation at left lower sternal edge.)
- 'I will now listen to your lower lungs.' (Pulmonary oedema – if appropriate from history.)
- Consider checking for liver edge and leg swelling. (Right-sided heart failure.)
- Consider checking for AAA and peripheral pulses. (Depending on age and history.)

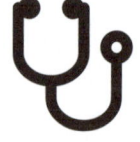

Examinations

Respiratory

Example description
'I'd like to **thoroughly** examine your chest and lungs in the chair and will ask you to take off your top, please. I'd also like to feel your pulse, check your breathing rate, oxygen levels, take your temperature and check a blowing test called the peak flow. This will help me look for signs of infection and check the airflow into lungs. Is that okay?'

Checklist
- 'I'd like to start by checking your pulse and oxygen saturations.'
- Then check breathing rate.
- 'Please may I see your hands and fingers?'
- 'Can you please stick out your tongue?' (Cyanosis.)
- 'I'm going to feel for lumps in the neck.' (Lymphadenopathy.)
- 'Big breath in for me.' (Expansion.)
- 'And say 99.' (Vocal resonance in quadrants.)
- 'And now some deep breaths in and out please.' (Auscultation.)
- 'I'm going to tap on your chest.' (Percussion.)
- 'Can I just check your legs for pain and swelling?' (DVT.)
- Consider temperature.
- Consider PEFR.
- Consider inhaler technique.

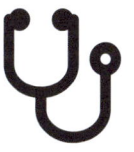

Examinations

Abdominal

Example description
'I'd like to **thoroughly** *examine your abdomen, by asking you to lie on the couch and lift up your top to under the breasts and undo the button on your trousers to look at your lower tummy. I would also like to take your pulse and temperature. This will help me to find the reason for your pain. Is that okay?'*

Checklist
- Consider taking: pulse, temperature and blood pressure. (Are they systemically unwell?)
- 'May I see your hands and fingers?' (E.g. liver disease.)
- 'I'm just going to have a close look at your face and eyes for colour change.'
- 'May I look in your mouth?'
- 'I'm just going to feel for any lumps above your collar bone.'
- 'Can you please lift your head off the bed and cough?' (Hernia.)
- 'Can you suck your tummy in?' (Peritonism.)
- 'Please tell me if you have any discomfort whilst I feel your tummy.' (Watch their face.)
- Check for rebound tenderness, McBurney's and Rovsing's signs.
- Palpate for hepatosplenomegaly.
- Then percuss for hepatosplenomegaly and consider shifting dullness for ascites.
- Auscultate.
- Consider offering: inguinal hernia, perineum, pelvic and rectal examinations.
- Consider requesting a urine sample for a pregnancy or urine dipstick test.

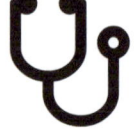

Examinations

Cranial Nerves

Example description
'I'd like to **thoroughly** examine the nerves in your brain by asking you to make some actions. I will sit opposite you. Is that okay?'

Checklist

II	'Can you read this chart covering each eye at a time.' (Snellen for acuity.)
	'Look at my finger at a distance and now close to your nose.' (Accommodation.)
	'Now I'll shine a light in your eye.' (Then the opposite eye for efferent/afferent pathway testing.)
	'Covering the left eye with your hand, look at my nose. Say *yes* when you see my fingers move.'
	'And now cover the other eye.' (Visual fields.)
	'Now with both eyes open how many fingers do you see?' (Double vision/4 quadrants.)
	Fundoscopy: 'Now I'd like to look at the back of your eyes. This involves shining a bright light into the eye. I will need to get close to your face, please try to keep looking straight forward – imagine you can see through me, and remember to breathe away normally.'
III, IV, VI	'Now keep your head still and follow my finger with your eyes.' (Eye movements and nystagmus.)
V	'Checking for sensation now: can you feel this on both sides?' (Upper, middle and lower face.)
VII	'Now I'm going to test the muscles. I will test the strength by resisting your movements.'
	'Please raise your eyebrows … now shut your eyes tight …'
	'Open your eyes and puff out your cheeks … and a big smile for me.'
VIII	'Can you hear me whisper a number?' Block the opposite ear, test each side at 1 m whisper.
	If not heard, try 1 m voice … if not heard try voice next to ear.
	Rinne/Weber if difficulty hearing (see ENT examinations).
IX	'Please swallow.'
X	'Open your mouth and say ah.' (Palatal rise.)
XI	'Shrug your shoulders and keep them up
	… and push your face against my hand' (Check sternocleidomastoid muscle strength.)
XII	'Please show me your tongue.'
Cerebellar	Acronym – DANISH: Dysdiadochokinesia. Ataxic gait. Nystagmus. Intention tremor.
	Slurred speech 'Baby hippopotamus' and heel-shin test (coordination).

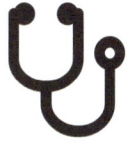

Examinations   Neurological

Example description

'I'd like to **thoroughly** *examine the nerves in your arms and legs by checking sensation and doing some movements. Is that okay?* Do you have any pain that I should be aware of when I examine you?'

Decide bed or chair – what do you do normally? Think about the exposure of the patient. It may be appropriate to leave clothes on if sensation can be tested easily through thin clothing.

Checklist

- 'Are you able to stand up without using your hands? … Now please walk across the room and back.' ('Get up and go' in the elderly to assess falls risk, gait and strength.)
- 'Can you stand feet together and then shut your eyes.' (Romberg's for proprioception – be ready to steady the patient should they lose balance!)
- 'And now with your feet comfortably apart again, close your eyes and touch your nose.'
- 'Can you walk heel-toe? … And now please lie down on the bed facing upwards.'
- Check arms +/– legs for wasting, scars, fasciculation.
- 'I'm going to check the tone by moving your arms.'
- 'Can we now check power … and reflexes?'
- 'And now your legs.'
- 'A scratch test on your feet now.' (Plantar reflexes and check clonus.)
- 'I'm going to test your sensation.' Demonstrate pins and cotton wool on the chest and then check all dermatomes.
- Test coordination – finger nose ataxia/heel against shin.
- Consider vibration sensation. (Peripheral neuropathy secondary to diabetes.)
- Consider cerebellar signs (DANISH – see CN examination)
- Consider testing for Parkinsonism features:
  Micrographia, each finger to thumb, hands open and closing for bradykinesia.

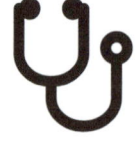

Examinations

Thyroid/Neck

Example description
'I'd like to **thoroughly** *examine your thyroid gland, which is in the neck, and also look at your hands and legs which can be affected by the thyroid, if I may?.'*

Patient in sitting position and expose neck fully.

Checklist
- 'May I start by looking at your hands?' (Tremor, warmth, palmar erythema, dry skin, clubbing.)
- 'And check your pulse?'
- 'Looking at your eyes now, can you look straight ahead … follow my finger up and down?' (Exophthalmos, lid retraction, lid lag, chemosis.)
- 'And now looking at your neck.' (Look from the front and side for scars and a visible thyroid.)
- 'Can you please stick out your tongue … and now swallow?'
- 'I'm going to feel your thyroid … and, if you can, please swallow again.' (Stand behind. ?asymmetry.)
- 'I'm going to listen.' (Bruit.)
- 'Now looking at your ankles for swelling. (Pre-tibial myxoedema.)
- 'And finally testing your reflexes.' (Slow relaxing reflexes.)
- 'May I check your weight now please?'

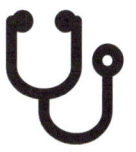

Examinations

Examinations

Shoulder/Cervical Spine

- Look → feel → move → power → sensation → function.
- Always examine the joint above and below for swelling, tenderness and ROM.

Example description

'I'd like to **thoroughly** *examine your shoulders, neck and elbow. May I ask you to take your shirt off please? Is that okay?'*

Checklist

- 'Can you please point to where you feel the pain?'
- Look for asymmetry, deformity, wasting, swelling or redness.
- 'Please tell me if you are tender or in pain when I examine you.' (Warmth/tenderness over C-spine, shoulder and elbow.)
- 'Can you move your neck and copy me?' (Test for full ROM of the neck.)
- Keeping your arms straight, can you lift the arms up in front of you … and now move the arms out to the sides and lift the arms into the air?' (Painful arc or frozen shoulder?)
- 'Put your arms out to the sides but just a little in front of you. Now imagine you are holding a can and emptying it onto the floor. Now please hold your arm in that position whilst I try to push your arm down.' (Jobe's test/empty can test = supraspinatus test.)
- 'Now glue both elbows into your waist but with your hands push my hands out to the sides.' (External rotation for teres minor test.)
- 'Can you hold your hand out so your thumb is up and tilted away from you? Now can you try and turn your hand further away from you against my resistance?' (Infraspinatus test.)
- 'Hands behind your back and push my hands backwards.' (Subscapularis test.)
- Then finally test power throughout the upper limb.
- Consider a neuro exam. 'Can you feel me touch your skin?' (Test all dermatomes.)
- 'How high up your spine can you reach there?' (Function.)
- 'Can you touch your head with both hands as if washing your hair?' (Function)
- 'Any issues checking your blind spot when driving?' (Function.)

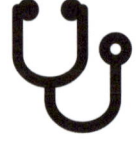

Examinations

Elbow

- Look → feel → move → power → sensation → function.
- Always examine joint above and joint below for swelling, tenderness and ROM.

Example description
'I'd like to **thoroughly** *examine your elbow as well as your shoulder and wrists. If I may ask you to remove your shirt – is that okay?'*

Checklist
- 'Please can you point to where you feel the pain?'
- 'Let's look at your elbow … and the other elbow.' (Swelling, redness, deformity.)
- 'Please tell me if you feel any pain when I examine your elbow now.' (Heat or tenderness over the epicondyles.)
- 'Now can you move your hands to touch your shoulder and straighten both your arms?'
- 'Can you place your palms up to the ceiling … and now down to the floor?' (Pronation/supination.)
- 'Now hold my hand as if you are going to shake it. Turn your hand as if twisting a handle and I will try to resist you.' (Use both of your hands to prevent injury to yourself!)
- 'And turn the other way.'
- 'Now with your arm outstretched, bend your wrist back towards you; if I resist you does that cause pain in your elbow?' (Lateral epicondylitis.)
- 'Now can you bend your wrist toward the floor? Does it hurt your elbow if I resist this movement?' (Medial epicondylitis)
- 'Can you feel me touch you at the elbow?'
- 'Can you reach both hands onto your head? Now can you reach your back?' (Function.)
- 'I want to have a look at the shoulder … and now feel your shoulder; is this painful? Keeping your arms straight, can you move the arms out to the sides and lift the arms into the air?'
- 'Now looking at your wrists, is there any tenderness? Can you move your wrists?'

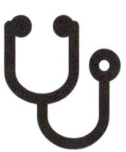

Examinations

Hands/Wrists

- Look → feel → move → power → sensation → function.
- Always examine joint above and joint below.

Example description

'I'd like to **thoroughly** *examine your hands, wrists and elbows. If you could please roll your sleeves above the elbow. Is that okay?'*

Checklist

- 'Let's put a pillow on your lap for your hands to rest on.'
- 'Please point to where you feel the pain.'
- 'Now let's look and see if there is any swelling or changes.'
- 'May I feel your skin for heat? ... And now, as I feel each joint in turn, let me know if you have any pain.' (Feel each finger joint, metacarpal, wrist and elbow joint in turn.)
- 'Are you able to copy the following movements?' (Make a fist, open and close hands, wrist full ROM and elbow full ROM.)
- 'Can you squeeze my fingers?'
- 'Now stretch your fingers out and keep them out' (Ulnar.)
- 'Lift your thumb to the ceiling and press against me' (Median.)
- Test sensation in ulnar and median distribution.
- 'Can you touch each finger against your thumb?' (Function.)
- 'Please copy me and place your hands like this. Hold the hands there and let me know if you feel any tingling.' (Phalen's test for carpal tunnel syndrome.)
- 'Now I will tap over your wrist. Tell me if you feel any tingling in the hand.' (Tinel's Test for carpal tunnel syndrome.)

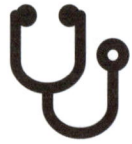

Examinations

Hips/Lumbar Spine

Example description
'I'd like to **thoroughly** *examine your back and hips, if I may, to find the cause of this pain.*'

Checklist
- 'Please point to where you feel the pain.'
- 'Please walk across the room.'
- 'Now with four fingers holding onto my hands, if you can please lift your right knee so you are standing on your left foot only. And now the other leg please.' (Trendelenburg's test.)
- 'Now please turn away from me and I'll look at your spine.' (Posture, lordosis, kyphosis.)
- 'As I feel your spine, please tell me if this is painful.' (Spine then paraspinal muscles.)
- 'Back to face me now … (step away) can you keep your legs straight and touch your toes?'
- 'And try leaning down each side and back.' (Flexion, extension, lateral flexion, rotation.)
- 'Now lift each leg out to each side.' (Hip abduction.)
- 'And leg behind you.' (Hip extension.)
- 'Onto the couch now; are you tender where I press on your hips?' (Greater trochanters.)
- 'Keep your leg straight and raise the leg one at a time.' (Hip flex and SLR – sciatica.)
- 'Can you bend your knee to your chest now?'
- 'Can I see if I can take that further? Now I'm going to check your hips.' (Int/ext rotations)
- Consider lower limb neurology testing.

Trendelenburg test: 'The sound side sags' when weight bearing on weak gluteals, i.e. if unable to hold pelvis level standing on one leg, the standing leg is the affected side.

Causes include: dislocated hip, # greater trochanter, subluxation of the upper femoral epiphysis (SUFE), muscle-wasting diseases – though can be positive in any painful hip condition.

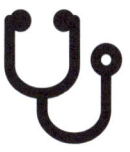

Examinations   Knee

Example description
'I'd like to **thoroughly** examine your knees as well as your hips and ankles as sometimes there is a problem with the adjacent joint. If I may ask you to remove your trousers/skirt (keep shorts on). Is that okay? If at any point you are in pain, please let me know.'

Checklist
- 'Facing me now, please, point to where you feel the pain.'
- Look for valgus/varus positioning of knees/ankles, deformity, wasting and swelling in the lower limb.
- 'Please turn to the side, now turn away from me, turn again and now back to face me.'
- 'Please walk across the room.'
- 'Now with four fingers, hold my hands and lift one knee up at a time.' (Trendelenburg test.)
- 'Lift each leg out to each side' (Hip abduction.) 'And leg behind you.' (Hip extension.)
- 'Please come over to the couch and lie facing upwards … with your knees slightly bent.'
- 'I'm just going to check for heat and tenderness now in the hip (greater trochanter) knee (joint lines) and ankle (malleolus).'
- 'Now straighten your leg and I will test for fluid.' Patellar tap and fluid test for effusion.
- 'Left side now, can you make this leg as straight as possible?' (Hyperextend knee.)
- 'Now lift your leg straight into the air.' (Hip flex). 'Bring your knee to your chest.' (Knee flex.)
- 'Now can I do the same and see if I can take that further?' (Feeling for crepitus.)
- 'I'm just going to test your hip movement.' (Internal and external rotation.)
- 'And now can you point your toes up and down, left and right?' (Ankle ROM.)
- 'Please bend your knee and I will pull and push, to test the ligaments in your knee.' (Anterior and posterior draw test for cruciates.)
- 'And now you will feel some pressure on the sides of the knees.' (Collateral ligaments.)
- 'And now as you straighten your knee I will move your ankle.' (McMurray's for meniscus tear.)

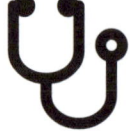

Examinations

Foot/Ankle

Example description

'I'd like to **thoroughly** *examine your foot and ankle as well as your knees as sometimes there is a problem with the adjacent joint. If I may ask you to remove your trousers/skirt (keep shorts on). Is that okay? If at any point you are in pain, please let me know.'*

Checklist

- 'Facing me now, please, point to where you feel the pain.'
- Look for valgus/varus positioning of knees/ankles, deformity, wasting and swelling in the lower limb.
- 'Please turn to the side, now turn away from me, turn again and now back to face me.'
- 'Please walk across the room … now walk on your tiptoes … and on your heels.'
- 'Please come over to the couch and lie facing upwards … with your knees slightly bent.'
- 'I'm just going to check for heat and tenderness now in the knee (joint lines) and ankle (malleolus) and foot (metatarsals).'
- 'Left side now, can you make this leg as straight as possible for me?' (Hyperextend knee.)
- 'Now lift your leg straight into the air.' (Hip flex.)
- 'Bend your knee to your chest.' (Knee flex.)
- 'Now can I do the same and see if I can take that further?' (Feeling for crepitus.)
- 'And now can you point your toes up and down, left and right?' (Ankle ROM.)
- 'Right side now please.' (Repeat.)
- 'Can you now turn over so you are facing the bed? I'm just going to squeeze your calf muscles.' (Achilles test.)
- 'And feel for pain under the foot.' (Plantar fasciitis.)
- 'Can you feel me touch your skin on the feet and toes?'

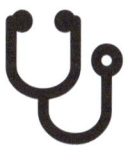

Examinations

ENT

Example description
'I'd like to **thoroughly** *examine your ears, nose and throat … is that okay?'*

Checklist
- 'First let's look at your ears.' Is there redness/swelling?
- 'Is it tender when I press on this bone?' (Mastoiditis.)
- 'Or pull slightly at your ear?' (Otitis externa.)
- 'What about when I press here?' (Tragus.) 'Now let's look inside the ears.'
- Ensure you hold the otoscope like a pen in the same hand as the ear which you are examining.
- 'Let's test your hearing.' (At 1 m whisper, then if required 1 m voice, then next to ear voice.)
- **Weber's test:** 'I'm going to place this tuning fork (512 Hz) on your forehead. Can you tell me where you hear the sound – in the middle or to one side?'
    - Conductive deafness: localises to the affected side.
    - Sensorineural deafness: localises to the unaffected side
- **Rinne's test:** 'Now I'm going to place the tuning fork behind your ear and then in front. Which is louder?'
    - Normal = air conduction (AC) >bone conduction (BC).
    - Conductive deafness = BC>AC.
    - Sensorineural deafness: AC>BC.
- 'Now can you tilt your head back? I'm going to look into the nose.'
- 'Now let's look at your throat.'
- 'And finally I want to see if you have any tenderness or lumps in your neck.'

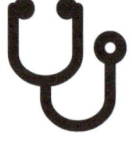

Examinations

Peripheral Vascular

Example description
'I'd like to **thoroughly** *examine your vessels in your tummy and legs. If I may ask you to remove your trousers so that I can feel your pulses. I'd also like to take your blood pressure if I may. Please lie on the couch facing up.*'

Checklist
- Inspect legs for hair loss, colour change and look around the feet for tissue damage/ulceration.
- 'I'm now going to feel your vessels.'
- 'May I start with your large vessel in your tummy?' (AAA.)
- 'And now the pulses starting in the groin please.'
    - Femoral, popliteal, posterior tibial and dorsalis pedis.
- 'Now I'd like you to lift this leg up; we are going to hold it (in reality for 45 seconds but not in the exam!) and watch for any colour change (pallor) … And now can you drop the leg over the edge of the bed.' (Reactive hyperaemia of Buerger's test.)
- Consider examining the heart, BP, lower limb sensation, offering a urine glucose test and ankle brachial pressure index (ABPI) checks.

If varicose veins are present, check with patient standing.
- Feel for tenderness in thrombophlebitis.
- Look for signs of DVT, oedema, tenderness along the greater saphenous vein (inner thigh).
- Measure calves from 10 cm below the tibial tuberosity.

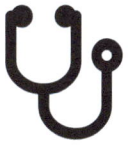

APPENDIX
Useful Resources

Updated at the Link Hub at CompleteCSA.co.uk

Information for GPs	Patient.co.uk and GP Notebook
PILs in different languages	http://www.nhs.uk/aboutNHSChoices/aboutnhschoices/accessibility/Pages/other-languages-section.aspx
DermNet	http://www.dermnetnz.org/
Primary care dermatology	http://www.pcds.org.uk/
Translated dermatology PILs	http://www.bad.org.uk/for-the-public/translated-patient-information-leaflets
Medicines in pregnancy	http://www.medicinesinpregnancy.org/
Medications in breastfeeding	http://toxnet.nlm.nih.gov/cgi-bin/sis/search2/f?./temp/~edzt0g:1
DVLA at a glance	https://www.gov.uk/government/publications/assessing-fitness-to-drive-a-guide-for-medical-professionals
Fitness to fly	https://www.caa.co.uk/Passengers/Before-you-fly/Am-I-fit-to-fly-/
Travel clinic	http://www.fitfortravel.nhs.uk/home.aspx
Drug monitoring requirements	http://www.seqo.nhs.uk/buckinghamshire/shared/images/files/ccg-prescribing/Clinical/Shared%20Care%20Protocols/4.%20Drug%20Monitoring%20Requirements%20for%20Shared%20Care%20Drugs%20%20-%20Jul.pdf
Parent advice	http://www.whenshouldiworry.com/
	The Incredible Years by Carolyn Webster-Stratton.
Oxford antimicrobial guidelines	http://www.oxfordshireccg.nhs.uk/wp-content/uploads/2013/08/Oxfordshire-ADULT-Antimicrobial-Prescribing-Guidelines-for-Primary-Care.pdf CHILD http://www.oxfordshireccg.nhs.uk/wp-content/uploads/2013/07/Oxfordshire-Antimicrobial-PAEDIATRIC-Guidelines-Primary-Care-v1.1-May-14.pdf

Useful guidance	Contraception	www.fsrh.org
	Green Top Guidelines	https://www.rcog.org.uk/guidelines
	SIGN	http://sign.ac.uk/
	NICE	https://www.nice.org.uk/guidance
	BTS	https://www.brit-thoracic.org.uk/guidelines-and-quality-standards/
Mental health	http://www.ntw.nhs.uk/pic/selfhelp/	
	http://www.oxfordmindfulness.org/about-mindfulness/	
	http://www.fearfighter.com/	
	https://moodgym.anu.edu.au/welcome	
	http://www.mind.org.uk/	

Antidepressant switches	http://www.mims.co.uk/antidepressants-guide-switching-withdrawing/mental-health/article/882430
Prescribing in psychiatry	*Maudsley Prescribing Guidelines in Psychiatry 2015* by Taylor and Paton.
CBT book for the keen reader	*Mindfulness: a practical guide to finding peace in a frantic world* by Mark Williams, Dr Danny Penman.
CBT – if struggling to concentrate	*Living in the Moment: with Mindfulness Meditations* by Anna Black.
Joint exercises	http://www.arthritisresearchuk.org/arthritis-information/exercises-to-manage-pain.aspx
Back screening tool	http://www.keele.ac.uk/sbst/
Osteoporosis assessment	http://www.shef.ac.uk/FRAX/
Physiotherapy websites:	http://www.sheffieldachesandpains.com/
Vitamin D guidelines – adults	http://www.ouh.nhs.uk/osteoporosis/useful-info/documents/VitaminDSupplementationinprimarycarev16.pdf
Vitamin D guidelines – children	http://www.neneccg.nhs.uk/resources/uploads/files/Vitamin%20D%20Deficiency%20in%20children%20and%20adolescents.pdf
Alcohol – useful information	www.talkingalcohol.com/files/pdfs/WHO_audit.pdf
Intellectual disability PILs	http://www.easyhealth.org.uk/categories/health-leaflets
	http://www.nhsinform.co.uk/easy-info/healthconditions/
	http://www.fairadvice.org.uk/free-downloads.php
Cardiovascular risk	http://qrisk.org/
Institute of Blind People	https://rnib.org.uk/
Deaf Association	http://www.bda.org.uk/
BMJs Easily Missed Series	http://www.bmj.com/specialties/easily-missed
	We recommend this exercise – for each 'easily missed' condition: 1. Consider what symptoms the patient may have presented with. 2. Then for each symptom think about what are the most likely diagnoses (common things are common!) and what is 'easily missed'?
E learning	http://elearning.rcgp.org.uk/
	http://www.pulse-learning.co.uk/
	http://www.gponline.com/education
Courses not to miss!	http://www.gp-update.co.uk/The-GP-Update-Course
	http://www.nbmedical.com/hot-topics-gp-update-courses
	http://www.rcgp.org.uk/learning/one-day-essentials.aspx
RCGP curriculum	http://www.rcgp.org.uk/training-exams/gp-curriculum-overview/online-curriculum.aspx
Conference not to miss!	http://www.rcgp.org.uk/annualconference
Consultation skills	*The Naked Consultation: a practical guide to primary care consultation skills* by Dr Liz Moulton.

Time out from revision … Watch a TED Talk for inspiration!

Useful Resources

Index

2WW (two weeks' wait) referral
    ENT, 381–2, 403
    gastrointestinal, 342, 346, 350
    gynaecology, 178, 186
    men's health, 212
5-alpha-reductase inhibitor, 221
6 S for success model, 10

A

AAA (abdominal aortic aneurysm), 58, 88, 312, 504, 544, 557
abbreviations, 28–31
ABCD2 score, 453, 470
abdominal pain, 85, 87
acamprosate, 360, 380
ACE inhibitors
    and angina, 326
    and diabetes, 438
    and heart failure, 330
    and hypertension, 334
    and kidney disease, 136
    and TIA, 470
ACL (anterior cruciate ligament) injuries, 499, 505–8
acne, 521–2, 527–30
    and contraception, 236, 244
    and PCOS, 179–82
ACS (acute coronary syndrome), 92
adapalene, 530
Addison's disease, 434, 534
adhesive capsulitis, 499, 520, 550
adrenaline, intramuscular, 100
agranulocytosis, 448–50
albuminuria, 50, 136, 222, 438
alcohol
    advice on consumption, 59
    and domestic violence, 370–1
    harmful drinking, 359–60, 368, 377–80
    and osteoporosis, 510–11
    and safeguarding, 359, 365–8
    useful resources on, 560
alcohol dependence, 359, 368, 378, 380
Alcoholics Anonymous (AA), 376, 378, 380
alendronate, 500, 510, 512
allergic reactions, 98–9
alpha blockers, 204, 220–1
Alzheimer's disease
    advanced, 145–8

and end-of-life care, 261–4
possible, 142–3
amblyopia, 414
ambulance, need for, 92, 96
amiodarone, 322, 450
amitriptyline, 418, 466
amlodipine
    and atrial fibrillation, 320–1
    and heart failure, 330
    and hypertension, 332
    and statins, 60
amoxicillin, 388–90, 397–8, 484, 490
AMTS (abbreviated mental test score), 475, 482–4
anaemia, iron deficiency, 350
anaphylaxis, 84, 98, 100, 171
angina, 313–14, 323–6
    and HCOM, 82
    and heart failure, 328–9
    and SVT, 94–5
angioedema, 83–4, 97–100
anhedonia, 277, 286
ankylosing spondylitis, 354, 504
antenatal check, 149–50, 155–8
antibiotics
    and blepharitis, 408–10
    in end-of-life planning, 252, 262–4
    and otitis media, 388–90
    and pneumonia, 484
    and sinusitis, 396–7
    and UTIs, 122
    and viral infections, 112–13
anticholinergics, 220
antidepressants, 154, 268, 276–9, 282, 560
antihistamines, 98, 100, 158, 362, 398, 538
antihyperglycaemics, 429–30, 438, 451–2
antioxidants, 420
antiplatelets, 313–18, 335, 438, 470
antipsychotics, 50, 204, 282, 286
anxiety, 269–73
    and chest pain, 92
    in consultation, 19, 27
    and erectile dysfunction, 204
    and hyperglycaemia, 101–3
    in palliative care, 268
anxiety disorder, generalised, 274
apixaban, 137–9, 320
ARMD (age-related macular degeneration), 405–6, 419–22
arteriosclerosis, 521, 542

arthritis
  palliative care for, 266-7
  rheumatoid, 516
  septic, 56, 508, 516
  see also osteoarthritis
Asian family origin, 54, 136
aspirin
  and angina, 326
  and atrial fibrillation, 320-1
  and cardiovascular problems, 90, 94-5, 313
  and colon cancer, 316-17
  and diabetes, 438
  indications for, 318
  and migraine, 466
  in pregnancy, 154, 164
  and stroke, 335
  and TIA, 468, 470
asthma
  acute, 475-6, 485-8
  diagnosis of, 475-80, 492, 497
ataxia, 466, 474, 547
atopy, 538
atrial fibrillation (AF), 313-14, 319-22
  and apixaban, 137, 139
  and palpitations, 96
atypical UTI, 122
autism, 36-8, 291, 301-3
autoimmune conditions, 358, 542
autosomal dominant disorders, 61, 74, 82
autosomal recessive disorders, 70
AVSD (atrioventricular septal defect), 64-5
azelaic acid, 530, 532

B

back pain, low, 499-504
bad news, breaking, 66
bedwetting, see nocturnal enuresis
Bell's palsy, 381-2, 384, 386
benzodiazepines, 274, 359, 363-4, 380
benzoyl peroxide, 530
best interests, 146-8, 232, 252, 262-4
beta-blockers, 96, 320, 322, 326, 330, 334, 442
biliary colic, 88
bisoprolol
  and angina, 324
  and atrial fibrillation, 322
  and SVT, 96
bisphosphonates, 512
bladder, overactive
  and bedwetting, 126
  in men, 199-200, 217-20
  in women, 173-4, 191-3

bladder outflow obstruction, 199, 203, 212, 222
bladder training, 192, 194, 218, 220
blepharitis, 405-6, 408-10
blood glucose lowering therapy, 430, 438
blood-thinning, 258-9, 320
borderline personality disorder, 269-70, 282
bowel cancer, 72, 273, 348-9
  screening for, 58, 312
  see also colon cancer; colorectal cancer
bowel habit, change in, 337-8, 346-50
BPH (benign prostatic hypertrophy), 199-200, 212, 220-1
BPPV (benign paroxysmal positional vertigo), 381-2, 399-402
brain tumour, 400-1, 464-5
Brandt-Daroff exercises, 402
breast cancer
  genetic testing for, 61, 75-8
  and HRT, 197
  references, 62
  screening, 58
breastfeeding, medicines in, 559

C

caffeine
  and atrial fibrillation, 320, 322
  and bedwetting, 126
  and dyspepsia, 340, 342
  and fatigue, 446
  and IBS, 346
  and incontinence, 192, 194, 220-1
  and menopause, 190
  and migraine, 464
calcipotriol, 542
calcium
  and hyperparathyroidism, 432-4
  and osteoporosis, 510-12
calcium channel blocker, 96, 322, 334
Calgary Cambridge model, 9
CAMHS (child and adolescent mental health), 301-3
cancer
  and intellectual disability, 294-5
  recognition and referral, 337, 350, 381
capacity, assessing, 140, 260
carbimazole, 447-50
cardiac syndrome X, 326
cardiovascular disease (CVD), risk of, 50, 59-60, 197, 318, 334, 560
cardiovascular examination checklist, 544
cardiovascular problems, 313-14
care homes, 127-8, 137-40, 143, 147-8, 262-3

cataracts, 300, 405–6, 414, 419–22, 426
cauda equina syndrome, 268, 458, 462, 504
CBT (cognitive behavioural therapy), 76, 269
    and anxiety, 272, 274
    for depression, 278
    and insomnia, 362
    and opiate abuse, 374, 376
    useful resources for, 560
cefalexin, 397
cerebral palsy, 125–6, 305–7
cervical cancer
    risk of, 40–2
    suspected, 57, 186
cervical cytology procedure, 42
cervical screening, 33–4, 39–42, 57, 300, 312
Cetraben, 539–41
chaperones, 543
chest pain
    angina, 324–5
    and anxiety, 273
    of recent onset, 83–4, 89–92
chest X-ray, 327, 482, 494, 496
chickenpox, 55, 149–50, 164, 171, 226
child consultation, 18
child protection, 372
chlamydia
    and fertility, 226–8
    and PID, 238, 240
cholesterol, high, 33–4, 47–50, 182, 356, 468
chronic conditions, 46, 410, 453
ciprofloxacin, 214, 216
cirrhosis, 356–8
citalopram, 190, 251
clinical management, 3–10, 13–15, 269–70
clinical modules, 3, 291
clopidogrel, 313, 318, 326, 335, 470
co-amoxiclav, 168, 249, 251, 484
co-codamol, 90–1, 347, 349
COCP (combined oral contraceptive pill), 230
    and acne, 190, 530
    and menorrhagia, 178
    and oligomenorrhea, 182
    postnatal, 170
    stopping, 246
co-cyprindiol, 182, 530
codeine, 91, 158, 258, 265–7, 348, 373–6, 502
colchicine, 515–16
colon cancer, 316–17, 346
colorectal cancer, 74, 337–8, 350
colposcopy, 40, 42, 178
Comfort milk, 109–10
community detox programmes, 380

confidentiality
    and eating disorders, 290
    and end-of-life care, 247, 256
conjunctivitis, 405, 407–10, 427–8, 450
Consultation Models, 6–13
consultation skills, useful resources for, 560
contact lenses, 408–10, 425, 427
continuity of care, 453
contraception, 223–4
    and intellectual disability, 309–12
    missed pill, 232, 236
    postnatal, 168–70
    and skin problems, 528, 534
    stopping, 224, 246
    for under-16s, 223, 229–32
    useful resources for, 559
    see also COCP; emergency contraception; LARC; POP
contraceptive coils, *see* IUD; IUS
contraceptive implant, *see* LARC
COPD (chronic obstructive pulmonary disease), 475–6, 488–92
    care plan, 46, 252
    and spirometry, 497
    and urine leakage, 219
copper coil, *see* IUD
corticosteroids, 50, 171, 398, 512, 516, 542
cough, 475–6, 493–6
    and viral infection, 112
    whooping, 56
counselling
    bereavement, 82
    for children, 44
    and depression, 277–9
    pre-pregnancy, 149, 166
    for PSA testing, 212, 221
    for sterilisation, 246
cow's milk protein allergy, 105, 108, 110
cranial nerve examination checklist, 547
CRB65 scores, 92, 475, 484
criminal activity, 282, 380
crisis teams, 104, 279–80
Crohn's disease, 338, 344–5, 354
CRP (C-reactive protein) testing, and pneumonia, 484
cryotherapy, 426, 526
CSA, assessment domains, 5–6
Cushing's syndrome, 429–30, 446
cystic fibrosis, 61, 67–9

D

dapagliflozin, 440, 442, 452

data gathering
　as assessment domain, 5–6
　as capability, 3–4
　in consultation models, 7–10
　on feedback card, 14
deafness
　sensorineural, 466, 556
　unilateral, 381, 403, 466
dehydration, 56, 220, 432, 434, 516
demanding patients, 529–30
dementia
　and hydrocephalus, 460, 462
　possible, 127–8, 141–4
depression, 269–70, 275–8
　and alcohol abuse, 378
　and back pain, 504
　and DNACPR, 249–51
　and erectile dysfunction, 204
　and heart pain, 324
　and intellectual disabilities, 306
　and opiate abuse, 373–5
　in palliative care, 268
　and personality disorder, 279–81
　postnatal, 19, 216, 269–70, 279, 282, 286
　and prostatitis, 216
　and psoriasis, 542
　and sleeping tablets, 364
　and weight loss, 51–3
dermatology, useful resources for, 559
DermNet NZ, 526, 534
Dermovate, 539–41
DESMOND Education programme, 436, 442
desmopressin, 126, 174, 194
desogestrel, 85, 87, 234, 236
DEXA scan, 509, 511–12
diabetes
　diagnosis, 429–30, 435–8
　and eyesight, 164, 423–5
　and frozen shoulder, 520
　in pregnancy, 149, 163–6
　review, 429–30, 439–42
diagnostic overshadowing, 291, 296
diaphragm, contraceptive, 234, 242
diazepam, 364, 502
diet advice, 59, 337
difficult questions from patients, 247, 264
digoxin, 322, 330
diltiazem, 320, 322, 326
dislocation, 300, 520
distress, medicalising, 269
disulfiram, 360, 380
diverticular disease, 348
Dix–Hallpike test, 381, 401–2

dizziness, recurrent, 402
DKA (diabetic ketoacidosis), 84, 102–3
DNACPR (do not attempt CPR) discussion, 247, 249–52, 260, 263, 268
doctor agenda, 27
domestic violence, 149, 152–4, 359, 369–72
domperidone, 466
Doublebase Dayleave, 536
Dovonex, 540, 542
Down syndrome, 61–6, 70, 291–2, 297–300
　screening for, 58, 66, 152–3
doxycycline, 250, 410, 484
driving
　and angina, 324–5
　and BPPV, 400
　and dementia, 143
　and eyesight, 420–2
　and OSA, 394
　and sleeping tablets, 362–3
　and TIA, 470
drug monitoring requirements, 559
Duac, 530
Duaklir, 490, 492
DUB (dysfunctional uterine bleeding), 173, 178
duloxetine, 194
dyspepsia, 313, 318, 337–42

E

easily missed conditions, 560
eating disorders, 269–70, 287–90
E. coli, 119, 121–2
eczema, 521–2, 535–7
　and allergies, 97–9
　and asthma, 477–80
　inheritance of, 542
　and reflux, 110
Edwards' syndrome, 58, 66
egg allergy, 98–100
elbow examination checklist, 551
elderly parents, 291–2, 296
e-learning, 560
emergency contraception, 223–4, 230, 232, 234, 236, 245
end-of-life care, discussion of, 247, 261–3
endometrial cancer, 186, 240
endometriosis, 173–4, 176–8, 195
endometritis, 149, 168, 170
ENT examination checklist, 556
EPDS (Edinburgh Postnatal Depression Scale), 170, 286
Epiduo, 179, 181, 528, 530
epiglottitis, 381, 403

EpiPens, 98–9
episcleritis, 354, 428
Epley manoeuvre, 381, 400, 402
erectile dysfunction, 199–204, 212
    and prostatitis, 215–16
erythromycin, 390, 398, 484
Eumovate, 535–7
Evra Patch, 232
examinations, 16, 543–57
exercise advice, 59

F

facial nerve palsy, 381–6, 474
facial pain, 381, 396–7
faecal calprotectin, 337–8, 346, 354
faecal occult blood test, 58, 350
familial adenomatous polyposis, 61, 71–4
feedback card, 14–15
fertility work-up, 223–8
fever, in under 5s, 114
fibroids, 176, 178, 184, 240
finasteride, 212, 221
fitness to fly, 559
fluoxetine, 154, 190, 279, 281
FOCUS Consultation Model, 1, 12–13, 16–17, 20, 27
FODMAPs, 344, 346
foetal movements, reduced, 149
folate, 144, 154, 456, 458
folic acid, 152–4, 164, 166, 226
foot/ankle examination checklist, 555
foot pain, 499–500, 514–16
Fostair, 490, 492
fragility fractures, 190, 499–500, 512
Fraser Guidelines, 232
FSH (follicle-stimulating hormone)
    and menopause, 246
        testing, 190
furosemide, 129–31, 136, 265, 267, 328

G

gallbladder polyp, 337, 342
gallstones, 86, 88, 340–1
gastrointestinal endoscopy, referral for, 342
genetic conditions, 61, 70
geratology, helpful resources in, 144
gestational diabetes, 150, 166, 170
glaucoma, acute, 405–6, 415–18, 428
gliclazide, 163–5, 439–41, 451
glitazone, 442, 452
goserelin, 221

gout, 428, 499, 508, 514–16
Grave's disease, *see* hyperthyroidism
grey areas, 21
gynaecology rule, 240
gynaecomastia, 199–200, 205–8, 221

H

haematemesis, 21, 88, 342
haematuria
    and CKD, 136
    in men, 199, 212, 222
    and polycystic kidney, 74
    and renal colic, 88
    and UTIs, 122
    in women, 186
haemoptysis, 92, 260, 495–6
haemorrhage, stomach, 146–7
hand/wrist examination checklist, 552
HAS-BLED score, 322, 335
hazardous drinking, 368
HbA1c targets, 429, 440–2
head injury
    in children and young people, 105–6, 115–18
    criteria for transfer to hospital, 118
health visitors, 44, 46, 107–9, 286, 412
heart attack
    and angina, 324–5
    antiplatelet therapy following, 318
    and chest pain, 90
    lowering risk of, 48, 53, 317
heart failure, 313–14, 327–30
    in older adults, 129–32
Helman, Cecil, 7
hip/lumbar spine examination checklist, 553
hirsutism, 182, 529
HNPCC (hereditary non-polyposis colon cancer), 74
HOCM (hypertrophic obstructive cardiomyopathy), 61, 74, 79–82, 96
HONK (hyperosmolar non-ketotic acidosis), 83, 104
hopelessness, 254, 277, 282, 286
hormone coil, *see* IUS
HRT (hormone replacement therapy), 173–4, 188–90, 197, 244, 246
hydrocephalus, normal pressure, 453, 459–62
hydrocortisone, 97, 99–100
hyperandrogenism, 182
hypercalcaemia, 268, 429–30, 434
hypercholesterolaemia, familial, 50, 74
hyperemesis, 149, 158
hyperglycaemia, 83–4, 101–4

hyperparathyroidism, 429–34, 512
hyperpigmentation, 530, 534
hypertension, 313–14, 331–4
    in pregnancy, 149
hyperthyroidism, 208, 322, 429–30, 447–50, 512
hypoglycaemic episodes, 164–6, 440–2, 452
hypotension, postural, 402, 458, 462
hypothyroidism, 58, 151, 153, 178, 182, 300

I

IBS (irritable bowel syndrome) 85, 87, 271, 273, 327, 337–8, 343–6, 501
    and prostatitis, 213, 215–16
    in women, 186
ibuprofen
    gel, 266
    and joint pain, 506, 514–15
    and kidney injury, 130–1, 134
    and melasma, 532–3
    and otitis media, 388–90
    see also NSAIDs
ICE (ideas, concerns, expectations), 7, 9, 11–13, 16, 20, 22–3
    in end-of-life discussions, 256
IHD (ischaemic heart disease), 318
IMB (intramenstrual bleeding), 178, 240
immunisation refusal, 33–8
immunisation schedules, 33, 38, 55
immunisation/vaccine preventable diseases, 56
inappropriate use of services, 33, 43–6
incontinence
    faecal, 344–5, 461
    urinary, 192, 220–1, 461–2
indapamide, and erectile dysfunction, 201–2
inflammatory bowel disease (IBD), 337–8, 346, 351–4, 358
information
    consent to disclose, 18
    parking, 19
information leaflets, 24, 180, 202, 400
informed consent, 11, 174, 360, 543
informed decisions, 21, 48, 258, 312, 362
insomnia, 361–3
insulin, 101–3, 164, 166, 436, 440–2, 451–2
intellectual disability (ID), 291–2
    adolescents with, 304
    annual health check, 300
    and Down syndrome, 152
    emotions and sexuality, 309–12
    need for procedure, 291–6
    presentation of illness in, 308
    useful resources for, 560

interpersonal skills, 5–10, 13–15
intimate examinations, 218, 543
IPSS (International Prostate Symptom Score), 214, 216, 220
isotretinoin, 528, 530
IUD (intrauterine device), 77, 170, 234, 242–6
    and acne, 528–9
    and menorrhagia, 178, 184–5
IUS (intrauterine system), 170, 178, 182, 190, 242, 244, 246; see also Mirena coil

J

jargon switch, 26
Jaydess, 244

K

ketones, 83, 102–4, 158, 164, 442
kidney disease, chronic (CKD), and AKI, 132
kidney injury, acute (AKI), 127–32, 452
    and CKD, 136
knee examination checklist, 554
knee pain, 52–3, 349, 499–500, 505–8

L

LABA (long-acting beta agonist), 492
lactic acidosis, 83, 104, 438, 451
LARC (long-acting reversible contraception), 195, 223–4, 231, 234, 241–4; see also IUD; IUS; Mirena coil
learning disabilities, see intellectual disability
learning disability register, 300
left ventricular systolic dysfunction, 330
levonorgestrel, 224, 236, 245
levothyroxine, 150–3
liver function tests (LFTs), abnormal, 337–8, 355–8
lumbar puncture, 460, 474
lung cancer, 208, 322, 326, 475–6, 494–6
lung disease, restrictive, 475
LUTS (lower urinary tract symptoms), 212, 216, 220
lymecycline, 528, 530
Lyme disease, 386, 458, 474

M

macrolides, 484
male hormone, excess, 528
management plan
    sharing, 12, 14
    structuring, 24

mebeverine, 271, 273, 346
medical complexity, 21
medication compliance, 104
melanoma, 426, 524
melasma, 521–2, 531–4
Melasma Area and Severity Index (MASI), 534
memory tests, 142–3, 378
menopause, 173–4, 184, 187–90, 246
    premature, 190
menorrhagia, 173–8, 183–5
mental capacity assessment, 140
mental health, 269–70
    and intellectual disability, 291–2, 306–8
    useful resources for, 559
mesalazine, 351–3
mesothelioma, 496
metformin
    and diabetes, 436–7, 442
    and PCOS, 180–2
    in pregnancy, 163–6
metoclopramide, 158, 253, 255, 464, 466
metoprolol, 96, 170
migraine, 453–4, 463–6
    focal, 234
    and melasma, 531–3
MIND, 272, 278, 302
Mirena coil, 168–9, 244, 246
    and HRT, 190
    and melasma, 532–3
    and menorrhagia, 176
mirtazapine, 279, 281
miscarriage, 152–4, 159–62
mitral regurgitation, 328, 544
MMR vaccination, 35–8
moisturiser, 532, 534, 536–8
motivational interview, 25, 33, 376
MRI
    and endometriosis, 195
    and knee pain, 507
    and opiate abuse, 373–5
    and TIA, 468, 470
multiple sclerosis, 453–4, 471–4

N

NAFLD (non-alcoholic fatty liver disease), 337, 356, 358
naltrexone, 360, 380
naproxen, 374, 502, 514, 516, 518
nasal decongestant, 392, 398
negative descriptors, 14
Neighbour model, 8
Neocate, 108–10

neurological examination checklist, 548
neuropathy, peripheral, 204, 438, 453, 455–8, 516, 548
newborns, screening for, 58
NHS screening programmes, 33, 58
NIH-CPSI (National Institutes of Health Chronic Prostatitis Symptom Index), 214, 216
nitrofurantoin, 119–20, 222, 261, 263
NOACs (novel oral anticoagulants), 313–14, 321–2, 335
nocturnal enuresis, 105–6, 123–6
norethisterone, 174, 178, 236
NSAIDs (non-steroidal anti-inflammatory drugs)
    and aspirin, 318
    and asthma, 480
    and hyperpigmentation, 534
    and joint pain, 516, 520
    and osteoarthritis, 508
    and prostatitis, 216
    and urinary incontinence, 195
nutrition, artificial, 264
Nuvaring, 232

O

obesity, 54
ofloxacin, 216, 238
Oilatum, 477, 479, 535–7
oligomenorrhoea, 182, 450
omeprazole
    and haemorrhage, 146
    and reflux, 110, 317, 340
ophthalmic emergency, 405, 418, 426–7
opiate abuse, 359–60, 373–6
orlistat, 52, 54, 182
OSA (obstructive sleep apnoea), 381, 394, 446, 466
osteoarthritis, 499, 508
    and shoulder pain, 520
    and weight loss, 51, 53
osteopenia, 512
osteoporosis, 190, 290, 499–500, 504, 509–12, 560
otitis media, 56, 381–2, 387–90, 402
Ottawa rules, 516
ovarian cancer, 41, 78, 186, 344, 346
ovarian cysts, 88, 173–4, 196, 240
overdose, 277, 279, 281, 376
Oxford antimicrobial guidelines, 559
oxybutynin, 194, 220

P

pain assessment, 268, 508
painful arc syndrome, 518, 520

pain relief, refusing, 266–7
palliative care symptoms, 247, 265–8
palpitations, assessment of, 83, 94–6
panic attacks, 272
paracetamol
    and joint pain, 506
    and morphine, 374
    and otitis media, 390
    overdose, 279
parent advice, 559
Parkinson's disease, 249–51, 453, 481–3
Patau's syndrome, 58, 66
patient autonomy, 260
patient needs, 27
PC (Presenting Complaint), instructions for, 1
PCDS (Primary Care Dermatology Society), 521, 526
PCOS (polycystic ovarian syndrome), 173–4, 179–82, 528
PE (pulmonary embolism), 56, 92, 247, 260, 268, 322
peanut allergy, 98–9
PEF (peak expiratory flow), 46, 475, 480
Pendleton model, 7
peptic ulcer, 88, 337
peripheral vascular examination checklist, 557
personality disorders, 269–70, 280–2
Pharmacy First, 44, 46
phenylephrine, 418
physiotherapy websites, 560
PID (pelvic inflammatory disease), 88, 178, 223–4, 237–40
PILs in different languages, 559
pioglitazone, 442, 452
plantar fasciitis, 499–500, 513–15, 555
PMB (post-menopausal bleeding), 173–4, 183–6
pneumococcal vaccine, 330, 490, 492
pneumonia, 475–6, 481–4
    aspiration, 249, 251, 484
    and COPD, 492
polycystic kidney, 74
POP (progesterone-only pill), 223–4, 233–5
    and HRT, 190
    postnatal, 170
postnatal check, 149–50, 167–70
postnatal psychosis, 269–70, 283–6
PPI (proton pump inhibitors), 313, 318, 335, 342, 375, 470
pre-diabetes, 430, 540–1
prednisolone, 386, 486, 488, 490, 497, 512
pre-eclampsia, 154, 158, 170, 182
pregnancy
    bleeding in, 149–50, 159–62

chickenpox in, 171
ectopic, 88, 160, 162, 234, 236, 242, 520
medicines in, 559
and melasma, 532
new, 149–50, 152–4
screening in, 58
prescriptions, in the exam, 19
professional modules, 3
progesterone injection, 170, 246
promethazine, 158, 362
propranolol, 274, 447, 450, 466
prostate, transurethral resection of, 221
prostate cancer, 199–200, 210–12
prostatitis, 199–200, 213–16, 222
proteinuria, 136, 158, 222
PSA (prostate-specific antigen) testing, 199–200, 204, 209–12, 221
psoriasis, 521–2, 539–42
psychiatry, prescribing in, 560
PTH (parathyroid hormone), 136, 429, 431–4, 512
pulse oximetry, 394, 475
pyelonephritis, 88, 216, 222, 504

Q

questions, open, 274

R

ramipril, 129–31, 440
RCGP, core statement capabilities, 3–5
RCGP curriculum, useful resources for, 560
recurrent UTI
    in children, 105–6, 119–22
    and fatigue, 443
    in men, 222
    and overactive bladder, 194
red eye, 405, 427–8
red flags
    in consultation, 11–14, 21
    for heart disease, 96
    in menorrhagia, 178
    and risk assessment, 274
referred pain, 92, 499, 504, 520
reflux
    in adults, 340, 342
    and alendronate, 510
    in babies, 105–10
    and peptic ulcer, 88, 92
refugees, 44–5, 413
relatives, discussion with, 247–8, 253–6, 264
renal colic, 88
resitting the exam, 27

respiratory examination checklist, 545
Restore, 302
resuscitation, 145, 250, 252, 264, 267; *see also* DNACPR
retinal detachment, 405–6, 423–6
retinoids, topical, 526, 530
reversibility testing, 475, 480, 492, 497
rhesus prophylaxis, anti-D, 149, 162
risedronate, 500, 512
risk assessment, 21, 154, 274, 326, 380
rotator cuff tendonitis, 499, 520

S

safeguarding, 291, 359–60, 366–8
safety netting
   in consultation models, 8–11
   in end-of-life discussions, 256
salbutamol, 322, 477, 479, 487–9, 492
sarcoidosis, 458, 474, 497
saxagliptin, 440, 451
SCC (squamous cell carcinoma), 524–6
sciatica, 373, 375, 502–3, 553
sedatives, 268, 282, 394
self-harm, 279, 281–2, 370
septicaemia, 56, 120–2
sertraline, 279–81, 343, 345
sexual abuse, 279–81
sexual health history, 203–4, 223, 238, 240
shampoo
   antidandruff, 410
   and eczema, 536
   and psoriasis, 539–42
shoulder, frozen, *see* adhesive capsulitis
shoulder/cervical spine examination checklist, 550
shoulder pain, 162, 499–500, 517–20
sick day rules, 132, 442
sinusitis, 56, 381–2, 395–8
skin lesion, 521–6, 532
sleeping tablets, weaning, 359, 361–3
smoking
   and hyperthyroidism, 448–9
   and lung cancer, 493–5
   and snoring, 392–4
smoking cessation, 318, 492
snoring, 381–2, 391–4
SNRI (selective noradrenaline reuptake inhibitors), 274
social prescribing, 376, 414
social services, 304, 366–8
SOCRATES, 268
solar keratosis, 521, 524, 526
spirometry, 330, 475–6, 480, 489, 492, 497
squint, 405–6, 411–14
SSRIs (selective serotonin reuptake inhibitors)
   and anxiety, 274
   and menopause, 190
   and contraception, 240
   in pregnancy, 154
statins, 34
   and cardiovascular disease, 60, 383, 385
   and cholesterol, 48–50
   and diabetes, 438
   and kidney disease, 134
   and liver disease, 358
   and TIA, 470
stepped care models, 274, 278
sterilisation, 223–4, 242–3, 246
steroids
   and asthma/COPD, 492
   and contraception, 240
   and eczema, 536–8
   and facial nerve palsy, 384
   and joint pain, 514, 518, 520
   and psoriasis, 540, 542
   see also corticosteroids
stools, black, 340–1, 344–5, 510
strabismus, 414, 450
stroke
   and contraceptive pill, 234
   and facial weakness, 384–6
   managing risk of, 320, 335
   risk of, 453
suicide
   and anxiety, 272
   and depression, 276–7, 279–81
   family history of, 73
sulfonylurea, 442, 451–2
sumatriptan, 464
summarising, in consultation models, 8, 10
support groups
   for anxiety, 272
   for carers, 104
   for depression, 278
   for relatives, 256
supraspinatus, 520
SVT (supraventricular tachycardia), 83–4, 93–6

T

tadalafil, 204, 221
tamoxifen, 77, 186, 190, 240
telephone consultations, 18
tendonitis, *see* painful arc syndrome
test results, providing answer to, 19
tetracyclines, oral, 410, 530

thiazides, 334, 434, 442, 470, 516
thoracic pain, referred, 92
thyroid/neck examination checklist, 549
TIA (transient ischaemic attack), 453–4, 467–70
time management, 17, 27
tiotropium, 489, 491–2
tired all the time, 430, 443–6
tolterodine, 194, 220
Top Tips, 17–21
tramadol, 266, 376
transition process model, 291–2, 302–4
treatment refusal, 247–8, 257–60
triglycerides, 50, 60
trimethoprim, 119–21, 216, 222, 263
triptans, 466
TVUSS (trans-vaginal ultrasound), 228, 236, 240

U
UC (ulcerative colitis), 338, 351–4
UPA (ulipristal acetate), 245
uric acid, 516
urinary incontinence, stress, 192–4, 220
useful phrases, 22–5
UTIs (urinary tract infection)
    in children, 105–6, 119–22
    and fatigue, 443–4
    and hydrocephalus, 460–2
    and hyperglycaemia, 102
    in men, 200, 212, 222
    in women, 154, 162
    see also atypical UTI; recurrent UTIs

V
vaginal discharge, 40, 102, 186
vaginal dryness, 188–90, 197, 236
varicella, see chickenpox

vasectomy, 242–3
Viagra, 202–3, 326
viral illness, in children and young people, 105–6, 111–13
viral wheeze, 478–9
visual acuity, 398, 426, 465, 473
vitamin B_{12} deficiency, 456, 458, 474
vitamin C, and ARMD, 420
vitamin D
    and hyperparathyroidism, 434
    and osteoporosis, 509–12
    in pregnancy, 152–4, 164
    and psoriasis, 542
    useful resources for, 560
VTE (venous thromboembolism), 92, 154, 178, 197

W
warfarin
    as anticholinergic, 220
    and atrial fibrillation, 320–1
    and contraception, 240
    refusing, 258
    and stroke, 335
weight, wanting to lose, 33–4, 51–3, 165, 227, 355, 392–3
well man check, 199, 203–4
Wells' score, 247, 260
Wilson's disease, 70, 358
wrists, cutting, see self-harm

X
X-linked genetic conditions, 70

Z
zopiclone, 361–4

CRC Press
Taylor & Francis Group
6000 Broken Sound Parkway NW, Suite 300
Boca Raton, FL 33487-2742

© 2017 by Taylor & Francis Group, LLC
CRC Press is an imprint of Taylor & Francis Group, an Informa business

No claim to original U.S. Government works

Printed on acid-free paper

International Standard Book Number-13: 978-1-4987-9646-0 (Hardback)

This book contains information obtained from authentic and highly regarded sources. While all reasonable efforts have been made to publish reliable data and information, neither the author[s] nor the publisher can accept any legal responsibility or liability for any errors or omissions that may be made. The publishers wish to make clear that any views or opinions expressed in this book by individual editors, authors or contributors are personal to them and do not necessarily reflect the views/opinions of the publishers. The information or guidance contained in this book is intended for use by medical, scientific or health-care professionals and is provided strictly as a supplement to the medical or other professional's own judgement, their knowledge of the patient's medical history, relevant manufacturer's instructions and the appropriate best practice guidelines. Because of the rapid advances in medical science, any information or advice on dosages, procedures or diagnoses should be independently verified. The reader is strongly urged to consult the relevant national drug formulary and the drug companies' and device or material manufacturers' printed instructions, and their websites, before administering or utilizing any of the drugs, devices or materials mentioned in this book. This book does not indicate whether a particular treatment is appropriate or suitable for a particular individual. Ultimately it is the sole responsibility of the medical professional to make his or her own professional judgements, so as to advise and treat patients appropriately. The authors and publishers have also attempted to trace the copyright holders of all material reproduced in this publication and apologize to copyright holders if permission to publish in this form has not been obtained. If any copyright material has not been acknowledged please write and let us know so we may rectify in any future reprint.

Except as permitted under U.S. Copyright Law, no part of this book may be reprinted, reproduced, transmitted, or utilized in any form by any electronic, mechanical, or other means, now known or hereafter invented, including photocopying, microfilming, and recording, or in any information storage or retrieval system, without written permission from the publishers.

For permission to photocopy or use material electronically from this work, please access www.copyright.com (http://www.copyright.com/) or contact the Copyright Clearance Center, Inc. (CCC), 222 Rosewood Drive, Danvers, MA 01923, 978-750-8400. CCC is a not-for-profit organization that provides licenses and registration for a variety of users. For organizations that have been granted a photocopy license by the CCC, a separate system of payment has been arranged.

Trademark Notice: Product or corporate names may be trademarks or registered trademarks, and are used only for identification and explanation without intent to infringe.

Library of Congress Cataloging-in-Publication Data

Names: Blount, Emily, author. | Kirby-Blount, Helen, author. | Moulton, Liz, author.
Title: The complete CSA casebook : 110 role plays and a comprehensive curriculum guide / Emily Blount, Helen Kirby-Blount, and Liz Moulton.
Description: Boca Raton : CRC Press, [2017]
Identifiers: LCCN 2016035528 | ISBN 9781498796460 (hardback binder : alk. paper)
Subjects: | MESH: Physical Examination--methods | General Practice--methods | Clinical Competence | Diagnosis | Great Britain | Outlines | Case Reports
Classification: LCC RC78.7.D53 | NLM WB 18.2 | DDC 616.07/54--dc23
LC record available at https://lccn.loc.gov/2016035528

Visit the Taylor & Francis Web site at
http://www.taylorandfrancis.com

and the CRC Press Web site at
http://www.crcpress.com

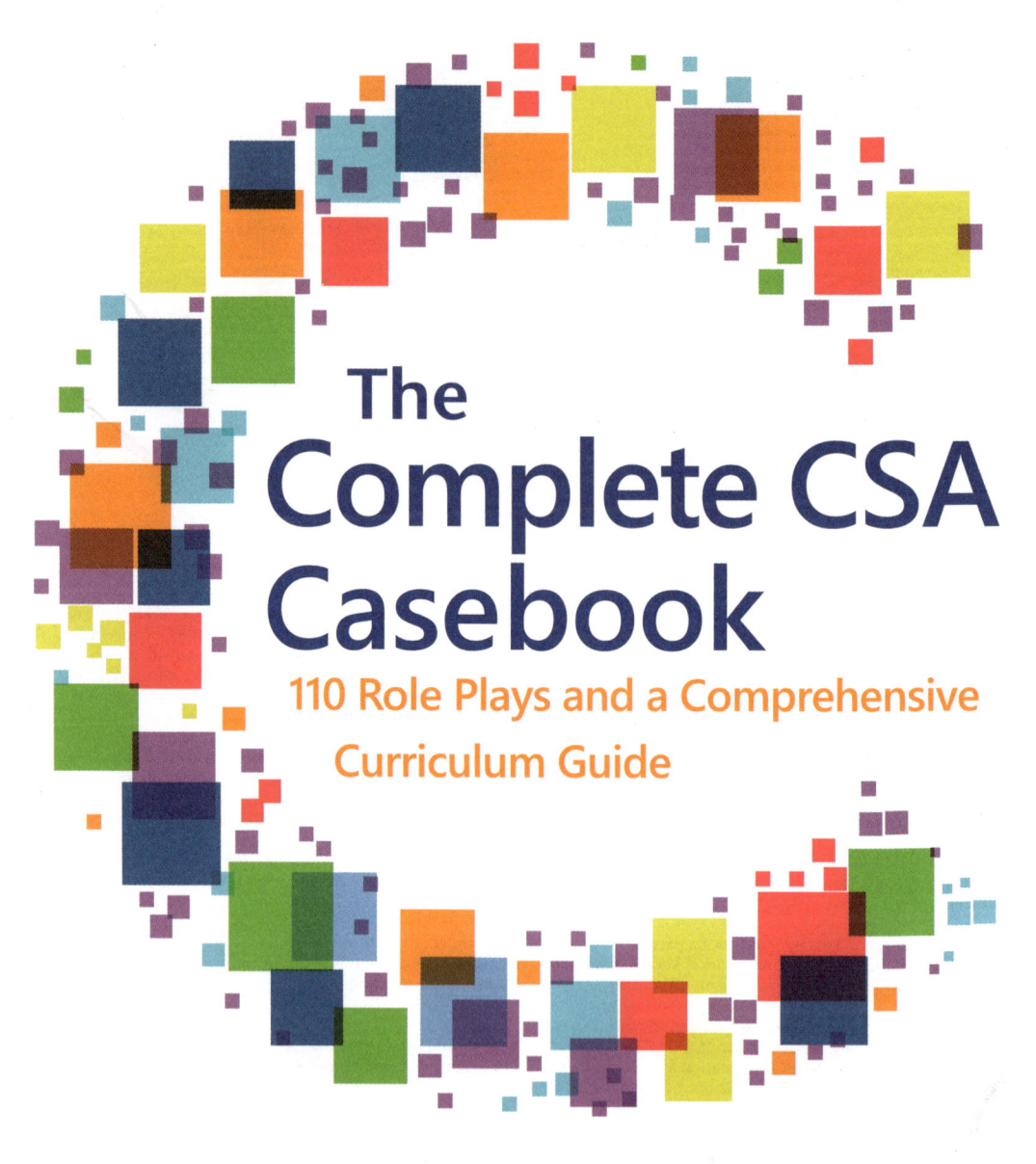

The Complete CSA Casebook

110 Role Plays and a Comprehensive Curriculum Guide

Emily Blount • Helen Kirby-Blount • Liz Moulton

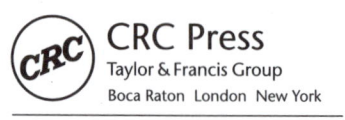

CRC Press
Taylor & Francis Group
Boca Raton London New York

CRC Press is an imprint of the
Taylor & Francis Group, an **informa** business